Evidence-based Management of HYPERTENSION

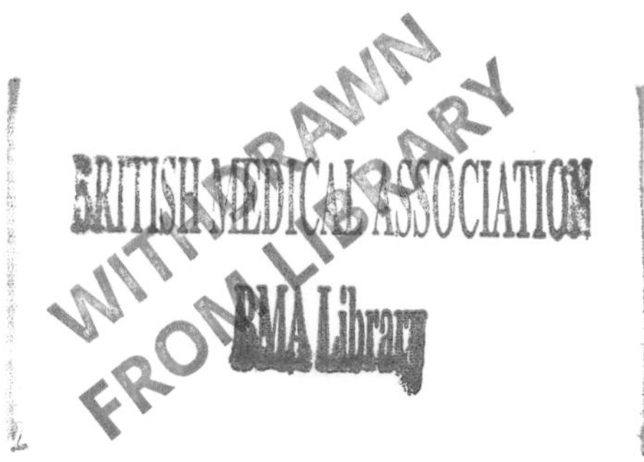

Matthew R. Weir

tfm Publishing Limited, Castle Hill Barns, Harley, Nr Shrewsbury, SY5 6LX, UK.
Tel: +44 (0)1952 510061; Fax: +44 (0)1952 510192
E-mail: nikki@tfmpublishing.com; Web site: www.tfmpublishing.com

Design & Typesetting: Nikki Bramhill BSc Hons Dip Law
First Edition: © August 2010
ISBN: 978 1 903378 72 4

Cover image: © 2010 3d4medical, www.3d4medical.com

Printed by Gutenberg Press Ltd., Gudja Road, Tarxien, PLA 19, Malta.
Tel: +356 21897037; Fax: +356 21800069.

Contents

Foreword

We are all on an age and genetically programmed slope of change of blood pressure. Environmental factors may also influence slope, but you cannot change your age or your parents. We use blood pressure as a continuous measure of risk for vascular disease. Consequently, important questions to consider are:

- how early should you start to modify the slope of change of blood pressure?
- who do we treat, and when?
- what therapies should you use?
- should we treat pre-hypertension?
- how does the choice of therapy change in the presence of comorbidities such as obesity, ischemic heart disease, left ventricular hypertrophy, diabetes or cerebrovascular disease?

These are some of the challenging questions which face us both professionally and personally. *Evidence-based Management of Hypertension* provides answers to these and many other questions, as the authors present an expert analysis of the available evidence and offer authoritative recommendations for treatment planning. In each chapter, tables highlight evidence from a variety of sources, and every chapter concludes with a series of key practice points that present a summary of evidence-based recommendations for best practice, graded according to the quality of that evidence.

For any clinician involved in the treatment of hypertension it is hoped that this evidence-based book will provide an important perspective.

Matthew R. Weir MD, Professor and Director
Division of Nephrology
University of Maryland School of Medicine
Baltimore, Maryland, USA

Contributors

Lawrence J. Appel MD MPH Professor of Medicine, Epidemiology and International Health (Human Nutrition), The Johns Hopkins University School of Medicine, The Welch Center for Prevention, Epidemiology and Clinical Research, and The Johns Hopkins Bloomberg School of Public Health, Johns Hopkins Medical Institutions, Baltimore, Maryland, USA

George Bakris MD Professor of Medicine; Director, Hypertensive Diseases Center, Section of Endocrinology, Diabetes and Metabolism, University of Chicago Pritzker School of Medicine, Chicago, Illinois, USA

Jan N. Basile MD Professor of Medicine, Seinsheimer Cardiovascular Health Program, Medical University of South Carolina, Ralph H. Johnson VA Medical Center, Charleston, South Carolina, USA

R. Michael Benitez MD FACC Associate Professor of Medicine, University of Maryland School of Medicine, Maryland, USA

Eric M. Brown MD Fellow, Division of Nephrology, University of Maryland School of Medicine, Baltimore, Maryland, USA

David A. Calhoun MD Professor of Medicine, Vascular Biology and Hypertension Program, University of Alabama at Birmingham, Birmingham, Alabama, USA

Lance D. Dworkin MD FACP FASN FAHA Professor of Medicine, Interim Chairman, Department of Medicine, Alpert Medical School of Brown University; Physician in Chief, Rhode Island & The Miriam Hospitals, Providence, Rhode Island, USA

William J. Elliott MD PhD Professor of Preventive Medicine, Internal Medicine and Pharmacology, Pacific Northwest University of Health Sciences, Yakima, Washington, USA

Deepashree Gupta MD PGY-3 Resident Physician, Department of Internal Medicine, University of Missouri-Columbia, Columbia, Missouri, USA

Joseph L. Izzo, Jr. MD Professor of Medicine and Pharmacology, State University of New York at Buffalo, New York, USA

Wallace R. Johnson, Jr, MD Assistant Professor of Medicine, University of Maryland School of Medicine, Maryland, USA

Rigas Kalaitzidis MD Senior Registrar in Nephrology, University Hospital of Ioannina, Ioannina, Greece

Radhika Kanthety MD MSHS Research Coordinator, Division of Nephrology and Hypertension, University Hospitals Case Medical Center, Cleveland, Ohio, USA

Guido Lastra MD Fellow, Department of Internal Medicine; Division of Endocrinology, Diabetes and Metabolism, University of Missouri-Columbia, Columbia, Missouri, USA

Camila Manrique MD Fellow, Department of Internal Medicine; Division of Endocrinology, Diabetes and Metabolism, University of Missouri-Columbia, Columbia, Missouri, USA

Mandeep R. Mehra MD Professor of Medicine and Head of Cardiology, University of Maryland School of Medicine, Division of Cardiology, Baltimore, Maryland, USA

Marvin Moser MD Professor of Medicine, Department of Medicine/Cardiology, Yale University School of Medicine, New Haven, Connecticut, USA

John W. O'Bell MD Assistant Professor of Medicine, Department of Medicine, Alpert Medical School of Brown University, Providence, Rhode Island, USA

Eduardo Pimenta MD Clinical Research Fellow, Endocrine Hypertension Research Centre and Clinical Centre of Research Excellence in Cardiovascular Disease and Metabolic Disorders, University of Queensland School of Medicine, Princess Alexandra Hospital, Brisbane, Australia

Mahboob Rahman MD MS Associate Professor of Medicine, Case Western Reserve University, Cleveland, Ohio, USA; Staff Nephrologist, Division of Nephrology and Hypertension, University Hospitals Case Medical Center, Cleveland, Ohio, USA and the Louis Stokes Cleveland VA Medical Center, Cleveland, Ohio, USA

C. Venkata S. Ram MD MACP FACC Clinical Professor of Internal Medicine, Texas Blood Pressure Institute, Dallas Nephrology Associates, University of Texas Southwestern Medical Center, Dallas, Texas, USA

Faisal Siddiqi MD Fellow, Cardiology, University of Maryland School of Medicine, Division of Cardiology, Baltimore, Maryland, USA

James R. Sowers MD Professor and Division Director of Endocrinology, Diabetes and Metabolism, Division of Endocrinology, Diabetes and Metabolism; Department of Internal Medicine, University of Missouri-Columbia, Columbia, Missouri, USA; Professor of Medicine, Physiology and Pharmacology, Department of Physiology and Pharmacology, University of Missouri-Columbia, Columbia, Missouri, USA

Kristin Thanavaro MD Resident, Internal Medicine, University of Maryland School of Medicine, Division of Cardiology, Baltimore, Maryland, USA

Raymond R. Townsend MD Director of the Hypertension Program, Department of Medicine, University of Pennsylvania, Philadelphia, USA

Sharon Turban MD MHS Assistant Professor of Medicine, Division of Nephrology, The Johns Hopkins University School of Medicine, Baltimore, Maryland, USA

Matthew R. Weir MD Professor and Director, Division of Nephrology, University of Maryland School of Medicine, Baltimore, Maryland, USA

Jackson T. Wright Jr. MD PhD Professor of Medicine, Case Western Reserve University, Cleveland, Ohio, USA; Program Director, William T. Dahms Clinical Research Unit, Clinical and Translational Science Collaborative; Director, Clinical Hypertension Program, Division of Nephrology and Hypertension, University Hospitals Case Medical Center, Cleveland, Ohio, USA

Acknowledgements

I am grateful to all of the contributors for taking on this important task and hope they will be proud to be part of a book which attempts to set out the evidence-based management of hypertension.

I also wish to acknowledge my best friend and wife of many years for allowing me the time to pursue my academic interests in the treatment of blood pressure and chronic kidney disease.

Using evidence-based medicine

The process of gathering evidence is a time-consuming task. One of the main reasons for supporting the use of evidence-based medicine, is the rate of change of new practices, and the increasing tendency for specialisation. Medical information is widely available from a variety of sources for clinicians but keeping up-to-date with current literature remains an almost impossible task for many with a busy clinical workload. *Evidence-based Management of Hypertension* has been written to aid this process. The chapters in this book have been written by internationally renowned experts who have applied the principles of evidence-based medicine and taken relevant clinical questions and examined the current evidence for the answers. The authors were asked to quote levels and grades of evidence for each major point, and to provide a summary of key points and their respective evidence levels at the end of each chapter. The levels of evidence and grades of evidence used in this book are shown in Tables 1 and 2 and are widely used in evidence-based medicine.

Table 1. Levels of evidence.

Level	Type of evidence
Ia	Evidence obtained from systematic review or meta-analysis of randomised controlled trials
Ib	Evidence obtained from at least one randomised controlled trial
IIa	Evidence obtained from at least one well-designed controlled study without randomisation
IIb	Evidence obtained from at least one other type of well-designed quasi-experimental study
III	Evidence obtained from well-designed non-experimental descriptive studies, such as comparative studies, correlation studies and case studies
IV	Evidence obtained from expert committee reports or opinions and/or clinical experience of respected authorities

Table 2. Grades of evidence.

Grade of evidence	Evidence
A	At least one randomised controlled trial as part of a body of literature of overall good quality and consistency addressing the specific recommendation (evidence levels Ia and Ib)
B	Well-conducted clinical studies but no randomised clinical trials on the topic of recommendation (evidence levels IIa, IIb, III)
C	Expert committee reports or opinions and/or clinical experience of respected authorities. This grading indicates that directly applicable clinical studies of good quality are absent (evidence level IV)

Chapter 1

Evidence-based management of hypertension: how much should you reduce blood pressure?

Jan N. Basile MD, Professor of Medicine
Seinsheimer Cardiovascular Health Program
Medical University of South Carolina
Ralph H. Johnson VA Medical Center
Charleston, South Carolina, USA

Marvin Moser MD, Professor of Medicine
Department of Medicine/Cardiology
Yale University School of Medicine
New Haven, Connecticut, USA

Introduction

Elevations in blood pressure exert a strong and continuous relationship with no threshold of risk for developing cardiovascular disease. Both systolic and diastolic blood pressure are independently related to cardiovascular risk [1]. For persons aged 40 to 70 years, the risk of cardiovascular disease begins at 115/75mm Hg and doubles with each 20/10mm Hg incremental increase up to 185/115mm Hg, although the number of events in people with blood pressure of 115/75 to 130-135/80-85 are relatively small [2]. For persons 50 years of age and older, a systolic blood pressure elevation is a more important risk factor for cardiovascular disease than an elevation in diastolic blood pressure [3, 4]. Currently, there are three targets for elevated blood pressure control: less than 140/90mm Hg for hypertensive individuals without evidence of diabetes or renal disease, less than 130/80mm Hg for patients with these diseases as well as those with ischemic heart disease or a Framingham risk score (FRS) of 10% or more for having a non-fatal MI or risk of death over the next 10 years, and less than 120/80mm Hg in patients with left ventricular dysfunction and ischemic heart disease [5] (Table 1). Only the standard target of lowering blood pressure below 140/90mm Hg is evidence-based in terms of reducing morbidity and mortality [6, 7]. When reducing systolic blood pressure to a goal of <140mm Hg, caution should be exercised if diastolic blood pressure is lowered to <55mm Hg in individuals without ischemic heart disease and <70mm Hg in people with ischemic heart disease [6].

Table 1. Consensus target blood pressure levels in the prevention and management of ischemic heart disease. American Heart Association (AHA) Scientific Statement. ***Adapted from Rosendorff et al*** [5].

Area of concern	BP target (mmHg)
General CAD prevention	<140/90
High CAD risk*	<130/80
Stable angina	<130/80
Unstable angina/NSTEMI	<130/80
STEMI	<130/80
LV dysfunction	<120/80

*High CAD risk = diabetes mellitus, chronic kidney disease, known CAD, CAD equivalent (carotid artery disease, peripheral artery disease, abdominal aortic aneurysm), or 10-year Framingham risk score >10%

Currently recommended blood pressure targets

More people today are aware of and are on therapy for hypertension than in previous years, but control rates, which are improving, were still achieved in only one in three people prior to 2003 [4]. A recent Harris survey suggests that about 50% of hypertensive subjects have their blood pressure controlled at <140/90mm Hg [8]. Since the late 1970s, the minimum goal for blood pressure reduction for most patients with hypertension has been less than 140/90mm Hg **(Ib/A)**. The National Heart Lung and Blood Institute has issued several reports on high blood pressure. In its Seventh report on the Prevention, Detection, Evaluation, and Treatment of High Blood Pressure (JNC 7), the panel recommended an even lower goal for higher-risk patients, (including diabetics and those with chronic renal impairment) to less than 130/80mm Hg [4] **(IV/C)**. Whereas the JNC VI in 1997 recommended a target blood pressure of less than 125/75mm Hg for patients with renal impairment and more than a gram per day of urinary protein, this goal, discussed below, is no longer recommended [9]. The most recent scientific statement from the American Heart Association has added patients with known coronary artery disease, carotid disease, peripheral arterial disease, or an abdominal aortic aneurysm, and those with a calculated 10-year FRS of 10% or more to the group of high-risk patients with a blood pressure target of <130/80mmHg. In addition, the guideline recommends that the clinician 'consider' a blood pressure target of <120/80mm Hg in patients with left ventricular systolic dysfunction of ischemic origin [5] **(IV/C)** (Table 1).

Clinical benefits of achieving blood pressure targets

Clinical trials over the past 35 years have proven the benefits of antihypertensive therapy in reducing the rates of stroke, heart failure and heart attack. But were the goals for blood pressure reduction currently recommended appropriately tested?

The first placebo-controlled co-operative hypertension trial, which targeted diastolic blood pressure reduction, was conducted in 1967 by the Veterans Administration (VA) [10]. The study, which enrolled 143 hospitalized US veterans with severe hypertension (supine diastolic blood pressure between 115-129mm Hg), was stopped prematurely without any statistical analysis because there was a major improvement in prognosis on active therapy (a diuretic, reserpine, and the vasodilator, hydralazine) compared to placebo. There were no deaths in patients on active therapy compared to four deaths on placebo when diastolic blood pressure was reduced to 105mm Hg. A follow-up study also under the direction of the VA showed that lowering the diastolic blood pressure to <90mm Hg further improved cardiovascular outcome. Several subsequent large, prospective placebo-controlled hypertension trials conducted in the 1970s, 1980s, and 1990s found a reduction in cardiovascular morbidity and mortality in treated compared to control patients. These have been summarized in several meta-analyses, which showed a 38% reduction in stroke, 16% reduction in heart attack, 52% reduction in heart failure, 21% reduction in cardiovascular death, and a 35% reduction in left ventricular hypertrophy in treated compared to placebo or control subject [11-14].

None of the clinical trials have achieved the recommended blood pressure goals of <130/80 or <120/80mm Hg recommended in recent clinical guidelines in high-risk hypertension subjects or in individuals in special populations **(IV/C)** [7, 15]. In non-diabetic patients with normal kidney function, guidelines continue to recommend <140/90mm Hg as the blood pressure target [16]. To investigate if a lower blood pressure goal was associated with less target organ damage, investigators from Italy recently randomized 1111 non-diabetic hypertensive patients to one of two systolic blood pressure goals: a goal of <130mm Hg (tight control) or <140mm Hg (usual control) [17]. Patients had at least one other cardiovascular risk factor and a baseline systolic blood pressure of greater than 150mm Hg (mean 163/90mm Hg) after being treated with antihypertensive therapy for at least 12 weeks. Treatment was open-label and individualized. The primary endpoint was prevalence of electrocardiographic left ventricular hypertrophy (LVH). At baseline, blood pressures were equal in the two groups, with roughly 20% of patients in each group having LVH. After 2 years, 27% and 72% of patients in the usual- and tight-control groups, respectively, had systolic blood pressures <130mm Hg. More patients in the usual-control group than in the tight-control group (17.0% vs. 11%) had LVH [odds ratio 0.63, 95% CI 0.43-0.91]. In addition, although few cardiovascular events occurred, significantly more patients in the usual-control group than in the tight-control group (9 % vs. 5%) reached a secondary composite endpoint [hazard ratio 0.50, CI 0.31-0.79] that consisted of any of nine adverse clinical cardiovascular outcomes. This is the first clinical trial to target a systolic blood pressure <130mm Hg in a non-diabetic population with normal renal function. LVH is a surrogate endpoint and studies powered to evaluate cardiovascular outcomes will be required before we can justify lowering the targeted blood pressure in this patient population to <130mm Hg.

Of note, it remains much easier to control diastolic blood pressure than systolic blood pressure in clinical practice [18]. In recent clinical trials, about 90% of hypertensive patients had their diastolic blood pressure reduced to <90mm Hg as in the Hypertension Optimal Treatment (HOT) trial [19], the Antihypertensive and Lipid-Lowering Treatment to Prevent Heart Attack Trial (ALLHAT) [20] and the Controlled Onset Verapamil Investigation of Cardiovascular Endpoints (CONVINCE) [21] trial, while only 60-80% of subjects had systolic blood pressure reduced to below 140mm Hg. In fact, most of the clinical trials failed to achieve an average systolic blood pressure goal <140mm Hg. Despite this, and based on epidemiologic data, a systolic goal of <140mm Hg and a diastolic blood pressure <90mm Hg appear to be a reasonable target.

Benefits of treating isolated systolic hypertension (ISH)

While the observed risk of an elevated systolic blood pressure on cardiovascular disease has been known for over 40 years, specific recommendations for treating ISH were first published in 1993 in the JNC V report [22]. Well-designed, randomized, placebo-controlled trials have shown benefit from drug treatment in elderly patients with ISH. In those patients with Stage 2 ISH (systolic blood pressure of >160mm Hg and a diastolic blood pressure <90 or 95mm Hg), a reduction in stroke, heart failure, coronary events, and mortality was found. Benefit occurred when systolic blood pressure was reduced by at least 20mm Hg below the entry systolic blood pressure, to either 150 or 160mm Hg [23, 24]. As noted, in many patients benefit was seen despite the fact that a blood pressure of <140mm Hg was not achieved (Table 2).

Table 2. Achieved blood pressure in elderly blood pressure trials.

	SHEP	Syst-Eur	HYVET
Subjects, n	4736	4695	3845
Inclusion BP criteria, mmHg	160-219/<90	160-219/<95	160-190/<110
Goal SBP, mmHg	<160	<150 or at least 20mm reduction	<150
BP reduction in active group compared to baseline, mmHg	27/9	23/7	30/13
Mean achieved BP, mmHg	143/68	151/79	144/78
Mean follow-up, yrs	4.5	2.0	1.8

A recent meta-analysis of eight placebo-controlled trials included 15,693 patients 60 years of age and older with ISH. It reported that active treatment over a 3.8-year period of time reduced coronary events by 23%, stroke by 30%, cardiovascular disease death by 18%, and overall mortality by 13% [25]. In patients older than 70 years of age, the absolute benefit was even greater. Treating 19 patients for 5 years prevented one major fatal or non-fatal cardiovascular event.

Most trials involving the elderly involve patients 60 to 80 years of age, but there are many in the over-80 age group. The placebo-controlled Hypertension in the Very Elderly Trial (HYVET) reported that lowering blood pressure in the 80 and older age group (1/3 of whom had ISH) even if not to a systolic blood pressure <140mm Hg (goal <150/80mm Hg; mean achieved 144/78mm Hg) (Table 2) reduced not only stroke and heart failure, but also reduced mortality by 21% [26]. This trial removed any doubt about the safety and benefits of treating hypertension in the very elderly.

Benefit of reducing blood pressure to <140mm Hg in the ISH patient

Is there actual clinical trial evidence to recommend a systolic blood pressure goal of <140mm Hg in patients with ISH? Only a few clinical trials have specifically attempted to randomize patients to different target levels of blood pressure as a primary intervention and no specific trial has targeted a blood pressure of <140mm Hg in individuals with ISH. In fact, most recommendations on the benefits of achieving a systolic blood pressure <140mm Hg come from epidemiologic observations or post hoc analyses of clinical trial data **(IV/C)**. One such post hoc analysis was published almost 10 years after the publication of the original results of the Systolic Hypertension in the Elderly Program (SHEP) trial [27]. In this analysis, the risk of stroke was calculated according to on-treatment blood pressure during follow-up. Patients who achieved the original goal of the trial, a systolic blood pressure <160mm Hg and at least a 20mm Hg reduction from baseline had a 33% reduction in stroke. The patients who achieved a systolic blood pressure <150mm Hg did even better with a 38% risk reduction in stroke. The group who achieved a systolic blood pressure <140mm Hg had a 22% reduction in stroke risk which did not reach statistical significance because of the smaller numbers of patients involved. These data do not mean that achieving a systolic blood pressure <140mm Hg is less beneficial than achieving a higher systolic blood pressure level. Rather, they suggest, that if systolic blood pressure is reduced at least 20mm Hg from baseline, even if not to the presently recommended goal of <140mm Hg, clinical outcome is still improved. Of note, no clinical trial has tested whether an improvement in outcome occurs in those with Stage 1 ISH (systolic blood pressure 140 to 159mm Hg and diastolic blood pressure <90mm Hg). On balance, most of the trials done indicate that benefit has been noted with an average decrease in blood pressure of 12/5mm Hg.

In summary, while none of the clinical trials in patients with ISH achieved a systolic blood pressure <140mm Hg, JNC 7 [4] and the most recent consensus statements from the National High Blood Pressure Education Program have continued to recommend a reduction in systolic blood pressure to less than 140mm Hg in patients with ISH **(IV/C)** [28].

Are there cardiovascular and renal benefits in reducing blood pressure to <130/80mm Hg in diabetic patients?

Diabetics are most likely to die of atherosclerotic vascular disease, the risk of which is accelerated by hypertension. The risk of stroke or any cardiovascular event is almost doubled in hypertensive patients with diabetes mellitus. In addition, diabetes is the number one cause of end-stage renal disease. There exists a nearly linear relationship between elevations in blood pressure and the rate of decline in kidney function. Current recommendations state that blood pressure should be reduced in diabetics to <130/80mm Hg and come from analyzing retrospective data suggesting a slower decline in renal function and greater cardiovascular disease risk reduction when blood pressure is lowered to these goals [4]. Is there sufficient clinical evidence to justify this recommendation?

The United Kingdom Prospective Diabetes Study (UKPDS) was performed in 1148 type 2 diabetics with hypertension [29]. It involved simultaneous randomizations to study both the effects of different initial antihypertensive medications (a treatment regimen comparing the angiotensin-converting enzyme inhibitor [ACE-I], captopril, to the β-blocker, atenolol), as well as two different blood pressure goals (blood pressure target of <150/85mm Hg compared to a target of <180/105mm Hg). There was no difference in outcome between the captopril and atenolol-based treatment groups after an average 8.4-year follow-up. However, the 758 patients randomized to the 'tight' blood pressure goal of <150/85mm Hg (who actually achieved an average blood pressure of 144/82mm Hg) experienced fewer cardiovascular events than the 390 randomized to the 'less tight' goal of <180/105mm Hg (who achieved an average blood pressure of 154/87mm Hg). Participants in the lower blood pressure group had a risk reduction of 32% in diabetes-related deaths, 24% reduction in diabetes-related endpoints (including amputations), 44% reduction in strokes and 37% reduction in microvascular complications (including nephropathy and advanced retinopathy requiring photocoagulation) (Table 3). Thus, a blood pressure difference of only -10/-5mm Hg resulted in a significant risk reduction in diabetes-related cardiovascular and microvascular (including renal) complications. While the achieved blood pressure difference was associated with benefit, the achieved average blood pressure was still more than 10mm Hg higher than the recommended goal of <130/80mm Hg.

If there is no clinical trial evidence for <130/80mm Hg in the diabetic, why is this goal recommended?

A post hoc analysis of the UKPDS found that for each 10mm Hg reduction in systolic blood pressure, additional risk reductions occurred in both macrovascular (atherosclerotic) and microvascular events: 15% for death related to diabetes, 11% for myocardial infarction, 12% for any complication related to diabetes and 13% for microvascular complications [30]. In this analysis, no threshold for lowering blood pressure was observed and the lowest risk of complications was found in diabetics whose systolic blood pressure was less than 120mm Hg. The authors concluded that while any reduction in systolic blood pressure reduces the risk of complications from diabetes, the greater the reduction in blood pressure the better the outcome.

Table 3. Comparative study of ace inhibitor- and β-blocker-based treatment program in UKPDS. *Adapted from United Kingdom Prospective Diabetes Study UKPDS* [29].
◆ Number of patients in study (non-insulin-dependent diabetics): 1148
◆ Tight blood pressure control; achieved blood pressure of 144/82mm Hg compared with group with blood pressures of 154/87mm Hg
◆ Reduction in cardiovascular risk – tight: less effective blood pressure control
◆ Reduction in events:
o strokes — 44%
o heart failure — 56%
o deaths related to diabetes — 32%
o microvascular disease — 37%
o myocardial infarction and sudden death — 21% (not significant)
◆ Difference in achieved blood pressure of -10/-5 mm Hg accounted for difference in outcome

Additional data on benefit from a reduction in systolic blood pressure on cardiovascular outcome were also reported in post hoc analyses of the diabetic cohorts within the SHEP [31] and Systolic Hypertension in Europe (Syst-Eur) trials [32]. Diabetics with a systolic blood pressure less than 140mm Hg had a greater cardiovascular disease risk reduction when compared to those with higher blood pressure levels, while those who achieved levels <130mm Hg had an even greater reduction in cardiovascular risk. Accordingly, the current recommendation for reducing systolic blood pressure to <130mm Hg in diabetics comes from post hoc and observational analysis **(IV/C)** [33].

What do the most recent trials suggest in patients with diabetes?

The Appropriate Blood Pressure Control in Diabetes (ABCD) trial randomized type 2 diabetic subjects with hypertension to different levels of blood pressure control in an attempt to answer the question of how low to go and does it make a difference in clinical outcome. This study found no difference between the groups in cardiovascular risk with a mean systolic blood pressure of 138mm Hg compared to 132mm Hg over a 5-year follow-up period [34].

The benefit in reducing diastolic blood pressure was tested in the Hypertension Optimal Treatment (HOT) trial [19]. Of 18,790 patients in the clinical trial, a sub-study evaluated 1501 type 2 diabetic patients randomized to one of three diastolic blood pressure goals: ≤90, ≤85, or ≤80mm Hg. After 3.8 years of follow-up, patients randomized to ≤80mm Hg had a 51% reduction in the total risk of heart attack, stroke, or death, the primary endpoint, compared to

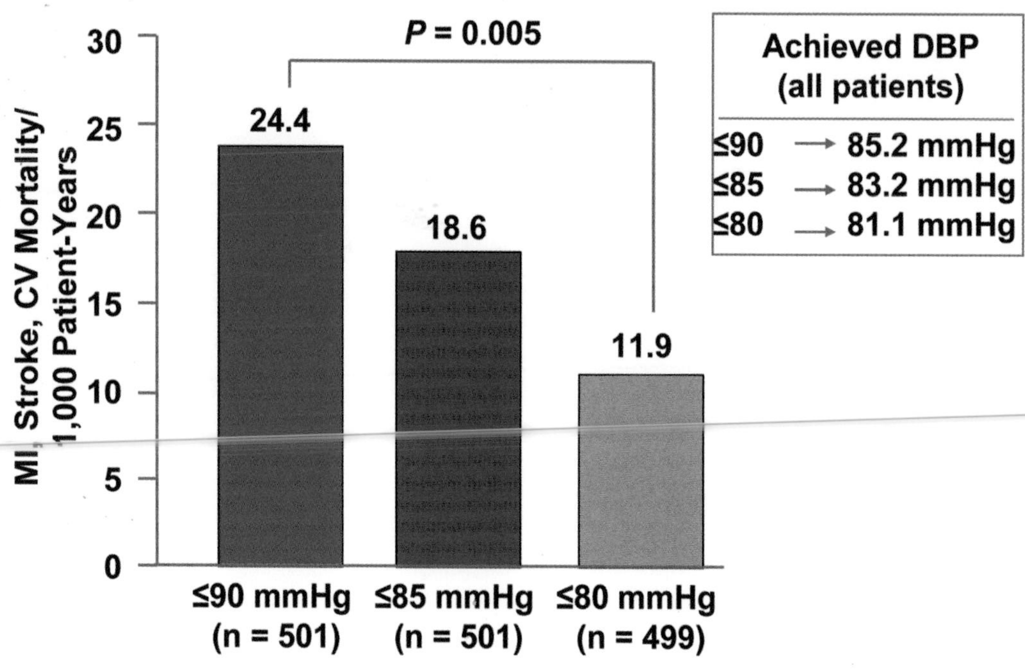

Figure 1. HOT Trial: blood pressure control reduces cardiovascular events (diabetes subgroup). DBP = diastolic blood pressure; HOT = hypertension optimal treatment. *Adapted from Hansson L, et al* [19].

those whose diastolic blood pressure was ≤90mm Hg (Figure 1). Mean achieved diastolic blood pressure in the two groups was 81 and 85mm Hg, respectively. Even when other endpoints were compared (e.g. including 'silent' myocardial infarction or cardiovascular death), the group randomized to the lowest diastolic blood pressure had the best prognosis. While the average achieved systolic blood pressure in this trial was 138mm Hg, lower trends in cardiovascular events were observed in individuals whose systolic blood pressure was <130mm Hg.

The Action in Diabetes and Vascular Disease Preterax and Diamicron-MR Controlled Evaluation (ADVANCE) was an industry-sponsored trial designed to determine whether there was a substantial benefit to using a combination of an ACE-I and a diuretic in patients with type 2 diabetes mellitus [35]. The mean age was 66 years (43% female) and approximately one third had a history of underlying cardiovascular disease. Of note, there was no specific blood pressure goal in randomization. The primary endpoint was a composite of major macrovascular events including cardiovascular death, non-fatal myocardial infarction or non-fatal stroke, and several types of microvascular events including new or worsening nephropathy or retinopathy. During a mean follow-up of 4.3 years, the mean blood pressure achieved was 135/75mm Hg in the active treatment arm and 140/77mm Hg in the placebo arm (difference in blood pressure of 5.6mm Hg systolic/2.2mm Hg diastolic). There was a reduction in the primary composite outcome that just met statistical significance. If we assume that 50-60% of subjects achieved their systolic goal blood pressure of 135mm Hg (which was not reported in the trial), this would have corresponded to having a goal blood pressure of <140mm Hg.

The Stop Atherosclerosis in Native Diabetics (SANDS) study compared standard versus aggressive therapy on the progression of subclinical atherosclerosis in 499 Native American adults with type 2 diabetes and no prior cardiovascular disease [36]. Patients were randomized to one of two levels of LDL-C (<100 versus <70mg/dL) and one of two levels of systolic blood pressure (<130 vs <115mm Hg). The primary endpoint was change in carotid intimal-medial thickness (c-IMT) and left ventricular mass reduction. Over the 3 years of the study, mean achieved LDL-C was 104 and 72mg/dL and mean achieved systolic blood pressure was 129 and 117mm Hg in the standard compared to aggressive group, respectively. The main finding was that in the more aggressively treated group, c-IMT actually regressed from baseline, while in the standard group c-IMT progressed, a difference that was statistically significant. In addition, a greater decrease in left ventricular mass occurred in those whose blood pressure was more aggressively treated. Because this study examined changes in a subclinical or surrogate atherosclerotic endpoint in a specific ethnic group and because clinical cardiovascular events did not differ significantly between groups, it remains unclear whether more aggressive treatment of LDL-C and specifically reduction of systolic blood pressure would result in an incremental benefit on cardiovascular events.

In summary, while epidemiologic data indicate that blood pressures of 120/80mm Hg or above are associated with an increase in chronic kidney disease progression as well as cardiovascular morbidity and mortality in persons with diabetes, the recommendation to lower blood pressure in the diabetic to less than 130/80mm Hg is at present evidence-based only for diastolic blood pressure **(Ib/A)** (HOT trial). Studies in patients with diabetes demonstrate that achieving a systolic blood pressure level around 135mm Hg markedly improves kidney disease outcome compared to levels above 140mm Hg [35]. Despite the lack of evidence, the European Society of Hypertension [16], American Diabetes Association [37], the National Kidney Foundation [33], the British Hypertension Society [38], and JNC 7 [4] still recommend a blood pressure of less than 130/80mm Hg in diabetic patients to reduce cardiovascular morbidity and mortality and to maximally preserve renal function **(IV/C)**. Whether achieving these lower levels of systolic blood pressure will reduce cardiovascular risk was evaluated in the Action to Control Cardiovascular Risk in Diabetes (ACCORD) trial, in which a systolic blood pressure of <120mm Hg (actually achieved 119mm Hg) was compared with a systolic blood pressure of <140mm Hg (actually achieved 133.5mm Hg) [38, 39]. Achieving lower blood pressures in ACCORD did not result in a significant reduction in overall cardiovascular events but reduced strokes (a secondary endpoint). The fact that few events occurred may have reduced the power of this trial to show results.

Benefits of reducing blood pressure to <130/80mm Hg in patients with renal disease

The sixth JNC report recommended a blood pressure of <125/75mm Hg for patients with more than 1g of proteinuria per day [40]. This was based on a post hoc analysis of the Modification of Diet in Renal Disease (MDRD) study whose primary purpose was to see if a lower intake of dietary protein would have a beneficial effect on the progression of renal impairment. All 585 subjects with chronic renal insufficiency were randomized to different levels of dietary protein intake and different blood pressure targets (mean arterial pressure [MAP] <107mm Hg or <92mm Hg, corresponding to cuff blood pressures of <140/90mm Hg or 125/75mm Hg). There were no significant differences in progression of renal disease, hospitalization, or death between randomized groups for either intervention [41]. Since the achieved MAP in the two randomized groups turned out to be only slightly different (93.0 ±7.3 vs. 97.7 ±7.7mm Hg), both blood pressure groups were pooled and stratified according to level of baseline proteinuria. For every 1mm Hg increase in MAP there was a 35% increase in the risk of hospitalization for cardiovascular disease [42]. Based on this post hoc analysis, JNC VI recommended a target blood pressure of <125/75mm Hg for patients with more than 1g per day of proteinuria **(IIb/B)**.

More recently, the African American Study on Kidney disease (AASK) was conducted in African-American non-diabetic patients with renal disease and hypertension [43]. Individuals were randomized to one of three antihypertensive agents and one of two blood pressure goals. African Americans with proteinuria randomized to the calcium antagonist, amlodipine, experienced more renal disease progression than those randomized to the ACE inhibitor, ramipril. Of interest, those randomized to the MAP of less than 92mm Hg (corresponding to a blood pressure <125/75mm Hg) had no further improvement in renal function compared to those randomized to the higher MAP between 102-107mm Hg (corresponding to a blood pressure of 140/90mm Hg). Most individuals, however, did not have greater than 1g of proteinuria at baseline. Based mostly on the AASK results, recommendations have changed; it is no longer recommended that blood pressure be reduced to <125/75mm Hg in patients with renal disease and without proteinuria. The recommended targeted blood pressure to protect against cardiovascular disease and nephropathy in diabetics and non-diabetics with underlying renal disease is now <130/80mm Hg. While data supporting a systolic blood pressure of <140mm Hg is overwhelming, the evidence to reduce the blood pressure to <130/80mm Hg based on prospective clinical trials is lacking [44]. The results of the recently completed ACCORD trial [39] in those with diabetes (see above) and the soon to be started Systolic Blood Pressure Intervention Trial (SPRINT) in those with hypertension, Stage 3 chronic kidney disease, but no diabetes, are comparing a systolic blood pressure goal of <120mm Hg with a systolic blood pressure of <140mm Hg on clinical cardiovascular and renal outcomes.

Are there any dangers of excessive blood pressure lowering?

While the lowering of elevated blood pressure can lead to an improvement in cardiovascular outcome, some studies have observed an increase in cardiovascular events when diastolic blood pressure was reduced below a critical value. This 'J-curve' hypotheses suggests that lowering diastolic blood pressure below a certain value in individuals with underlying cardiovascular disease may increase the risk of cardiovascular death. This has not been observed with reductions in systolic blood pressure.

The HOT study was designed to test this question. As stated above, this was a prospective, randomized, open with blinded endpoint (PROBE) trial which assigned 18,790 hypertensive patients from 26 countries (mean age, 61.5 years) to a target diastolic blood pressure of less than 80mm Hg, less than 85mm Hg, or less than 90mm Hg. After an average 3.8 years of follow-up, only a small 2mm Hg difference (less than the expected 5mm Hg difference) was achieved among the three groups (81, 83 and 85mm Hg, respectively). While no benefit was seen in the overall group that achieved the lowest diastolic blood pressure, except in diabetes, no increase in cardiovascular events occurred either at the achieved diastolic blood pressure 81mm Hg compared to achieved 85mm Hg. The 'optimum' blood pressure to prevent cardiovascular events was 138.5/82.6mm Hg [18].

While the HOT study found no evidence of a J-curve, a retrospective analysis of the SHEP trial found that in the few patients whose diastolic blood pressure was lowered to less than 55mm Hg, no benefit in outcome occurred compared with those in the placebo group. Furthermore, an analysis of The International Verapamil-Trandolapril Study (INVEST) found that in patients with hypertension and coronary artery disease, reducing blood pressure to lower than 70mm Hg was associated with outcomes similar to those with diastolic blood pressure readings above 100mm Hg [6]. Until further prospective trials examine this question, it appears prudent to exercise caution in reducing diastolic blood pressure to less than 55mm Hg in older individuals with ISH [45] and to less than 70mm Hg in people with hypertension and underlying coronary artery disease [6]. Fortunately, it is uncommon to achieve a blood pressure below 55mm Hg as systolic blood pressure is lowered.

Conclusions

Treating and controlling hypertension is associated with less cardiovascular and renal disease than if blood pressure remains uncontrolled. Despite the fact that many patients who experienced benefit in clinical trials did not achieve the recommended blood pressure goals, there is evidence to recommend a blood pressure goal of <140/90mm Hg in patients with uncomplicated hypertension and a diastolic blood pressure goal of <80mm Hg in individuals with diabetes (keeping the systolic blood pressure goal at <140mm Hg) **(Ib/A)**. Although a goal of <130/80mm Hg is recommended for patients with chronic renal disease and diabetes, there is no good clinical trial-based evidence to support this **(IV/C)**. Finally, the recommendation to achieve a blood pressure of <120/80mm Hg in people with heart failure of ischemic origin is also without good clinical trial evidence of benefit **(IV/C)**. The results of the ACCORD trial suggest that setting a goal toward a systolic blood pressure to below 120mm Hg rather than <140mm Hg will not reduce cardiovascular events but will further reduce strokes, a secondary endpoint. The SPRINT trial will provide more clinical-trial data on the benefit of treating to a more aggressive systolic blood pressure goal especially in those with chronic kidney disease.

Key points	Evidence level
◆ While current guidelines suggest that the minimum goal for blood pressure reduction is a systolic blood pressure <140mm Hg and a diastolic blood pressure <90mm Hg, there is more evidence for the diastolic goal from clinical trials.	Ib/A
◆ While the current guidelines suggest that systolic blood pressure be lowered to <140mm Hg in patients with ISH, clinical trial evidence suggests that cardiovascular benefit occurs when systolic blood pressure is reduced by 15-20mm Hg below the baseline systolic blood pressure, even if not to the recommended goal.	IV/C
◆ The guideline recommendation to lower blood pressure in the diabetic to <130/80mm Hg is evidence-based only for diastolic blood pressure. The ACCORD trial found that achieving a systolic BP goal <120mm Hg did not result in a significant reduction in overall cardiovascular events compared to a systolic BP goal <140mm Hg.	IV/C
◆ Based mostly on the AASK trial, the current evidenced-based goal for blood pressure reduction both to protect against cardiovascular disease and progressive nephropathy in patients with underlying renal disease should be <140/90mm Hg.	Ib/A
◆ Until prospective trials examine the question further, it seems prudent to exercise caution when lowering diastolic blood pressure to less than 55mm Hg in older individuals with ISH and to no less than 70mm Hg in those with underlying ischemic heart disease.	IV/C

References

1. Kannel WB. Elevated systolic blood pressure as a cardiovascular risk factor. *Am J Cardiol* 2000; 15: 251-5.
2. Lewington S, Clarke R,Qizilbash N, *et al.* Age-specific relevance of usual blood pressure to vascular mortality. *Lancet* 2002; 360: 1903-13.
3. Kannel WB, Schwartz MJ, McNamara PM. Blood pressure and risk of coronary heart disease. The Framingham Study. *Dis Chest* 1969; 56: 43-62.
4. The Seventh Report of the Joint National Committee on Prevention, Detection, Evaluation, and Treatment of High Blood Pressure The JNC 7 Report. *JAMA* 2003; 289: 2560-72.
5. Rosendorff C, Black HR, Cannon CP, *et al.* Treatment of hypertension in the prevention and management of ischemic heart disease: a scientific statement from the American Heart Association Council for High Blood Pressure Research and the Councils on Clinical Cardiology and Epidemiology and Prevention. *Circulation* 2007; 115: 2761-88.
6. Messerli FH, Mancia G, Conti CR, *et al.* Dogma disputed: can aggressively lowering blood pressure in hypertensive patients with coronary artery disease be dangerous? *Ann Intern Med* 2006; 144: 884-93.
7. Arguedas JA, Perez MI, Wright JM. Treatment blood pressure targets for hypertension. *Cochrane Database Syst Rev* 2009; 3: CD004349.

8. Moser M, Franklin SS. Hypertension Management Results of a National Survey for the Hypertensive Foundation. Harris Interactive. *J Clin Hypertension* 2007; 9 (5): 316-22.
9. The Sixth report of the Joint National Committee on Prevention, Detection, Evaluation, and Treatment of High Blood Pressure (JNC VI). *Arch Intern Med* 1997; 157: 2413-46.
10. Veterans Administration Cooperative Study Group on Antihypertensive Agents. Effects of treatment on morbidity in hypertension: results in patients with diastolic blood pressure averaging 115 through 129 mm Hg. *JAMA* 1967; 202: 1028-34.
11. Moser M, Hebert PR. Prevention of disease progression, left ventricular hypertrophy and congestive heart failure in hypertension treatment trials. *J Am Coll Cardiol* 1996; 27: 1214-8.
12. Psaty BM, Smith NL, Siscovick DS, *et al.* Health outcomes associated with antihypertensive therapies used as first-line agents: a systematic review and meta-analysis. *JAMA* 1997; 277: 739-45.
13. Blood Pressure Lowering Treatment Trialists' Collaborative. Effects of ACE-inhibitors, calcium antagonists, and other blood-pressure-lowering drugs: results of prospectively designed overviews of randomised trials. *Lancet* 2000; 356: 1955-64.
14. Hebert PR, Moser M, Mayer J, Hennekens CH. Recent evidence on drug therapy of mild to moderate hypertension and decreased risk of coronary heart disease. *Arch Intern Med* 1993; 153: 578-81.
15. Staessen JA, Li Y, Thijs L, *et al.* Blood pressure reduction and cardiovascular prevention: an update including the 2003-2004 secondary prevention trials. *Hypertens Res* 2005; 28 (5): 385-407.
16. The task force for the management of arterial hypertension of the European Society of Hypertension (ESH) and of the European Society of Cardiology (ESC). 2007 guidelines for the management of arterial hypertension. *J Hypertens* 2007; 25: 1105-87.
17. Verdecchia P, Staessen JA, Angeli F, *et al*, on behalf of the Cardio-Sis investigators. Usual versus tight control of systolic blood pressure in non-diabetic patients with hypertension (Cardio-Sis): an open-label randomised trial. *Lancet* 2009; 374: 525.
18. Lloyd-Jones DM, Evans JC, Larson MG, *et al.* Differential control of systolic and diastolic blood pressure. Factors asssociated with lack of blood pressure control in the community. *Hypertension* 2000; 36: 504-9.
19. Hansson L, Zanchetti A, Carruthers SG, *et al.* Effects of intensive blood-pressure lowering and low-dose aspirin in patients with hypertension: principal results of the Hypertension Optimal Treatment (HOT) randomized trial. HOT Study Group. *Lancet* 1998; 351: 1755-62.
20. Major outcomes in high-risk hypertensive patients randomized to angiotensin-converting enzyme inhibitor or calcium channel blocker vs diuretic. The Antihypertensive and Lipid-Lowering Treatment to Prevent Heart Attack Trial (ALLHAT). *JAMA* 2002; 288: 2981-97.
21. Black HR, Elliot WJ, Grandist G, Grambsch P, Lucente T, White WB, *et al*, for the CONVINCE Research Group. Principal results of the Controlled Onset Verapamil Investigation of Cardiovascular Endpoints (CONVINCE) trial. *JAMA* 2003; 289: 2073-82.
22. The Fifth Report of the Joint National Committee on Prevention, Detection, Evaluation, and Treatment of High Blood Pressure (JNC V). *Arch Intern Med* 1993; 153: 154-83.
23. SHEP Cooperative Research Group. Prevention of stroke by antihypertensive drug treatment in older persons with isolated systolic hypertension. *JAMA* 1991; 265(4): 3255-64.
24. Staessen JA, Fagard R, Thijs L, *et al.* Morbidity and mortality in the placebo controlled European trial on isolated systolic hypertension (Syst-Eur) in the elderly. *Lancet* 1997; 350: 757-64.
25. Staessen JA, Gasowski J, Wang JC, *et al.* Risk of untreated and treated isolated systolic hypertension in the elderly: meta-analysis of outcome trials. *Lancet* 2000; 355: 865-72.
26. Beckett NS, Peters R, Fletcher AE, *et al*, for the HYVET Study group. Treatment of hypertension in patients 80 years of age or older. *N Engl J Med* 2008; 359: 2417-28.
27. Perry HM Jr, Davis BR, Price TR, *et al.* Effect of treating isolated systolic hypertension on the risk of developing various types and subtypes of stroke. The Systolic Hypertension in the Elderly Program (SHEP). *JAMA* 2000; 284: 465-71.
28. Izzo J, Levy D, Black HR. Clinical Advisory Statement. Importance of systolic blood pressure in older Americans. *Hypertension* 2000; 35: 1021-4.
29. Turner R, Holman R, Stratton I, *et al*, for the United Kingdom Prospective Diabetes Study Group. Tight blood pressure control and risk of macrovascular and microvascular complications in type 2 diabetes: UKPDS 38. *BMJ* 1998; 317: 707-13.

30. Adler AI, Stratton IM, Neil HA, *et al.* Association of systolic blood pressure with macrovascular or microvascular complications of type 2 diabetes (UKPDS 36) *BMJ* 2000; 312(7258): 412-9.
31. Curb JD, Pressel SL, Cutler JA, *et al.* Effect of diuretic-based antihypertensive treatment on cardiovascular disease risk in older diabetic patients with isolated systolic hypertension. Systolic Hypertension in the Elderly Program Cooperative Research Group. *JAMA* 1996; 276 (23): 1886-92.
32. Tuomilehto J, Rastenyte D, Birkenhager WH, *et al.* Effects of calcium-channel blockade in older patients with diabetes and systolic hypertension. Systolic Hypertension in Europe Trial Investigators. *N Engl J Med* 1999; 340(9): 677-84.
33. Bakris GL, Williams M, Dworkin L, *et al.* Preserving renal function in adults with hypertension and diabetes: a consensus approach. National Kidney Foundation Hypertension and Diabetes Executive Committees working group. *Am J Kidney Diseases* 2000; 36(3): 646-61.
34. Estacio RO, Jeffers BW, Gifford N, Schrier RW. Effect of blood pressure control on diabetic microvascular complications in patients with hypertension and type 2 diabetes. *Diabetes Care* 2000; Suppl 2: B54-64.
35. Patel A, *et al*, for the ADVANCE Collaborative Group. Effects of a fixed combination of perindopril and indapamide on macrovascular and microvascular outcomes in patients with type 2 diabetes mellitus (the ADVANCE trial): a randomised controlled trial. *Lancet* 2007; 370: 829.
36. Howard BV, Roman MJ, Devereux RB, *et al.* Effect of lower targets for blood pressure and LDL cholesterol on atherosclerosis in diabetes: the SANDS randomized trial. *JAMA* 2008; 299: 1678-89.
37. American Diabetes Association: Summary Statement 2009. *Diabetes Care* 2009; 32 Suppl 1: S1-147.
38. Ramsay LE, Williams B, Johnston GD, *et al.* British Hypertension Society Guidelines for hypertension management 1999: Summary. *BMJ* 1999; 319: 630-5.
39. Cushman WC, Evans GW, Byington RP, *et al*, for the ACCORD Study Group. The effects of intensive blood pressure control in type 2 diabetes mellitus. Epub - published on March 14, 2010, www.nejm.org.
40. The Sixth report of the Joint National Committee on Prevention, Detection, Evaluation, and Treatment of High Blood Pressure (JNC VI). *Arch Intern Med* 1997; 157: 2413-46.
41. Klahr S, Levey AS, Beck GJ, *et al.* The effects of dietary protein restriction and blood-pressure control on the progression of chronic renal disease: Modification of Diet in Renal Disease Study Group. *N Engl J Med* 1994; 330: 877-84.
42. Lazarus JM, Bourgoignie JJ, Buckalew VM, *et al*, for the Modification of Diet in Renal Disease Study Group. Achievement and safety of a low blood pressure goal in chronic renal disease: the Modification of Diet in Renal Disease Study Group. *Hypertension* 1997; 29: 641-50.
43. Wright JT Jr, Bakris G, Greene T, *et al.* African American Study of Kidney Disease and Hypertension (AASK) Study Group. Effect of blood pressure lowering and antihypertensive drug class on progression of hypertensive kidney disease. *JAMA* 2002; 288: 2421-31.
44. Kalaitzidis R, Bakris G. Lower blood pressure goals for cardiovascular and renal risk reduction: are they defensible? *J Clin Hypertension* 2009; 2(7): 345-7.
45. Somes G, Pahor M, Shorr RI, *et al.* The role of diastolic blood pressure when treating isolated systolic hypertension. *Arch Intern Med* 1999; 159: 2004-9.

Chapter 2

The effects of sodium and potassium intake on blood pressure

Sharon Turban MD MHS, Assistant Professor of Medicine, Division of Nephrology, The Johns Hopkins University School of Medicine, Baltimore, Maryland, USA

Lawrence J. Appel MD MPH, Professor of Medicine, Epidemiology and International Health (Human Nutrition)
The Johns Hopkins University School of Medicine, The Welch Center for Prevention, Epidemiology and Clinical Research, and The Johns Hopkins Bloomberg School of Public Health, Johns Hopkins Medical Institutions, Baltimore, Maryland, USA

Introduction

The earliest known comment on the relationship of dietary salt intake with blood pressure was from a Chinese physician who in approximately 1700 BC stated that "if large amounts of salt are taken, the pulse will stiffen and harden" [1]. In 1904, two French scientists noted that increased sodium intake raised blood pressure in non-hypertensive individuals [2]. In the 1920s, several investigators found that reducing sodium intake in hypertensive patients led to an improvement in blood pressure [3]. Evidence continued to mount, including the results of large-scale epidemiologic studies [4] and well-done clinical trials [5]. Currently, virtually all major health organizations now advocate sodium reduction as a means to lower blood pressure.

Although most attention has focused on lowering dietary sodium intake, a large body of evidence suggests that increased potassium intake also lowers blood pressure. As early as the 1920s, increased intake of dietary potassium was recommended as a means to lower blood pressure. In the 1960s-1970s, animal studies were performed which suggested that potassium lowers the rise in blood pressure caused by high sodium intake. The first controlled trial of increased potassium intake in humans took place in the 1980s.

What are the recommended and actual sodium and potassium intake in the U.S. and what are common forms of sodium and potassium?

Table 1 shows the recommended intake of sodium and potassium for adults in the general population (from the Institute of Medicine), the estimated median daily U.S. intake (from the National Health and Nutrition Examination Survey [NHANES] III survey) [6], and common sources of these nutrients. As seen in the table, the estimated daily U.S. intake of sodium vastly exceeds recommended intake levels. For dietary potassium, estimated intake is much lower than what is recommended. Note that the recommendations for potassium intake differ in certain populations such as those with chronic kidney disease. Although there is no specific recommendation for the urinary sodium-to-potassium ratio, the typical ratio in the U.S. is approximately 2.5, which is much higher than would be expected with a recommended sodium and potassium intake.

Most sodium (likely >90%) is consumed as sodium chloride, while potassium from foods is accompanied by bicarbonate or bicarbonate precursors (e.g. citrate). Potassium chloride, the common form of potassium supplements, does not occur naturally in foods.

How are sodium and potassium intake estimated in humans?

Sodium and potassium intake are typically estimated by dietary recall questionnaires (e.g. food frequency questionnaires or repeated 24-hour dietary recall) or measurement of 24-hour urinary sodium and potassium excretion. All methods of assessment have limitations because of the high day-to-day variation in sodium and potassium intake. In addition, questionnaires are limited because they are based on recall. Urinary electrolyte excretion is a better estimator of intake than questionnaires, but it only reflects recent consumption, and is often inaccurate because of incomplete urine collections. Furthermore, urinary potassium excretion appears to more poorly reflect dietary intake than does urinary sodium excretion (the reported percentage of dietary potassium excreted in the urine is quite variable).

The urinary sodium-to-potassium ratio predicts blood pressure [4] and cardiovascular disease [7] more strongly and consistently than urinary sodium and urinary potassium alone **(III/B)**. This ratio simultaneously takes into account the effects of both sodium and potassium and 'corrects' for incomplete urine collections.

What are potential adverse effects of sodium?

Animal and human studies have shown that sodium chloride consumption increases blood pressure **(Ia/A)**. In aggregate, the evidence strongly supports the hypothesis that high levels of sodium consumption are etiologically related to the development of hypertension, which is a major risk factor for cardiovascular and renal disease. The effects of sodium will be discussed further below. In addition, sodium may have blood pressure-dependent and independent adverse cardiovascular effects **(Ib/A)**, including increased stroke risk. For example, studies have shown a direct relationship between increased sodium intake and left

Table 1. Recommended and typical intake of sodium and potassium in the U.S. along with common forms and sources.

	Recommended minimum/maximum intake for the general population*	Estimated median daily U.S. intake**	Forms and sources
Sodium	*Upper Intake Level (UL):* No more than 2.3g/d (100mmol/day) (1.5g/d for certain populations, such as hypertensives, chronic kidney disease, diabetics, and African-Americans) *Adequate intake (AI)* • young adults: 1.5g (65mmol)/day • ages 50-70: 1.3g (55mmol)/day • age >70: 1.2g (50mmol)/day	Men: 3.1-4.7g (135-204mmol)/day Women: 2.3-3.1g (100-135mmol)/day	• Sodium chloride (table salt): found naturally in some foods (e.g. meats, nuts, and grains), but most intake is from preserved and processed foods (e.g. sandwich meats, soups, cheeses, fast food) • Monosodium glutamate (MSG): common seasoning • Disodium phosphate: in quick-cooking cereals and processed cheeses • Sodium bicarbonate: baking soda • Sodium benzoate: common condiment preservative • Sodium nitrite: in cured meats • Sodium sulfite: dried fruit preservative • Sodium propionate: mold inhibitor (in pasteurized cheeses, breads, and cakes) • Sodium alginate: in chocolate milks and ice creams
Potassium	*Adequate intake (AI)* At least 4.7g (120mmol)/day (no upper limit established)	Men: 2.8-3.3g (72-84mmol) Women: 2.2-2.4g (56-61mmol)	• Potassium citrate and potassium phosphate: food sources high in potassium (>400mg/serving) include raisins, baked potatoes, prunes, beans, papayas, bananas, melons • Potassium chloride: salt substitutes • Potassium chloride, potassium citrate, potassium bicarbonate: potassium supplements

* Recommended by the Institutes of Medicine of the National Academies [6]

** The estimated median daily U.S. intake of potassium is based on the National Health and Nutrition Examination Survey (NHANES) III data for adults (1998-1994) [6]

ventricular mass which persists even after adjustment for blood pressure [8, 9]. A randomized controlled trial in hypertensive individuals [10] showed that a low-sodium intervention

* Footnotes: *To convert g sodium to mmol sodium, divide by 0.023; to convert g potassium to mmol (or mEq) potassium, divide by 0.0391.*

significantly reduced left ventricular mass. Animal studies and human epidemiological studies suggest that a high sodium diet may lead to strokes, both independent of and additive to its effect on blood pressure. An analysis of the INTERSALT study found a positive correlation between 24-hour urinary sodium excretion and stroke mortality [11]. A low sodium diet may also have positive renal benefits, including a decrease in proteinuria [12, 13] **(Ib/A)** and reduced risk of kidney stones. A study in post-menopausal women showed that, at 2 years, the loss of hip bone density was positively associated with baseline 24-hour urinary sodium excretion [14] **(III/B)**. The effects of sodium on kidney stones and bones are likely due to the increased intestinal calcium absorption, increased urinary calcium excretion, and increased mobilization of calcium from bone associated with a high sodium intake.

What are potential beneficial effects of potassium?

Potassium deficiency has been shown to have multiple negative cardiovascular and renal effects, while potassium supplementation has been shown to have multiple benefits in animal and human studies. Adverse cardiovascular effects of potassium depletion include arrhythmias [15, 16], impaired myocardial performance [17], and increased morbidity and mortality in patients with congestive heart failure. Renal consequences of potassium depletion include elevated blood pressure, cyst formation, hypercalciuria, nephrolithiasis, and deterioration of kidney function via tubulointerstitial, glomerular, and vascular renal injury. Low serum potassium has also been associated with glucose intolerance.

A major benefit of potassium demonstrated in multiple studies includes lowering blood pressure in hypertensive and non-hypertensive individuals **(Ia/A)**. Diets rich in potassium may also have cardiovascular benefits [18] **(Ib/A)** including reduction of arrhythmias, myocardial fibrosis, and strokes, and improvement in left ventricular function. Other potential benefits include improvement in endothelial function and arterial compliance [19]. An increase in potassium intake may also decrease calcium excretion, which may lead to a reduction in nephrolithiasis and bone demineralization **(Ib/A)**. In children on a ketogenic diet, the use of potassium citrate was associated with a reduction in kidney stones [20]. Similarly, a retrospective analysis showed that potassium citrate was associated with a decrease in the rate of kidney stone formation [21]. Potassium bicarbonate reduced bone turnover in small studies of postmenopausal women [22] and mild hypertensives [19]. In patients with medullary sponge kidney, retrospective analyses revealed that long-term potassium citrate use was associated with an improvement in bone density [23]. In addition, animal studies have shown that increased potassium intake may protect against kidney damage, and, therefore, may potentially retard the progression of kidney disease [24-29]. These cardiovascular and renal effects may be mediated via both blood pressure-dependent and blood pressure-independent mechanisms.

What are the potential mechanisms by which sodium and potassium affect blood pressure?

The effects of sodium intake appear to be modulated by dietary potassium intake, and vice versa. Prehistoric diets were extremely low in sodium and concomitantly high in potassium.

In this setting, humans evolved to conserve sodium and excrete potassium. In contrast to prehistoric diets, the modern Western diet is high in sodium and low in potassium. Low-potassium diets have been shown to lead to renal sodium retention, while high sodium intake can cause an increase in urinary potassium excretion.

There appears to be an interdependency of sodium and potassium in influencing blood pressure. There are several mechanisms by which high dietary sodium intake and low potassium intake might raise blood pressure. A high sodium intake may lead to extracellular volume expansion and an increased expression of the renal sodium pump via release of a digitalis-like factor. Increased activity of the renal sodium pump, also stimulated by long-term potassium depletion, promotes sodium retention. Both high sodium and potassium depletion also have effects on vascular smooth muscle cell contraction, leading to increased peripheral vascular resistance and increased blood pressure.

Potassium may lower blood pressure via several potential mechanisms, including natriuresis (although this is likely an acute effect), and vasodilation (via direct and indirect effects, including those mediated by angiotensin II and nitric oxide). Other potential mechanisms have been hypothesized, including effects of prostaglandins, endothelin, kallikrein, and atrial natriuretic peptides. Animal studies suggest that potassium has multiple beneficial vascular effects as well.

What do observational studies in humans reveal about the association between sodium and potassium intake and blood pressure?

Animal studies demonstrate that increased sodium intake increases blood pressure. Multiple observational studies within and across human populations around the world have supported a direct relationship between sodium intake and blood pressure as well as an inverse relationship between potassium intake and blood pressure. Blood pressure and rates of hypertension are lower in populations known to have a low sodium and high potassium intake, although this association has not been confirmed in all studies.

The INTERSALT study [4] was one of the largest (10,079 participants in 32 countries) observational studies that investigated the relationship between sodium and potassium intake and blood pressure. In that study, urinary sodium excretion ranged from 4.6mg (0.20mmol)/day (Yanomamo Indians of Brazil) to 5.6g (242mmol)/day (Northern Chinese population). A positive relationship between urinary sodium excretion (and urinary sodium-to-potassium ratio) and systolic blood pressure and a negative association between urinary potassium excretion and blood pressure were found in individual subjects.

Is there an association between the age-related rise in blood pressure and sodium/potassium?

In most populations, blood pressure rises as individuals age. There are, however, several isolated populations around the world in which an age-related rise in blood pressure is not seen or is minimal. Sodium intake in these populations is very low, while potassium intake is high. Figure 1 from the INTERSALT study [4] demonstrates that the slope of systolic blood pressure with age is higher in populations with a higher urinary sodium excretion. For

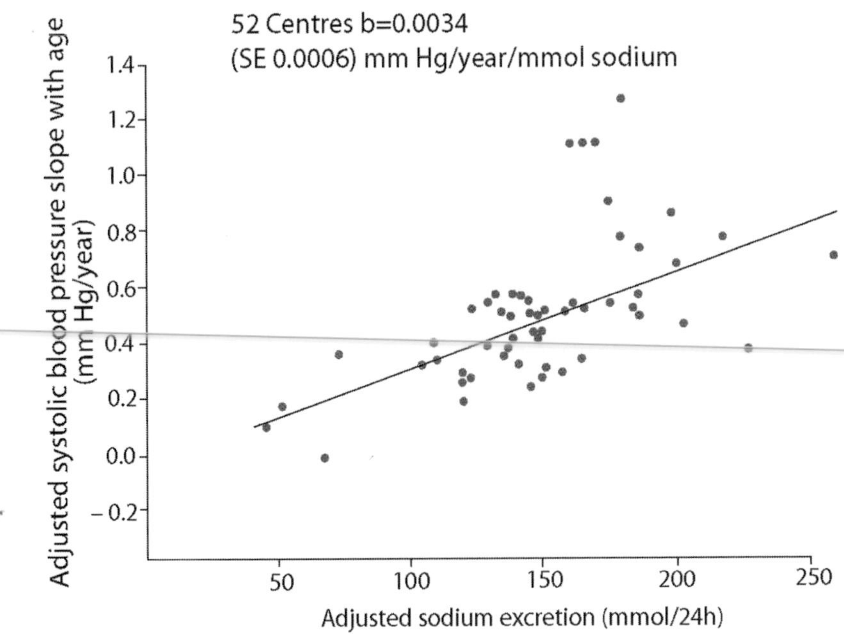

Figure 1. Slope of systolic blood pressure with age and urinary sodium excretion in the INTERSALT study [4]. *Reproduced with permission from the BMJ Publishing Group Ltd., © 1988.*

example, the Yanomamo Indians do not experience an age-related rise in blood pressure. As mentioned above, in the INTERSALT study, their mean sodium intake was less than 1mmol per day. This absence of a rise in blood pressure with age that is seen in certain populations has been attributed to their low sodium intake. However, there may be other factors involved, such as the increased potassium intake which is often present in low-sodium diets, as well as genetic and other environmental factors.

What do migratory studies reveal about sodium and potassium and blood pressure?

Populations that migrate from one geographic area to another commonly adopt the dietary pattern of the new environment. Such events provide an opportunity to examine genetic versus environmental determinants of blood pressure, because migration occurs rapidly without an opportunity for genetic changes. In one migration study, farmers in Kenya who ate a low-sodium/high potassium diet at baseline and subsequently migrated to an urban community, thereby increasing their sodium intake and decreasing their potassium intake, were found to have a significantly higher mean systolic blood pressure than farmers who did not move [30]. Although the study did not account for other changes that occurred during the move, this and other migratory studies suggest that changes in sodium and potassium intake are among the lifestyle changes that lead to higher blood pressure when individuals migrate from a rural area to an urban area.

What are some drawbacks of observational studies?

Observational studies, while providing strong evidence for an association of sodium and potassium intake with blood pressure, nonetheless have limitations. Because of suboptimal measurement techniques, assessment of sodium intake is often inaccurate. In addition, measurements of sodium intake are often imprecise because of the large day-to-day variability in sodium intake. Also, it is difficult in these studies to separate the effects of sodium and potassium, because potassium intake typically is high in low-sodium diets, and vice-versa. Other confounding variables related to genes, other dietary factors, and other potential determinants of blood pressure are often not measured. For these reasons, investigators have conducted clinical trials, including feeding studies, to assess the impact of a dietary factor, manipulated in isolation, while holding other factors constant.

What do intervention studies of sodium intake and blood pressure demonstrate?

Multiple clinical trials in humans have investigated the association between sodium intake and blood pressure. Several meta-analyses of intervention trials of sodium reduction have been performed. In general, these analyses document that sodium reduction lowers blood pressure. Some of the meta-analyses included studies of limited public health relevance, such as trials with extremely short duration or which studied levels of sodium intake that will unlikely be achieved (e.g. <10mmol/d). Residual debate pertains to the strength of the association and its implications for public health. He and MacGregor published a relevant meta-analysis of modest sodium reduction which only included trials that lasted at least one month [31]. In this meta-analysis, a 2.3g (100mmol)/day decrease in sodium intake was associated with an average decrease in systolic/diastolic blood pressure of 7.1/3.9mmHg ($p<0.001$ for both) in hypertensive individuals and a 3.6/1.7mm Hg decrease ($p<0.001$ and <0.05, respectively) in non-hypertensives.

Of the available trials, two dose-response trials have been particularly influential [32, 33]. The Dietary Approaches to Stop Hypertension (DASH) – Sodium study [33] was a multi-center randomized, controlled feeding trial that tested the effects of three levels of dietary sodium on blood pressure in individuals with and without hypertension in the setting of two different diets. As shown in Figure 2, in the setting of a control (low potassium; typical American) diet, there was a progressive reduction in systolic blood pressure as sodium intake was lowered from 3.4g (150mmol) to 2.3g (100mmol) to 1.1g (50mmol)/day. Importantly, the dose-response was non-linear; a greater blood pressure reduction occurred when sodium was reduced from 100 to 50mmol/d than when it was lowered from 150 to 100mmol/d. A similar pattern of results occurred in hypertensives and non-hypertensives. The dose-response trial by MacGregor [32], conducted in hypertensive individuals, demonstrated a similar, potentially non-linear dose-response relationship.

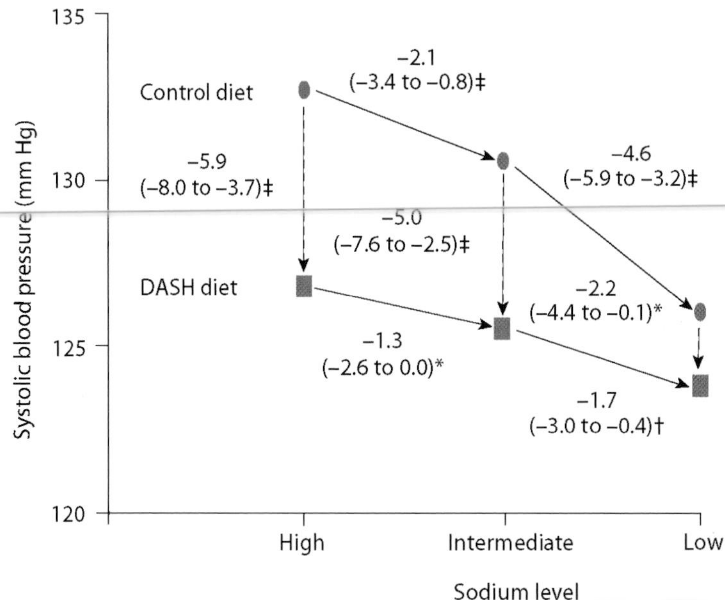

Figure 2. The effect of the DASH diet and various levels of dietary sodium intake on systolic blood pressure [33]. *Reproduced with permission from the Massachusetts Medical Society.*

Does altering potassium intake in intervention studies affect blood pressure?

Intervention trials avoid many problems faced in observational studies, in which it can be difficult to tease apart the effects of potassium from other nutrients and confounding variables. Trials of potassium intake include potassium supplement trials and trials that test potassium-rich diets, such as diets that emphasize fruits and vegetables. Several trials have evaluated the effect of potassium on blood pressure. However, many of these trials were small, brief, and had other design limitations. Most supplement trials tested potassium chloride rather than potassium with a bicarbonate precursor, the most common form of potassium in our diet. Also, most supplement trials did not control dietary potassium intake.

A meta-analysis of potassium supplement trials by Whelton *et al* [34] demonstrated that (excluding one study) potassium supplementation lowered blood pressure by 4.4mm Hg in hypertensives (95% CI 2.2, 6.6) and 1.8mm Hg in normotensive individuals (95% CI 0.6, 2.9). Corresponding values for diastolic blood pressure were 2.5mm Hg (95% CI 0.1, 4.9) and 1.0mm Hg (0.0, 2.1), respectively. The median increase in urinary potassium excretion was 2g (50mmol)/day. Although some meta-analyses did not detect a significant effect of potassium on blood pressure, non-significant trends were typically observed. Available evidence also suggests that the effects of potassium on blood pressure are more evident in the setting of a low baseline intake and in African-Americans.

In a potassium depletion trial [35], 10 healthy, normotensive men were given a baseline diet of 0.39g (10mmol) potassium per day, and received potassium chloride supplementation (3.1g [80mmol] potassium per day) or placebo in a crossover design study. Mean arterial blood pressure was significantly higher after 9 days on the low potassium diet than after 9 days on the standard potassium diet.

Diets rich in potassium have been shown to lower blood pressure. For example, the DASH diet which is rich in fruits, vegetables and low-fat dairy products and reduced in total fat, saturated fat, and cholesterol lowered systolic and diastolic blood pressure by 5.5 and 3.0mm Hg, respectively, in comparison to a control diet in the DASH trial [36]. The DASH diet provided 4.4g potassium/day, while the control diet provided 1.7g potassium/day. The DASH-Sodium trial further documented that the DASH diet, compared to a control diet, lowers BP at three different sodium levels [33]. Nonetheless, it should be recognized that potassium was one of several differences between the DASH and control diets and that the DASH and DASH-Sodium trials were not designed to assess the effects of potassium, *per se*, on blood pressure.

What are the outcomes of population-wide campaigns to lower sodium intake?

Results of community-based intervention projects and trials suggest that such interventions can have a beneficial impact in broad populations. In 1969, a campaign in Belgium to lower sodium intake was conducted. The mean systolic blood pressure decreased in elderly individuals followed in Belgium between 1967 and 1986. There were associated mean reductions in urinary sodium excretion of 77mmol/day in men and 48mmol/day in women [37]. In Portugal, a successful intervention study was carried out in two similar villages with a high incidence of hypertension [38]. One community received vigorous health education about sodium reduction. In this community, sodium intake decreased and was associated with a highly significant improvement in blood pressure control at 1 and 2 years. After 2 years, the control community had a small rise in systolic blood pressure. Other successful population-based intervention programs, such as those in Finland and Asia, have been associated with decreases in blood pressure, stroke, and mortality [39, 40].

What are the long-term effects of reduced sodium intake and/or increased potassium intake?

In contrast to clinical trials that test the effects of antihypertensive medications, few trials have tested the long-term effects of reduced sodium or increased potassium intake on clinical outcomes. There are large, if not insurmountable, obstacles to the conduct of trials that test the effects of dietary changes on clinical outcomes. Nonetheless, the few available trials each suggest beneficial long-term effects from a reduced sodium and/or increased potassium intake **(Ib/A)**.

The long-term follow-up of the Trials of Hypertension Prevention (TOHP) I [41] and II [42] trials suggested that interventions aimed at lowering sodium intake may reduce the long-term risk of cardiovascular events [43]. In those studies, a higher urinary sodium-to-potassium excretion ratio was associated with a higher risk of subsequent cardiovascular disease [7]. Furthermore, a study of almost 2000 elderly Taiwanese veterans demonstrated a long-term beneficial effect on cardiovascular mortality associated with a switch from regular salt to potassium-enriched salt [18]. In aggregate, these trials reinforce dietary recommendations to lower sodium intake as a means of preventing cardiovascular disease in the general population.

Are there arguments against lowering sodium intake?

Although there is widespread support for a population-wide decrease in sodium intake, some scientists have expressed concerns that the long-term effects of such a change are not known and could be harmful. Although the U.S. Food and Drug Administration concluded that "no convincing evidence has been presented that a moderate but significant reduction in salt intake would have any adverse health effects" [44], some individuals have argued that sodium reduction should not be universally recommended. Concerns about activation of the renin-angiotensin and sympathetic nervous systems have been expressed. However, in contrast to the effects on blood pressure, the clinical relevance of an activated renin-angiotensin system or sympathetic nervous system is unknown.

Based on all of the above, what should we recommend for our patients?

In aggregate, a diverse body of evidence strongly supports recommendations for population-wide consumption of a diet that is low in sodium and rich in potassium. Such diets should lower blood pressure, retard the age-related rise in blood pressure, and thereby prevent blood pressure-related as well as blood pressure-independent cardiovascular and renal disease. A seemingly small reduction in blood pressure may actually have substantial implications on a population level. According to Stamler [45], a reduction in systolic blood pressure of 3 to 5mm Hg could lead to a reduction in stroke mortality of 8 to 14% and a reduction in total mortality of 4 to 7% on a population level. Importantly, there is no compelling evidence that a reduced sodium intake is harmful, especially at levels that might be consumed given the current food supply. A high potassium intake in the setting of advanced kidney disease or in the setting of other factors (e.g. certain medications) that may predispose to hyperkalemia might be harmful, but these individuals represent a small fraction of the general population; they should be kept under close medical supervision.

To reduce sodium intake, consumers should choose foods low in sodium and limit the amount of salt added to food. However, because over 75% of consumed salt comes from processed foods, any meaningful strategy to reduce salt intake must involve the efforts of food manufacturers and food service operations, which should progressively reduce the salt added to foods by at least 50%. Several economic studies [46, 47] have demonstrated that a population-wide reduction in sodium intake would be extremely cost-effective, potentially resulting in a net saving of several hundred million to billions of dollars per year, along with a potential reduction in cases of hypertension by 11 million in the United States. To increase their potassium intake, individuals will need to select potassium-rich foods such as many fruits and vegetables. Despite the obvious challenges of decreasing sodium and increasing potassium, the potential benefits are substantial and warrant major public health efforts to accomplish these goals.

Conclusions

Current evidence suggests:

- sodium chloride consumption increases blood pressure;
- other negative effects of high sodium chloride intake include hypercalciuria and calcium nephrolithiasis;
- the benefits of a low-sodium intake include improved blood pressure and may include cardiovascular, renal, and bone-related benefits;
- increased potassium intake decreases blood pressure, may have multiple cardiovascular benefits, including decreased stroke risk, and may have beneficial effects on the kidney (including decreased stone formation) and on bone health.

Key points	Evidence level
◆ Reduced sodium intake lowers blood pressure.	Ia/A
◆ Reduced sodium intake likely prevents cardiovascular disease.	Ib/A
◆ Reduced sodium intake lowers proteinuria.	Ib/A
◆ Increased potassium intake lowers blood pressure.	Ia/A
◆ Increased potassium intake likely prevents cardiovascular disease.	Ib/A
◆ Increased potassium intake may prevent kidney stones.	Ib/A
◆ Increased potassium intake may have beneficial effects on bone health.	Ib/A
◆ The urinary sodium-to-potassium ratio predicts blood pressure and cardiovascular events more strongly than urinary sodium or urinary potassium alone.	III/B

References

1. MacGregor GA, deWardener HE. *Salt, Diet, and Health: Neptune's Poisoned Chalice: The Origins of High Blood Pressure*. Cambridge, UK: Cambridge University Press, 1998.
2. Ambard LBE. Causes de l'hypertension arterielle. *Arch Gen Med* 1904; I: 520-33.
3. Allen FM, SherrilL JW. The treatment of arterial hypertension. *J Metab Res* 1925; 2: 429-545.
4. Rose G, Stamler J, Stamler R, *et al.* Intersalt: an international study of electrolyte excretion and blood pressure. Results for 24 hour urinary sodium and potassium excretion. Intersalt Cooperative Research Group. *BMJ* 1988; 297(6644): 319-28.
5. MacGregor GA, Markandu ND, Best FE, *et al.* Double-blind randomised crossover trial of moderate sodium restriction in essential hypertension. *Lancet* 1982; 1(8268): 351-55.
6. Panel on Dietary Reference Intakes for Electrolytes and Water, Standing Committee on the Scientific Evaluation of Dietary Reference Intakes. Institutes of Medicine of the National Academies. Dietary references intakes for water, potassium, sodium, chloride, and sulfate, 2004: 186-268.
7. Cook NR, Obarzanek E, Cutler JA, *et al.* Joint effects of sodium and potassium intake on subsequent cardiovascular disease: the Trials of Hypertension Prevention follow-up study. *Arch Intern Med* 2009; 169(1): 32-40.
8. du Cailar G, Ribstein J, Grolleau R, Mimran A. Influence of sodium intake on left ventricular structure in untreated essential hypertensives. *J Hypertens Suppl* 1989; 7(6): S258-9.
9. Liebson PR, Grandits G, Prineas R, *et al.* Echocardiographic correlates of left ventricular structure among 844 mildly hypertensive men and women in the Treatment of Mild Hypertension Study (TOMHS). *Circulation* 1993; 87(2): 476-86.
10. Jula AM, Karanko HM. Effects on left ventricular hypertrophy of long-term nonpharmacological treatment with sodium restriction in mild-to-moderate essential hypertension. *Circulation* 1994; 89(3): 1023-31.
11. Perry IJ, Beevers DG. Salt intake and stroke: a possible direct effect. *J Hum Hypertens* 1992; 6(1): 23-5.
12. He FJ, Marciniak M, Visagie E, *et al.* Effect of modest salt reduction on blood pressure, urinary albumin, and pulse wave velocity in white, black, and Asian mild hypertensives. *Hypertension* 2009; 54(3): 447-8.
13. Swift PA, Markandu ND, Sagnella GA, He FJ, MacGregor GA. Modest salt reduction reduces blood pressure and urine protein excretion in black hypertensives: a randomized control trial. *Hypertension* 2005; 46(2): 308-12.
14. Devine A, Criddle RA, Dick IM, Kerr DA, Prince RL. A longitudinal study of the effect of sodium and calcium intakes on regional bone density in postmenopausal women. *Am J Clin Nutr* 1995; 62(4): 740-5.
15. Evans SJ, Levi AJ, Jones JV. Wall stress induced arrhythmia is enhanced by low potassium and early left ventricular hypertrophy in the working rat heart. *Cardiovasc Res* 1995; 29(4): 555-62.
16. Nordrehaug JE, Johannessen KA, von der Lippe G. Serum potassium concentration as a risk factor of ventricular arrhythmias early in acute myocardial infarction. *Circulation* 1985; 71(4): 645-9.
17. Srivastava TN, Young DB. Impairment of cardiac function by moderate potassium depletion. *J Card Fail* 1995; 1(3): 195-200.
18. Chang HY, Hu YW, Yue CS, *et al.* Effect of potassium-enriched salt on cardiovascular mortality and medical expenses of elderly men. *Am J Clin Nutr* 2006; 83(6): 1289-96.
19. He FJ, Marciniak M, Carney C, Markandu ND, Anand V, Fraser WD, Dalton RN, Kaski JC, MacGregor GA. Effects of potassium chloride and potassium bicarbonate on endothelial function, cardiovascular risk factors, and bone turnover in mild hypertensives. *Hypertension* 2010; 55(3): 681-8.
20. McNally MA, Pyzik PL, Rubenstein JE, Hamdy RF, Kossoff EH. Empiric use of potassium citrate reduces kidney-stone incidence with the ketogenic diet. *Pediatrics* 2009; 124(2): e300-4.
21. Robinson MR, Leitao VA, Haleblian GE, *et al.* Impact of long-term potassium citrate therapy on urinary profiles and recurrent stone formation. *J Urol* 2009; 181(3): 1145-50.
22. Sebastian A, Harris ST, Ottaway JH, Todd KM, Morris RC, Jr. Improved mineral balance and skeletal metabolism in postmenopausal women treated with potassium bicarbonate. *N Engl J Med* 1994; 330: 1776-81.
23. Fabris A, Bernich P, Abaterusso C, *et al.* Bone disease in medullary sponge kidney and effect of potassium citrate treatment. *Clin J Am Soc Nephrol* 2009; 4(12): 1974-9.
24. Ellis D, Banner B, Janosky JE, Feig PU. Potassium supplementation attenuates experimental hypertensive renal injury. *J Am Soc Nephrol* 1992; 2(10): 1529-37.

25. Pere AK, Krogerus L, Mervaala EM, Karppanen H, Ahonen J, Lindgren L. Beneficial effects of dietary magnesium and potassium on cardiac and renal morphologic features in cyclosporin A-induced damage in spontaneously hypertensive rats. *Surgery* 2000; 128(1): 67-75.
26. Pere AK, Lindgren L, Tuomainen P, *et al.* Dietary potassium and magnesium supplementation in cyclosporine-induced hypertension and nephrotoxicity. *Kidney Int* 2000; 58(6): 2462-72.
27. Tobian L, MacNeill D, Johnson MA, Ganguli MC, Iwai J. Potassium protects against renal tubule lesions in NaCl-fed hypertensive Dahl S rats. *Trans Assoc Am Physicians* 1983; 96: 417-25.
28. Tobian L, MacNeill D, Johnson MA, Ganguli MC, Iwai J. Potassium protection against lesions of the renal tubules, arteries, and glomeruli and nephron loss in salt-loaded hypertensive Dahl S rats. *Hypertension* 1984; 6(2 Pt 2): I170-6.
29. Wang W, Soltero L, Zhang P, Huang XR, Lan HY, Adrogue HJ. Renal inflammation is modulated by potassium in chronic kidney disease: possible role of Smad7. *Am J Physiol Renal Physiol* 2007; 293(4): F1123-30.
30. Poulter NR, Khaw KT, Hopwood BE, *et al.* The Kenyan Luo migration study: observations on the initiation of a rise in blood pressure. *BMJ* 1990; 300(6730): 967-72.
31. He FJ, MacGregor GA. Effect of modest salt reduction on blood pressure: a meta-analysis of randomized trials. Implications for public health. *J Hum Hypertens* 2002; 16(11): 761-70.
32. MacGregor GA, Markandu ND, Sagnella GA, Singer DR, Cappuccio FP. Double-blind study of three sodium intakes and long-term effects of sodium restriction in essential hypertension. *Lancet* 1989; 2(8674): 1244-7.
33. Sacks FM, Svetkey LP, Vollmer WM, *et al.* Effects on blood pressure of reduced dietary sodium and the Dietary Approaches to Stop Hypertension (DASH) diet. DASH-Sodium Collaborative Research Group. *N Engl J Med* 2001; 344(1): 3-10.
34. Whelton PK, He J, Cutler JA, *et al.* Effects of oral potassium on blood pressure. Meta-analysis of randomized controlled clinical trials. *JAMA* 1997; 277(20): 1624-32.
35. Krishna GG, Miller E, Kapoor S. Increased blood pressure during potassium depletion in normotensive men. *N Engl J Med* 1989; 320(18): 1177-82.
36. Appel LJ, Moore TJ, Obarzanek E, *et al.* A clinical trial of the effects of dietary patterns on blood pressure. DASH Collaborative Research Group. *N Engl J Med* 1997; 336(16): 1117-24.
37. Joossens JV, Kesteloot H. Trends in systolic blood pressure, 24-hour sodium excretion, and stroke mortality in the elderly in Belgium. *Am J Med* 1991; 90(3A): 5S-11.
38. Forte JG, Miguel JM, Miguel MJ, de Padua F, Rose G. Salt and blood pressure: a community trial. *J Hum Hypertens* 1989; 3(3): 179-84.
39. Laatikainen T, Pietinen P, Valsta L, Sundvall J, Reinivuo H, Tuomilehto J. Sodium in the Finnish diet: 20-year trends in urinary sodium excretion among the adult population. *Eur J Clin Nutr* 2006; 60(8): 965-70.
40. Tanaka H, Tanaka Y, Hayashi M, *et al.* Secular trends in mortality for cerebrovascular diseases in Japan, 1960 to 1979. *Stroke* 1982; 13(5): 574-81.
41. The effects of nonpharmacologic interventions on blood pressure of persons with high normal levels. Results of the Trials of Hypertension Prevention, Phase I. *JAMA* 1992; 267(9): 1213-20.
42. Effects of weight loss and sodium reduction intervention on blood pressure and hypertension incidence in overweight people with high-normal blood pressure. The Trials of Hypertension Prevention, Phase II. The Trials of Hypertension Prevention Collaborative Research Group. *Arch Intern Med* 1997; 157(6): 657-67.
43. Cook NR, Cutler JA, Obarzanek E, *et al.* Long-term effects of dietary sodium reduction on cardiovascular disease outcomes: observational follow-up of the trials of hypertension prevention (TOHP). *BMJ* 2007; 334(7599): 885-8.
44. Food labelling: declaration of sodium content of food and label claims for foods on the basis of sodium content. Department of Health and Human Services. Food and Drug Administration. 21 CFR, parts 101 and 105. *Fed Reg* 1984; 76: 15510.
45. Stamler R. Implications of the INTERSALT study. *Hypertension* 1991; 17(1 Suppl): I16-20.
46. Joffres MR, Campbell NR, Manns B, Tu K. Estimate of the benefits of a population-based reduction in dietary sodium additives on hypertension and its related health care costs in Canada. *Can J Cardiol* 2007; 23(6): 437-43.
47. Palar K, Sturm R. Potential societal savings from reduced sodium consumption in the U.S. adult population. *Am J Health Promot* 2009; 24(1): 49-57.

Chapter 3

What is the optimal treatment in obesity-related hypertension?

Eric M. Brown MD, Fellow
Matthew R. Weir MD, Professor and Director
Division of Nephrology
University of Maryland School of Medicine
Baltimore, Maryland, USA

Introduction

Hypertension has been recognized as a leading global risk factor for mortality by the Global Burden of Disease study [1] **(IIa/B)**. In the United States, hypertension affects 29.3% of the population [2] **(IIa/B)**. Similarly, 32.9% of the US population is obese according to the report of the National Health and Nutrition Examination Survey (NHANES 2003-2004) [3] **(Ib/A)**. However, over 70% of hypertensive individuals have been shown to be overweight or obese with the prevalence of high blood pressure rising progressively with increasing body mass index (BMI) [3] **(Ib/A)**, suggesting a link between these two conditions. This chapter will review the link between hypertension and obesity from a mechanistic standpoint as well as examine non-pharmacologic and pharmacologic treatment approaches that serve to best benefit this population.

Pathophysiology

Multiple pathophysiologic mechanisms have been proposed to be responsible for obesity-related hypertension with derangements occurring at the level of major organ systems as well as at the molecular level (Figure 1). There is marked activation of the renin-angiotensin-aldosterone system (RAAS) as well as the sympathetic nervous system (SNS), both of which contribute to increased renal sodium reabsorption and subsequent chronic volume expansion. Moreover, obstructive sleep apnea (OSA), a comorbid condition of obese individuals, is associated with essential hypertension. Imbalances in bioactive molecules such as leptin, adiponectin, resistin, insulin, and endothelin appear to play an additional role.

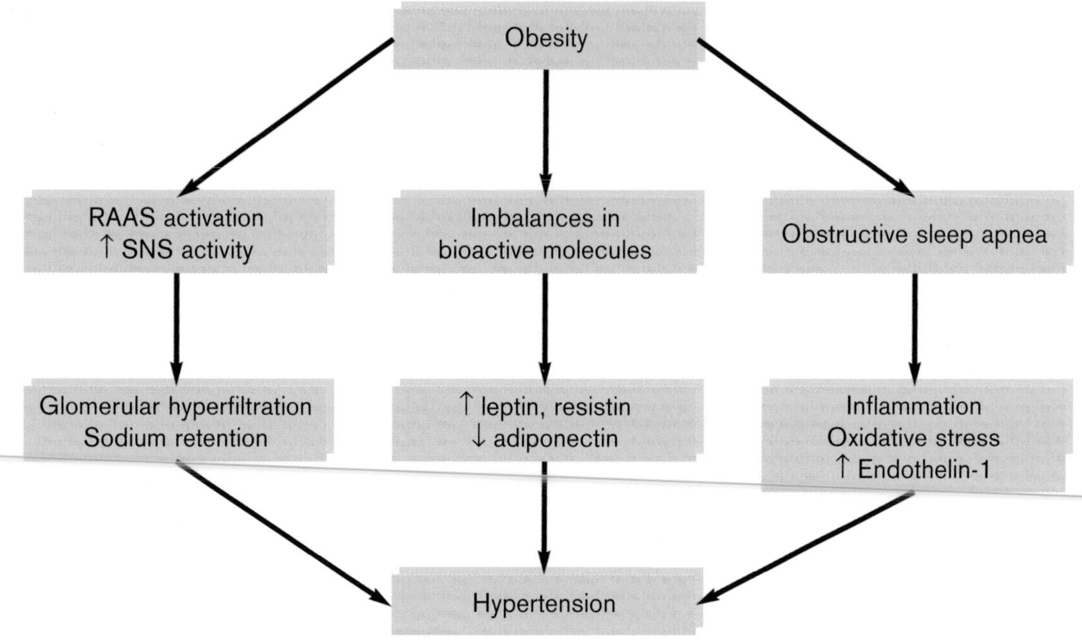

Figure 1. Pathophysiologic mechanisms leading to hypertension in the obese population. RAAS = renin-angiotensin-aldosterone system; SNS = sympathetic nervous system. *Adapted from Kurukulasuriya LR, et al* [75].

Renin-angiotensin-aldosterone system

Numerous studies have shown that the RAAS is upregulated in obese subjects [4] **(IIb/B)**, [5] **(II/B)**, [6] **(IIIb/B)**, [7] **(IIb/B)**. In an animal model of acquired obesity, rats who became obese after being fed a high-fat diet for 11 weeks had plasma levels of angiotensinogen and angiotensin drawn and compared to lean rats fed standard chow. There were significant elevations in both angiotensinogen and angiotensin II, the latter of which correlated directly to an increase in mean arterial pressure (MAP) [8]. Similar findings have been confirmed in humans as well. In a study of 38 post-menopausal women, plasma renin, angiotensinogen, angiotensinogen-converting enzyme, angiotensin II, and aldosterone levels were shown to be elevated in obese individuals when compared to their lean counterparts [3]. Moreover, when a 5% weight loss was achieved in these individuals, there was a statistically significant corresponding decline in all aforementioned factors of the RAAS cascade. Several other studies have reproduced this finding that weight loss decreases one or more elements of the RAAS [9-11] **(II/B)**.

Activation of the systemic RAAS in obese individuals is, in part, linked directly to adipose tissue mass. Adipocytes have been shown to produce angiotensinogen in both animal and human models [12,13]. This production of angiotensinogen appears to be nutritionally regulated; that is, there is gene upregulation in obesity and downregulation in starvation [14] **(II/B)**. More importantly, there is evidence that selective production of angiotensinogen in adipose tissue significantly increases circulating plasma levels of both angiotensinogen and angiotensin II, leading to systemic RAAS activation and hypertension [15].

Sympathetic nervous system

Sympathetic nervous system (SNS) activity has been shown to be increased in obesity, especially in models of visceral obesity [16]. Measures of muscle sympathetic nerve activity, which accounts for approximately 20% of total-body norepinephrine release to plasma [17], are approximately 55% higher in men with elevated visceral fat compared to age-, total fat mass-, BMI- and abdominal subcutaneous fat-matched controls with lower visceral fat [18] **(II/B)**, [19] **(IIb/B)**. However, the increase in SNS activity appears to be regionally differentiated with increased activity seen in skeletal muscle and kidney but decreased activity in cardiac muscle [20]. Experimental models suggest that this increased renal SNS activation may serve as a primary mechanism of hypertension in obese individuals by inducing a sodium avid state. In one study, when the renal sympathetic nerve efferents were denervated in obese dogs, there was attenuation of sodium and water reabsorption when compared to normal controls fed the same high-fat diet [21]. As may be expected, the control animals in this study had a rise in MAP of approximately 15% while the denervated animals showed no significant increase from baseline.

Although it is evident that there is activation of the SNS in obesity, the factors that mediate this activity have not been clearly identified. One proposed molecule that links SNS activation to obesity is leptin. Secreted by adipocytes, leptin acts to suppress appetite and increase energy expenditure [22] **(IV/C)**. With infusion in rats, leptin has been shown to impair pressure natiuresis; presumably, this effect takes place via stimulation of renal sympathetic nerves as it is not observed when adrenergic blockade is co-administered [23]. Chronic infusion of leptin has also been shown to result in gradual elevations in MAP and heart rate that are similarly reversed with adrenergic blockade [23]. Additional molecules such as adiponectin, resistin, insulin, and angiotensin II have been implicated in obesity-associated SNS activation but require further investigation to unmistakably define their roles.

Obstructive sleep apnea

According to recent data, approximately 85% of obese individuals also carry the diagnosis of obstructive sleep apnea (OSA) [24] **(II/B)**. Hypertension is a well-studied manifestion of OSA, occurring via several proposed mechanisms. Intermittent hypoxia, the hallmark of OSA, has been demonstrated to raise systolic blood pressure (SBP) both acutely and chronically [25] **(II/B)**, [26] **(IV/C)**. Patients with OSA have also been shown to have enhanced SNS activity with elevation in both plasma and urine norepinephrine and in baseline MSNA [27] **(II/B)**, [28] **(II/B)**. Vascular endothelial function is impaired in those with OSA as there is loss of endothelium-mediated vasodilation of resistance vessels [29] **(II/B)**. Additionally, endothelin-1 (ET-1) levels were found to be elevated in those with OSA; changes in ET-1 correlated with the severity of OSA and hypertension [30] **(II/B)**. Adding more evidence that OSA is directly responsible for the aforementioned pathophysiologic changes is the finding each resolves with the administration of nocturnal continuous positive airway pressure (CPAP).

Treatment

Non-pharmacologic therapies

Weight loss

Of all therapeutic strategies to treat obesity-related hypertension, weight loss is by far the most important as it is the most effective [31] **(Ia/A)**. Evidence displays that, with weight loss, the previously discussed pathophysiologic derangements found in obese hypertensives are corrected. There is a reduction in plasma renin activity, angiotensin-converting enzyme, angiotensin II, aldosterone, sympathetic nerve activity, insulin, and leptin [7, 13, 32] **(IIb/B)**. As a result, there is a decline in stroke volume, cardiac output, left ventricular mass, and blood volume leading to a drop in blood pressure [33] **(IIa/B)**. Even modest reductions in weight have been shown to improve blood pressure with one study suggesting the average decrease in SBP and DBP per kilogram of weight loss is 1-4mm Hg and 1-2mm Hg, respectively [34] **(II/B)**. However, successful weight reduction can be difficult to achieve for many patients. Non-pharmacologic interventions to reduce weight include dietary changes, exercise, and bariatric surgery.

Dietary interventions

Several dietary strategies are effective in decreasing blood pressure in the obese population. The Dietary Approaches to Stop Hypertension (DASH) diet, which is rich in fruits, vegetables, and low-fat dairy products, has been shown to be especially effective in blood pressure reduction in obese patients as compared to lean individuals on the same diet [35] **(IIb/B)**. Low sodium diets have been shown to reduce the risk of cardiovascular disease and hypertension in some individuals [36] **(Ib/A)**, [37] **(IIa/B)**, with new data supporting beneficial effects of sodium restriction in an obese subset of the population. A recent animal study indicates that there is an increase in salt-sensitive hypertension in obese subjects [38]. Moreover, another study suggests that the decrease in blood pressure seen in obese patients who have lost weight is determined by the salt-sensitivity of the patient (i.e. only salt-sensitive patients exhibit decreases in BP with weight loss) [39] **(II/B)**. If obese patients are, in fact, more prone to have a salt-sensitive phenotype, sodium restriction should be advocated to promote more effective blood pressure control.

Despite evidence to support the benefits of the DASH diet and sodium restriction, it is important to emphasize that sustained weight loss achieved by reduction in caloric intake is most effective in lowering blood pressure. When patients are randomized to weight loss versus sodium restriction, weight loss has, time and again, proved to be more effective in contolling blood pressure [40] **(Ib/A)**, [41] **(Ib/A)**, [38]. It is recommended that caloric consumption should be reduced by 500 to 1000 kilocalories daily with total fat accounting for less than 30% of caloric intake [42] **(IV/C)**.

Exercise

Physical activity, particularly aerobic exercise, has clearly been shown to lower blood pressure with one meta-analysis showing average reductions in SBP and DBP of 3.84 and 2.58mm Hg, respectively [43] **(IIa/B)**. When added to caloric restriction, regular physical activity has been shown to augment and accelerate weight loss [44] **(IIb/B)**. Most importantly, individuals who continue to exercise can better avoid regaining the weight they have lost [45] **(IIa/B)**.

Bariatric surgery

Bariatric surgery is typically recommended for individuals with a BMI ≥40 or ≥35 with one or more comorbid conditions related to obesity (cardiovascular disease, uncontrolled diabetes, or OSA) who have failed a trial of weight loss with dietary intervention [46] **(IV/C)**. As may be expected, bariatric surgery has been shown to be extremely effective in improving blood pressure and, in 45-70% of cases, resolves hypertension altogether [47] **(II/B)**, [48] **(II/B)**. Observed reductions in blood pressure are directly related to percentage of excess weight lost; because of this fact, maintenance of a normotensive state is sustained as most subjects continue to lose weight up to 2 years following surgery [49] **(II/B)**. Moreover, bariatric surgery is increasingly being recognized as a safe alternative to weight loss with little peri-operative morbidity or mortality [50] **(IIb/B)**.

Treatment of obstructive sleep apnea

As previously discussed, OSA is thought to cause hypertension via multiple mechanisms. The prevalence of hypertension in those with OSA has been reported to be as high as 70% [51] **(Ib/A)**. Numerous studies have been performed to evaluate the efficacy of nocturnal CPAP, the treatment of OSA, in reducing blood pressure. A recent meta-analysis pooled the results of these studies and found that there are significant decreases in SBP, DBP, and MAP in patients with OSA treated with CPAP versus untreated controls [52] **(Ia/A)**.

Pharmacologic therapies (Table 1)

RAAS blockade

ACE inhibitors (ACE-I), angiotensin receptor blockers (ARB), renin inhibitors, and aldosterone blockers specifically target one of the major pathogenic mechanisms, RAAS activation, leading to hypertension in the obese population. The positive physiologic and

Table 1. Metabolic effects of antihypertensive agents. *Adapted from Wofford MR, et al* [42].

Drug class	Metabolic effects
RAAS blockers (ACE inhibitors and ARBs)	↓plasma insulin ↑insulin sensitivity ↓plasma norepinephrine ↓plasma leptin ↓BMI
β-blockers	↓insulin sensitivity ↑triglycerides ↑weight gain
α-blockers	↓plasma insulin ↑insulin sensitivity ↓plasma leptin ↓total cholesterol
Diuretics	↓insulin sensitivity ↑LDL cholesterol ↑triglycerides Redistribution of fat to visceral regions
CCBs	↑sympathetic activity ↑insulin sensitivity ↓plasma insulin ↓plasma leptin

RAAS = renin-angiotensin-aldosterone system; ACE = angiotensin-converting enzyme; ARB = angiotensin receptor blocker; BMI = body mass index; LDL = low-density lipoprotein; CCB = calcium channel blocker

metabolic effects of RAAS blockade are well described and include improvement in insulin sensitivity, a reduction of proteinuria, a decrease in left ventricular mass, promotion of natiuresis, and reduction in circulating norepinephrine, leptin, and insulin levels [53]. However, the amount of large randomized studies that examine the efficacy of RAAS blockers to treat hypertension in an obese population are limited.

One such trial that investigated this question was the Treatment of Obese Patients with Hypertension (TROPHY) trial in which lisinopril was compared to hydrochlorothiazide (HCTZ) for the treatment of obese hypertensive subjects. Whereas blood pressure control was similar in both groups, the lisinopril arm achieved target blood pressure at lower doses

(10mg vs 50mg in the HCTZ arm) [54] **(Ib/A)**. Moreover, the HCTZ arm had an increased incidence of plasma glucose elevation, whereas the lisinopril arm displayed no adverse metabolic effects [54].

Head to head trials of the renin inhibitor, aliskiren, and ARBs against other drugs for the initial treatment of obesity-mediated hypertension have not been performed. However, one study examined the effect of adding aliskiren or irbesartan to the antihypertensive regimen of obese patients who had uncontrolled hypertension on HCTZ monotherapy; additional comparison arms included addition of amlodipine (a calcium channel blocker) and placebo [55] **(Ib/A)**. Blood pressure control in all treatment arms was similar. However, the arms taking aliskiren and irbesartan reported fever adverse treatment effects than those taking amlodipine, namely secondary to the high rate of peripheral edema seen in this arm [55].

Aldosterone blockers also have not been specifically studied in an obese population. Nevertheless, there is an increasing body of data showing that the addition of aldosterone blockade is highly efficacious in treating multi-drug resistant hypertension [56] **(II/B)**, [57] **(IIa/B)**, [58] **(IIb/B)**, [59] **(II/B)**. In addition to hypertensive and sodium retentive effects of elevated aldosterone, new research shows that hyperaldosteronism is associated with multiple adverse metabolic effects, namely glucose intolerance and decreased insulin sensitivity [60]. These effects are due to a direct action of aldosterone on the mineralocorticoid receptor [60], suggesting that blockade of this interaction in an obese subset of patients would be especially beneficial.

SNS blockade

In theory, drugs that target blockade of SNS activation would be highly efficacious in reducing blood pressure in obese individuals given the marked SNS upregulation seen in this state. However, α-1 blockers, α-2 agonists, and β-blockers, have limited use in obesity-mediated hypertension due to their adverse side effects or metabolic profiles.

α-1 blockers have been shown, in conjunction with β-blockers, to be efficacious agents in treating obese hypertensives when compared to lean individuals [61] **(II/B)**. They also have positive metabolic effects as they have been shown to improve lipid profiles, insulin resistance, and endothelial-mediated vasomotor function in subjects with the metabolic syndrome [62]. In spite of this, α-1 blockers have fallen out of favor for use as first-line treatment for hypertension due to the high rate of heart failure in the doxazosin arm of the Antihypertensive Lipid-Lowering Treatment to Prevent Heart Attack Trial (ALLHAT) [63] **(Ib/A)**.

Centrally acting α-2 agonists work well to reduce sympathetic outflow; several studies have displayed that clonidine reduces norepinephrine release [64, 65]. Nonetheless, compliance with α-2 agonists is reduced due to multiple side effects including dry mouth, sedation, and difficulty concentrating. Thus, they are not considered optimal first-line antihypertensive agents [42].

Classic β-blockers (metoprolol, atenolol, etc), of all agents targeted to attenuate SNS activation, have the most adverse metabolic effects. They have been shown to cause dyslipidemia, insulin resistance, and subsequent weight gain [66] **(II/B)**. Moreover, studies that examine the use of classic β-blockers in obese hypertensive subjects do not show consistent reductions in blood pressure [67] **(Ib/A)**, [68] **(Ib/A)**.

Conversely, some of the more newly developed vasodilating β-blockers such as carvedilol and nebivolol may prove to be more effective in treating hypertension in an obese population due to their favorable metabolic profiles. These agents have been shown to have favorable effects on lipids and do not influence glucose metabolism or promote insulin resistance [69]. Although promising, trials have not yet been performed to support the use of these drugs in obese patients.

Diuretics

As discussed above, there is an impaired natriuresis in the obese hypertensive patient due to multiple mechanisms. Thus, because of their natriuretic effects, diuretics are valuable antihypertensive drugs in the obese population as confirmed by the aforementioned TROPHY study [40]. However, diuretics have a deleterious metabolic profile at higher doses. HCTZ has been shown to be associated with insulin resistance and a redistribution of fat to visceral regions [70] **(Ib/A)**; furosemide has similarly been found to impair glucose tolerance by causing inflammation in pancreatic islet cells [71] **(IV/C)**. As a result, the role of diuretics in the obese hypertensive patient has been suggested to be for use as a second- or third-step therapy [53] **(IV/C)**.

Calcium channel blockers

Calcium channel blockers (CCB) do not specifically target any of the pathophysiologic derangements observed in obesity-mediated hypertension and have not been shown to be more proficient in reducing blood pressure in obese as compared to non-obese patients [72] **(II/B)**. However, this should not diminish their role as effective antihypertensives as multiple studies have shown significant reductions in SBP and DBP with the use of CCBs in overweight or obese populations [72, 73] **(IIb/B)**. In addition to their action to reduce peripheral resistance, CCBs have a mild natriuretic and diuretic effect which is potentially beneficial [74]. Moreover, CCBs have a positive metabolic profile given that they improve insulin sensitivity [73].

Conclusions

In summary, weight loss, achieved by diet and exercise is the most effective intervention to lower blood pressure in the obese hypertensive **(Ia/A)**. Even modest reduction in weight can help reduce blood pressure. Based on tolerability, metabolic neutrality, and its physiologic target, drugs that block the RAAS should be considered first-line therapy in obese hypertensives unless there are therapeutic contraindications **(Ib/A)**. CCBs and or diuretics can be added to facilitate achievement of goal blood pressure.

Key points	Evidence level
◆ Treatment of hypertension in the obese patient should be directed at the various pathophysiologic mechanisms that raise blood pressure. Weight loss, achieved by diet and exercise, is clearly the most effective intervention to lower blood pressure in this population; patients should be counseled that even mild decreases in weight can result in blood pressure reduction.	Ia/A
◆ When instituting pharmacotherapy, agents should be chosen based not only on their physiologic targets and antihypertensive actions but on their metabolic profiles (Table 1). For this reason, ACE-Is and ARBs should be considered first-line drugs for treatment of obesity-mediated hypertension.	Ib/A
◆ If target blood pressure is not achieved with ACE-I or ARB monotherapy, addition of a CCB or diuretic is advised.	Ib/A
◆ With further study, aldosterone blockade may also prove to be extremely effective and may also be advocated as second-line therapy.	IIa/B
◆ If β-blockade is indicated for a comorbid condition, vasodilating β-blockers should be prescribed (Ib/A). Otherwise, ß-blockers should be excluded as first-line agents (II/B) due to their negative metabolic profile; the same can be said about α1-blockers and α2-agonists due to their side effects.	Ib/A & II/B
◆ Treatment of comorbid conditions such as OSA and diabetes is indicated in all patients and may further augment reductions in blood pressure.	Ib/A
◆ If a trial of non-invasive lifestyle modifications and pharmacologic treatment fails, bariatric surgery should be considered in patients who meet BMI criteria for operative intervention.	IV/C

References

1. Ezzati M, Lopez AD, Rodgers A, *et al.* Selected major risk factors and global and regional burden of disease. *Lancet* 2002; 360: 1347-60.
2. Ong KL, Cheung BM, Man YB, *et al.* Prevalence, awareness, treatment, and control of hypertension among United States adults 1999-2004. *Hypertension* 2007; 49: 69-75.
3. Ogden CL, Carroll MD, Curtin LR, *et al.* Prevalence of overweight and obesity in the United States, 1999-2004. *JAMA* 2006; 295(13): 1549-55.
4. Tuck ML, Sowers J, Dornfield L, Kledzik G, Maxwell M. The effect of weight reduction on blood pressure plasma renin activity and plasma aldosterone level in obese patients. *N Engl J Med* 1981; 304: 930-3.
5. Goodfriend TL, Kelley DE, Goodpaster BH, Winters SJ. Visceral obesity and insulin resistance are associated with plasma aldosterone levels in women. *Obes Res* 1999; 7: 355-62.
6. Engeli S, Bohnke J, Gorzelniak K, Janke J, Schiling P, Bader M, *et al.* Weight loss and the renin-angiotensin-aldosterone system. *Hypertension* 2005; 45: 356-62.

7. Cooper R, McFarlane-Anderson N, Bennett FI, Wilks R, Puras A, Tesksbury D, Ward R, Forrester T. ACE, angiotensinogen and obesity: a potential pathway leading to hypertension. *Journal of Human Hypertension* 1997; 11: 107-11.
8. Boustany CM, Bharadwaj K, Daugherty A, Brown DR, Randall DC, Cassis LA. Activation of the systemic and adipose renin-angiotensin system in rats with diet-induced obesity and hypertension. *Am J Physiol Regul Integr Comp Physiol* 2004; 287: R943-9.
9. Engeli S, Boschmann M, Frings P, Beck L, Janke J, Titze J, *et al.* Influence of salt intake on renin-angiotensin and natriuretic peptide system genes in human adipose tissue. *Hypertension* 2006; 48: 1103-8.
10. Ho JT, Keogh JB, Bornstein SR, Ehrhart-Bornstein M, Lewis JG, Clifton PM, Torpy DJ. Moderate weight loss reduces renin and aldosterone but does not influence basal or stimulated pituitary-adrenal axis function. *Horm Metab Res* 2007; 39(9): 694-9.
11. Harp JB, Henry SA, DiGirolamo M. Dietary weight loss decreases serum angiotensin-converting enzyme activity in obese adults. *Obes Res* 2002; 10: 985-90.
12. Cassis LA, Saye J, Peach MJ. Location and regulation of rat angiotensinogen messenger RNA. *Hypertension* 1988; 11: 591-6.
13. Engeli S, Gorzelniak K, Kreutz R, Runkel N, Distler A, Sharma AM. Co-expression of renin-angiotensin system genes in human adipose tissue. *J Hypertens* 1999; 17: 555-60.
14. Frederich, RC Jr, Kahn BB, Peach MJ, Flier JS. Tissue-specific nutritional regulation of angiotensinogen in adipose tissue. *Hypertension* 1992; 19: 339-44.
15. Massiera F, Bloch-Faure M, Ceiler D, Murakami K, Fukamizu A, Gasc JM, Quignard-Boulange A, Negrel R, Ailhaud G, Seydoux J, Meneton P, Teboul M. Adipose angiotensinogen is involved in adipose tissue growth and blood pressure regulation. *FASEB J* 2001; 15: 2727-9.
16. Davy KP, Orr JS. Sympathetic nervous system behavior in human obesity. *Neurosci Biobehav Rev* 2009; 33: 116-24.
17. Straznicky NE, Eikelis N, Lambert EA, *et al.* Mediators of sympathetic activation in metabolic syndrome obesity. *Curr Hypertens Rep* 2008; 10: 440-7.
18. Alvarez GE, Beske SD, Ballard TP, *et al.* Sympathetic neural activation in visceral obesity. *Circulation* 2002; 106(20): 2533-6.
19. Grassi G, Dell'Oro R, Facchini A, *et al.* Effect of central and peripheral obesity body fat distribution on sympathetic and baroreflex function in obese normotensives. *J Hypertens* 2004; 22: 2363-9.
20. Vaz M, Jennings G, Turner A, *et al.* Regional sympathetic nervous activity and oxygen consumption in obese normotensive human subjects. *Circulation* 1997; 96: 3423-9.
21. Kassab S, Kato T, Wilkins C, *et al.* Renal denervation attenuates the sodium retention and hypertension associated with obesity. *Hypertension* 1995; 25: 893-7.
22. Schwartz MW, Woods SC, Porte D Jr, *et al.* Central nervous system control of food intake. *Nature* 2000; 404: 661-71.
23. Carlyle M, Jones OB, Kuo JJ, Hall JE. Chronic cardiovascular and renal actions of leptin: role of adrenergic activity. *Hypertension* 2002; 39: 496-501.
24. Foster GD, Sanders MH, Millman R, *et al.* Obstructive sleep apnea among obese patients with type 2 diabetes. *Diabetes Care* 2009; 32: 1017-9.
25. Davies RJ, Crosby J, Vardi-Visy K, *et al.* Non-invasive beat to beat arterial blood pressure during non-REM sleep in obstructive sleep apnoea and snoring. *Thorax* 1994; 49(4): 335-9.
26. Lesske J, Fletcher EC, Bao G, *et al.* Hypertension caused by chronic intermittent hypoxia-influence of chemoreceptors and sympathetic nervous system. *J Hypertens* 1997; 15(12 Pt 2): 1593-603.
27. Dimsdale JE, Coy T, Ziegler MG, *et al.* The effect of sleep apnea on plasma and urinary catecholamines. *Sleep* 1995; 18(5): 377-81.
28. Narkiewicz K, Pesek CA, Kato M, *et al.* Baroreflex control of sympathetic activity and heart rate in obstructive sleep apnea. *Hypertension* 1998; 32(6): 1039-43.
29. Kato M, Roberts-Thomson P, Phillips BG, *et al.* Impairment of endothelium-dependent vasodilation of resistance vessels in patients with obstructive sleep apnea. *Circulation* 2000; 102(21): 2607-10.
30. Gjorup PH, Sadauskiene L, Wessels J, *et al.* Abnormally increased endothelin-1 in plasma during the night in obstructive sleep apnea: relation to blood pressure and severity of disease. *Am J Hypertens* 2007; 20(1): 44-52.

31. Chobanian AV, Bakris G, Black HR, *et al.* The Seventh Report of the Joint National Committee on Prevention, Detection, Evaluation, and Treatment of High Blood Pressure. The JNC 7 Report. *JAMA* 2003; 289(19): 2560.
32. Straznicky NE, Lambert EA, Lambert GW, *et al.* Effects of dietary weight loss on sympathetic activity and cardiac risk factors associated with the metabolic syndrome. *The Journal of Clinical Endocrinology & Metabolism* 2005; 90(11): 5998-6005.
33. Poirier P, Giles TD, Bray GA, *et al.* Obesity and cardiovascular disease: pathophysiology, evaluation, and effect of weight loss. *Circulation* 2006, 113: 898-918.
34. Schotte DE, Stunkard AJ. The effects of weight reduction on blood pressure in 301 obese patients. *Arch Intern Med* 1990; 150: 1701-4.
35. Lopes HF, Martin KL, Nashar K, *et al.* DASH diet lowers blood pressure and lipid-induced oxidative stress in obesity. *Hypertension* 2003; 41: 422-430.
36. He J, Whelton PD, Appel LJ, *et al.* Long-term effects of weight loss and dietary sodium reduction on incidence of hypertension. *Hypertension* 2000; 35: 544-9.
37. Appel LJ, Brands MW, Daniels SR, *et al.* Dietary approaches to prevent and treat hypertension: a scientific statement for the American Heart Association. *Hypertension* 2006; 47: 296-308.
38. Morrison RG, Mills C, Moran AL, Walton CE, Sadek MH, Mangiarua EI, Wehner PS, McCumbee WD. A moderately high fat diet promotes salt-sensitive hypertension in obese zucker rats by impairing nitric oxide production. *Clin Exp Hypertens* 2007; 29(6): 369-81.
39. Hoffmann IS, Alfieri AB, Cubeddu LX. Salt-resistant and salt-sensitive phenotypes determine the sensitivity of blood pressure to weight loss in overweight/obese patients. *J Clin Hypertens* 2008; 10(5): 355-61.
40. Gillum RF, Prineas RJ, Jeffery RW, *et al.* Nonpharmacologic therapy of hypertension: the independent effects of weight reduction and sodium restriction in overweight borderline hypertensive patients. *Am Heart J* 1983; 105(1): 128-33.
41. Whelton PK, Appel LJ, Espeland MA, *et al.* Sodium reduction and weight loss in the treatment of hypertension in older persons: a randomized controlled trial of nonpharmacologic interventions in the elderly (TONE). TONE Collaborative Research Group. *JAMA* 1998; 279(11): 839-46.
42. Wofford MR, Smith G, Minor DS. The treatment of hypertension in obese patient. *Current Hypertension Reports* 2008; 10: 143-50.
43. Whelton SP, Chin A, Xin X, *et al.* Effect of aerobic exercise on blood pressure; a meta-analysis of randomized, controlled trials. *Ann Intern Med* 2002; 136: 493-503.
44. Blair SM, Goodyear NN, Gibbons LW, Copper KH. Physical fitness and incidence of hypertension in healthy normotensive men and women. *JAMA* 1984; 52: 487-90.
45. National Institutes of Health, National Heart, Lung, and Blood Institutes: Clinical guidelines on the identification, evaluation, and treatment of overweight and obesity in adults: the evidence report. *Obes Res* 1998; 6(Suppl 2): 51S-209S.
46. Consensus Development Conference Panel. Gastrointestinal surgery for severe obesity. *Ann Int Med* 1991; 115: 956-61.
47. Hinojosa MW, Varela JE, Smith BR, Che F, Nguyen NT. Resolution of systemic hypertension after laparoscopic gastric bypass. *J Gastrointest Surg* 2009; 13: 793-7.
48. Sugerman HJ, Wolfe LG, Sica DA, Clore JF. Diabetes and hypertension in severe obesity and effects of gastric bypass-induced weight loss. *Ann of Surgery* 2003; 237(6): 751-8.
49. Carson JL, Ruddy ME, Duff AE, *et al.* The effect of gastric bypass surgery on hypertension in morbidly obese patients. *Arch Intern Med* 1994; 154: 193-200.
50. Longitudinal Assessment of Bariatric Surgery (LABS) Consortium. Perioperative safety in the longitudinal assessment of bariatric surgery. *N Engl J Med* 2009; 361: 445-54.
51. Kiely JL, McNicholas WT. Cardiovascular risk factors in patients with obstructive sleep apnoea syndrome. *Eur Respir J* 2000; 16: 128-33.
52. Bazzano LA, Khan Z, Reynolds K, He J. Effect of nocturnal nasal continuous positive airway pressure on blood pressure in obstructive sleep apnea. *Hypertension* 2007; 50: 417-23.
53. Reisin E, Jack AV. Obesity and hypertension: mechanisms, cardio-renal consequences, and therapeutic approaches. *Med Clin N Am* 2009; 93: 733-51.
54. Reisin E, Weir MR, Falkner B, *et al.* Lisinopril versus hydrochlorothiazide in obese hypertensive patients: a multicenter placebo-controlled trial. Treatment in Obese Patients With Hypertension (TROPHY) Study Group. *Hypertension* 1997; 30(1 Pt 1): 140-5.

55. Jordan J, Engeli S, Boye SW, Le Breton S, Keefe DL. Direct renin inhibition with aliskiren in obese patients with arterial hypertension. *Hypertension* 2007; 49: 1047-55.
56. Ouzan J, Pérault C, Lincoff AM, Carré E, Mertes M. The role of spironolactone in the treatment of patients with refractory hypertension. *Am J Hypertens* 2002; 15: 333-9.
57. Jansen PM, Danser AH, Imholz BP, van den Meiracker AH. Aldosterone-receptor antagonism in hypertension. *Journal of Hypertension* 2009; 27: 680-91.
58. Sharabi Y, Adler E, Shamis A, Nussinovitch N, Markovitz A, Grossman E. Efficacy of add-on aldosterone receptor blocker in uncontrolled hypertension. *Am J Hypertens* 2006; 19: 750-5.
59. Chapman N, Dobson J, Wilson S, Dahlöf B, Sever PS, Wedel H, Poulter NR. Effect of spironolactone on blood pressure in subjects with resistant hypertension. *Hypertension* 2007; 49: 839-45.
60. Sowers JR, Whaley-Connell A, Epstein M. Narrative review: the emerging clinical implications of the role of aldosterone in the metabolic syndrome and resistant hypertension. *Ann Intern Med* 2009; 150(11): 776-83.
61. Wofford MR, Anderson DC Jr, Brown CA, *et al.* Antihypertensive effect of alpha and beta-adrenergic blockade in obese and lean hypertensive subjects. *Am J Hypertens* 2001; 14(7 Pt 1): 694-8.
62. Dell'Omo G, Penno G, Pucci L, Pellegrini G, Scotti A, Del Prato S, Pedrinelli R. The vascular effects of doxazosin in hypertension complicated by metabolic syndrome. *Coron Artery Dis* 2005; 16(1): 67-73.
63. ALLHAT Collaborative Research Group. Major cardiovascular events in hypertensive patients randomized to doxazosin vs chlorthalidone: the Antihypertensive and Lipid-lowering Treatment to Prevent Heart Attack Trial (ALLHAT). *JAMA* 2000; 283(15): 1967-75.
64. Tuck ML. Obesity, the sympathetic nervous system, and essential hypertension. *Hypertension* 1992; 19(1 Suppl): I67-77.
65. Jarrott B,Conway EL,Maccarrone C, *et al.* Clonidine: understanding its disposition, sites and mechanism of action. *Clin Exp Pharmacol Physiol* 1987; 14(5): 471-9.
66. Gress TW, Neito FJ, Shahar E, *et al.* Hypertension and antihypertensive therapy as risk factors for type 2 diabetes mellitus. Atherosclerosis Risk in Communities Study. *N Engl J Med* 2000; 342: 905-12.
67. MacMahon SW, Macdonald GJ, Bernstein L, *et al.* Comparison of weight reduction with metoprolol in treatment of hypertension in young overweight patients. *Lancet* 1985; 1(8440): 1233-6.
68. Fagerberg B, Berglund A, Andersson OK, *et al.* Cardiovascular effects of weight reduction versus antihypertensive drug treatment: a comparative, randomized, 1-year study of obese men with mild hypertension. *J Hypertens* 1991; 9(5): 431-9.
69. Sarafidis PA, Bakris GL. Do the metabolic effects of beta blockers make them leading or supporting antihypertensive agents in the treatment of hypertension? *J Clin Hypertens* (Greenwich) 2006; 8(5): 351-6.
70. Eriksson JW, Jansson PA, Carlberg B, Hägg A, Kurland L, Svensson MK, Ahlström H, Ström C, Lönn L, Ojbrandt K, Johansson L, Lind L. Hydrochlorothiazide, but not Candesartan, aggravates insulin resistance and causes visceral and hepatic fat accumulation: the Mechanisms for the Diabetes Preventing Effect of Candesartan (MEDICA) Study. *Hypertension* 2008; 52: 1030-7.
71. Sandström PE, Sehlin J, Amark K. Furosemide treatment causes age-dependent glucose intolerance and islet damage in obese-hyperglycaemic mice. *Pharmacol Toxicol* 1993; 72(4-5): 304-9.
72. Tuck ML, Bravo EL, Krakoff LR, *et al.* Endocrine and renal effects of nifedipine gastrointestinal therapeutic system in patients with essential hypertension. Results of a multicenter trial. The Modern Approach to the Treatment of Hypertension Study Group. *Am J Hypertens* 1990; 3(12 Pt 2): 333S-41.
73. Fogari R, Preti P, Zoppi A, Mugellini A, Corradi L, Lazzari P, Santoro T, Derosa G. Effect of valsartan addition to amlodipine on insulin sensitivity in overweight-obese hypertensive patients. *Intern Med* 2008; 47(21): 1851-7.
74. Richards RJ, Thakur V, Reisin E. Obesity-related hypertension: its physiological basis and pharmacological approaches to its treatment. *J Hum Hypertens* 1996; 10(Suppl 3): S59-64.
75. Kurukulasuriya LR, Stas S, Lastra G, Manrique C, Sowers JR. Hypertension in obesity. *Endocrinol Metab Clin N Am* 2008; 37: 647-62.

Chapter 4

Medical management of renal artery stenosis

John W. O'Bell MD, Assistant Professor of Medicine
Department of Medicine, Alpert Medical School of Brown University
Providence, Rhode Island, USA

Lance D. Dworkin MD FACP FASN FAHA, Professor of Medicine
Interim Chairman, Department of Medicine
Alpert Medical School of Brown University
Physician in Chief, Rhode Island & The Miriam Hospitals
Providence, Rhode Island, USA

Introduction

Renal artery stenosis (RAS) is a relatively common clinical finding often felt to contribute to refractory hypertension, loss of kidney function and cardiovascular morbidity and mortality. Although RAS is easily identified in varying degrees of severity using modern techniques of medical imaging, the magnitude of stenosis required to produce hypertension, fluid retention and possible renal dysfunction is unclear. In clinical practice, some perform interventions on lesions with a 50% or greater luminal narrowing [1], while others define clinically significant stenosis as 80% or greater [2]. Other parameters including kidney size, renal resistive index by ultrasound, or pressure gradients across the lesion stenosis have been suggested as means to identify functionally significant lesions; however, none of these have proven predictive value.

RAS can occur as a result of fibromuscular dysplasia (FMD) or atherosclerotic disease. Patients with FMD tend to be younger and female, with lesions typically in the middle segment of the renal artery. Although these patients can be cured of their hypertension with an interventional approach, they do not typically develop azotemia as a complication of their disease. By contrast, patients with atherosclerotic renal artery stenosis (ARAS) tend to be older, with ostial lesions, and typically develop worsening renal function over time.

Patients with FMD as the cause of their renal artery stenosis represent a distinct population with a very different natural history of their disease. Intervention can provide a cure for hypertension over 50% of the time [3]. Predictors of a beneficial response to intervention include younger age, duration of hypertension of less than 5 years, and less severe (Stage 1) hypertension. Because of the general lack of progression to azotemia, a medical management may be a reasonable approach in patients that lack these positive predictors. Because of the dramatically different patient characteristics and clinical course, most research on the management of renal artery stenosis focuses on patients with atherosclerotic disease.

Reasons for treatment

Clinically, there have been three major justifications for revascularization in patients with atherosclerotic renal artery stenosis:

- in patients with severe or resistant hypertension in order to achieve better blood pressure control;
- in patients with impaired or declining renal function in order to prevent progression to end-stage renal disease; and
- in patients with severe congestive heart failure in order to reduce the number of hospitalizations for that condition.

Reviewed elsewhere, convincing data demonstrating that revascularization is superior to medical management in each of these clinical settings are lacking. Furthermore, patients with atherosclerotic RAS typically have multiple risk factors for cardiovascular disease and poor outcomes [4]. Therefore, regardless of whether an intervention is performed, these patients should receive an intensive medical regimen aimed at reducing their cardiovascular risk.

Control of hypertension

Traditionally, hypertension in patients with atherosclerotic renal vascular disease was felt to be severe and difficult to control with medications. Successful control of blood pressure typically requires multiple agents from different classes, a condition which often persists even after a successful revascularization [5]. With the increasing number of antihypertensive classes and agents, achievement of blood pressure targets is increasingly feasible using a medical approach alone.

Prolonged exposure to hypertension in the non-stenotic kidney may lead to irreversible changes in architecture and physiologic responses. Animal studies convincingly demonstrate alterations in structure and function of the non-stenotic kidney [6,7], and these data have been supported by non-invasive techniques in human populations as well [8]. This may be the explanation for the observation that even after a successful intervention to correct RAS, the majority of patients still require antihypertensive therapy, frequently with multiple agents [5,9].

Preservation of renal function

Ischemic renal injury from progressive RAS was once thought to be a major contributor to end-stage renal disease. The most recent USRDS data from 2008 show that renovascular disease (including RAS, renal artery occlusion and cholesterol emboli) account for 2.3% of incident dialysis patients although this may be an under-representation of the actual amount [10].

Atherosclerotic disease tends to be progressive and for this reason there has been concern that untreated RAS will ultimately progress to cause clinically significant renal dysfunction or failure; however, population-based studies have demonstrated that this occurs less frequently than previously thought. One population-based study of patients with cardiovascular risk factors undergoing sequential duplex imaging of the renal arteries found that only 4% progressed to clinically significant disease over 8 years of follow-up with no patients progressing to complete occlusion [11].

Reduction in cardiovascular events

It remains unclear whether clinically significant RAS is an independent contributor to cardiovascular morbidity/mortality or whether it represents a marker for overall burden of atherosclerotic disease. There are compelling observational data about cardiovascular morbidity and mortality. In one community-based screening study, the presence of adverse cardiovascular events was three-fold higher in patients with incidentally discovered RAS; a two-fold increase in risk was observed even after adjusting for other cardiovascular risk factors [12]. Long-term mortality risk has been observed to be two- to three-fold higher in patients in whom significant RAS was discovered at the time of coronary or peripheral angiography and appears to be proportional to the severity of stenosis [13, 14].

Pathophysiology

Intrinsic autoregulation and the renin-angiotensin-aldosterone system are two major factors regulating renal perfusion. Under normal circumstances, autoregulation maintains stable renal perfusion across a wide range of blood pressures. Mechanistically, a drop in perfusion pressure leads to dilation of the afferent arteriole which tends to maintain renal plasma flow and glomerular capillary pressure. Endothelially-derived factors are felt to play a contributory role to maintaining renal perfusion in this setting, and disruption of these mechanisms has been implicated in renovascular hypertension [6]. Activation of the renin-angiotensin-aldosterone axis with a resultant increase in angiotensin II production preferentially constricts the post-glomerular, efferent arteriole which also serves to maintain glomerular capillary pressure, filtration fraction and glomerular filtration rate (GFR) during periods of decreased perfusion.

While renin-angiotensin-aldosterone activity is clearly responsible for the initial elevation in blood pressure in the setting of renal artery stenosis [15, 16], in the long term, other factors including increased sodium retention [17], endothelial dysfunction, vascular remodeling and intrinsic kidney damage also contribute to the maintenance of hypertension [6]. Patients with prolonged duration of hypertension preceding intervention are typically not cured of their hypertension [18, 19].

Therapeutic targets/previous studies

There is considerable controversy regarding whether revascularization provides superior outcomes in terms of blood pressure control, preservation of kidney function, or cardiovascular morbidity and mortality for patients with atherosclerotic RAS as compared to a pharmacologic approach. The few randomized controlled trials of medical versus surgical therapy that have been performed have been limited by study design, low numbers of patients, and absence of well-defined medical management strategies. None of the three most well-known randomized trials prescribed ACE inhibitors or ARBs by protocol [1, 20, 21]. A recent meta-analysis of randomized and non-randomized trials in renal artery stenosis made the following observations: there was no conclusive evidence to support medical versus interventional strategy with regard to cardiovascular outcomes and no study truly assessed the value of aggressive medical intervention [5]. To date there are no studies that have compared different types of medical therapy on outcomes in patients with RAS. In fact, the vast majority of patients are treated medically and whether or not an intervention is performed, patients with atherosclerotic RAS require an intensive medical regimen aimed at reducing their cardiovascular risk.

Targeted medical approach

A rational approach to management of renal artery stenosis includes an understanding of the underlying pathophysiology as well as an appreciation for other factors contributing to overall morbidity and mortality. Given the concurrent burden of systemic and cardiac atherosclerosis, a treatment approach, whether surgical or medical, that focuses solely on the renovascular lesion and ignores other systemic factors, is unlikely to provide significant overall benefit. For this reason, an approach that includes blood pressure reduction with targeted classes of agents as well as interventions that reduce overall cardiovascular risk, is advocated. As has been previously mentioned, achievement of blood pressure targets will typically require multiple agents from different classes, and a stepwise approach with appropriate monitoring and follow-up is ideal.

An algorithm for medical management of atherosclerotic RAS is presented in Figure 1. Blood pressure targets have not been specifically developed for patients with RAS. Although there is the concern that a drop in blood pressure below a critical threshold could induce azotemia, this event tends to be reversible when it occurs [22]. Extrapolation of blood pressure targets from the JNC 7 and K-DOQI guidelines suggests a treatment goal of 140/90mm Hg or lower for patients with normal kidney function, and 130/80mm Hg for patients with chronic kidney disease (CKD) or diabetes [23] **(Ia/A for HTN and CKD, IV/C for RAS)**. Other interventions including management of hyperlipidemia, smoking cessation and glycemic control are also considered important and crucial to a successful multifaceted management strategy.

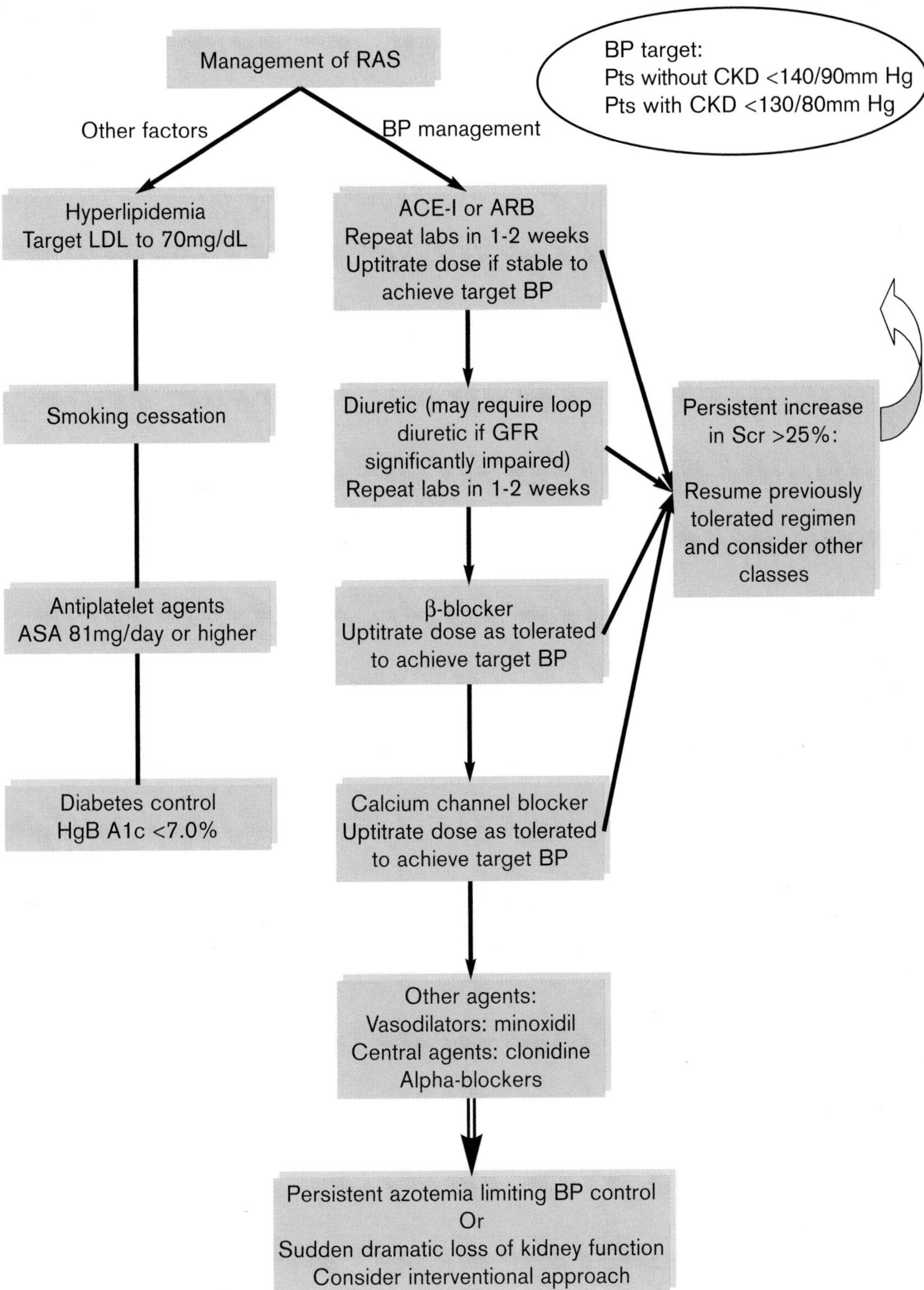

Figure 1. An algorithm for the medical management of atherosclerotic RAS. Scr=serum creatinine; ASA=aspirin; CKD=chronic kidney disease.

Specific agents for treatment

ACE inhibitors/angiotensin receptor blockers

In the Goldblatt 2 kidney, 1 clip (2K,1C) model of RAS, hypertension is mediated, at least in the initial stages, by activation of the renin-angiotensin axis [15, 16]. Interruption of this axis appears to be a rational approach to therapy. Efferent arteriolar vasodilatation in the post-stenotic kidney in unilateral RAS or in both kidneys in bilateral RAS has led to concern among practitioners about precipitating acute renal failure and/or irreversible renal ischemia and atrophy. In clinical practice, ischemia and atrophy of the post-stenotic kidney have been observed [24]; however, the salutary effects on renal perfusion pressure in the contralateral kidney appear to compensate [25], and numerous animal studies have found a mortality benefit for the use of ACE inhibitors or ARBs for the control of renovascular hypertension [26]. The mortality benefit persists even when the result of long-term ACE inhibition is atrophy and fibrosis of the post-stenotic kidney [27].

When acute kidney injury develops in the 1K 1C model (equivalent to bilateral RAS), it is typically entirely reversible with discontinuation of the medication. Over time there appears to be an adaptive response and stabilization of kidney function even with continued exposure to the medication [28].

The beneficial effects of RAAS-blocking agents may extend beyond their effects on blood pressure control and protection of the non-stenotic kidney. Effects on left ventricular hypertrophy and vascular remodeling may also play a role and have been demonstrated in animal models [29-31]. In humans, a 5-year follow-up study (non-randomized) of revascularization of RAS versus medical management failed to find a benefit to revascularization, but use of ACE inhibition was associated with a reduction in overall mortality [32] **(IIa/B)**.

Most clinicians use ACE inhibitors and angiotensin receptor blockers (ARBs) interchangeably, frequently employing the more expensive ARBs for patients who experience intolerable side effects with ACE inhibitors. There are no data in humans supporting the use of one agent over the other for renal artery stenosis. There have been interesting observations in the 2K 1C rat models where, despite similar drops in mean arterial pressure, GFR was better preserved with an ARB, losartan, than with enalapril, an ACE inhibitor. This difference was lessened by the infusion of a bradykinin receptor antagonist, leading the authors to suspect that the differential effect on GFR may be from the elevated bradykinin levels associated with administration of the ACE inhibitor [33]. It is not clear whether this occurs in humans or would have significant long-term consequences on kidney function or cardiovascular outcomes.

Because of the potential for causing azotemia, particularly in the presence of bilateral RAS, or when used concurrently with diuretics, introduction of these classes of agents or change in dose should be accompanied by laboratory assessment of serum creatinine and serum potassium, usually within 1 to 2 weeks of initiation of the drug or a change in dose.

Diuretics

Sodium retention contributes substantially to hypertension in RAS, particularly in patients with bilateral disease. Although diuretics in combination with blockade of the renin-angiotensin-aldosterone axis may be more likely to result in azotemia [22], when used cautiously, diuretics are an effective and often essential component of antihypertensive therapy **(IV/C)**. Again, because of the potential for worsening renal function with the combination of RAAS blockade and diuretic therapy, addition of or change in the dose of a diuretic should prompt follow-up and laboratory assessment within 1 to 2 weeks.

β-blockers

β-blockers are known to decrease renin activity and are therefore a rational choice to control hypertension in RAS. Additionally, β-blockade can help counter the expected increase in renin secretion that can be induced by diuretic therapy. To date there has not been a well-controlled trial investigating the use of β-blockers in RAS, but β-blockade has been a part of most regimens for control of renovascular hypertension for many years **(IV/C)**.

Calcium channel blockers

Whereas ACE inhibitors result in hypoperfusion of the post-stenotic kidney, calcium channel blockers dilate the afferent arteriole [34], resulting in increased perfusion of the post-stenotic kidney when compared to ACE inhibition [35, 36]. This has not been linked to clinical benefit. Furthermore, there may be adverse hemodynamic effects on the contralateral kidney, which may already be exposed to increased intraglomerular pressures from hypertension and relative vasodilation of the renal microvasculature. It is unclear whether this increased perfusion may accelerate fibrosis and loss of renal function in the long run. In animal studies, calcium channel blockade has been associated with nephrosclerosis of the contralateral kidney when compared with ACE inhibitor therapy; however, this has also not been confirmed in man [25]. Because of their potent blood pressure lowering effects and the need for multiple antihypertensives, calcium channel blockers are frequently employed in the management of hypertension due to RAS **(IV/C)**.

Other factors

Hyperlipidemia

Controlling dyslipidemia would be expected to help slow progression of atherosclerotic renal disease although direct human evidence is lacking. Renal artery stenosis is considered to be a coronary artery disease (CAD) equivalent according to most established guidelines [37]. As such, the recommended target LDL cholesterol should be 70mg/dL [37-39] **(Ia/A for CAD, IV/C for RAS)**. There are some interesting animal models suggesting a role for statin therapy to help slow fibrosis and promote angiogenesis in the ischemic kidney [40, 41]. There is also the potential for stabilization or perhaps regression of atheromatous plaques in the renal arteries with aggressive lipid-lowering therapy; however, this has not been demonstrated to alter outcomes for patients with RAS [42].

Smoking cessation

Tobacco use clearly contributes to progression of atherosclerotic disease and renovascular disease in particular. A thorough approach to medical management of RAS should include aggressive interventions targeted to smoking cessation. Moreover, tobacco use has clearly been implicated as a major contributor to declining renal function in patients with CKD, possibly due to effects on endothelial function and vasoactive factors [43] **(III/B)**.

Antiplatelet agents

There are no direct data supporting the use of antiplatelet agents in atherosclerotic renal artery stenosis. There is a strong correlation between the presence of coronary disease, peripheral arterial disease and RAS [13, 14], and as has been mentioned, RAS is considered a CAD equivalent [37]. Extrapolating from studies in patients with CAD and in patients with hypertension and risk factors for CAD, most recommend the use of at least 75mg/day of aspirin in patients with atherosclerotic RAS [44, 45] **(Ia/A for CAD, IV/C for RAS)**.

Diabetes control

The importance of good glycemic control on both microvascular and macrovascular complications of diabetes mellitus has been well-established [46, 47]. An apparent increase in cardiovascular mortality was noted in a recent trial of intensive glycemic control (HgB A1c 6.0% or less) and has recently generated controversy [48]; however, achieving a target of 7.0% or lower for glycated hemoglobin is still advised and is the current recommendation from the American Diabetes Association, American Heart Association and American College of Cardiology Foundation [49].

Revascularization

Despite the potential success of a multifaceted medical management approach, there may remain a subset of patients who benefit from interventional therapy. The rationale and possible indications for intervening in RAS are discussed elsewhere.

Conclusions

The increasing frequency with which RAS is being discovered as well as the widespread use of interventional therapies such as angioplasty and stenting are tempting reasons to attempt an interventional 'cure' for renovascular disease. Unfortunately, the bulk of the literature demonstrates the systemic nature of atherosclerotic renal artery stenosis and, regardless of whether an intervention is performed, treatment should include a broad-based medical approach aimed at reducing the risk of adverse cardiovascular and renal events.

A stepwise algorithm should be employed in order to reach recommended blood pressure targets based on current clinical practice guidelines for patients with hypertension and comorbidities such as diabetes and chronic kidney disease which are prevalent in this population. The use of agents that interrupt the renin-angiotensin system is rational, based on the underlying pathophysiology, as well as data on cardiovascular and renal outcomes in other related conditions. Interventions to address the systemic component of atherosclerotic disease are also advised. Based on the current body of literature and the potential complications of an interventional approach, the medical management strategy may provide at least equal outcomes in terms of overall morbidity/mortality and cardiovascular events, and is a reasonable option for most patients. Large multicenter trials that are currently underway may provide additional data in support of one strategy over the other.

Key points	**Evidence level**
◆ Blood pressure should be reduced to a target of 140/90mm Hg for patients without CKD, 130/80mm Hg for patients with CKD. *(No direct evidence in RAS [IV/C], but Ia/A evidence from HTN and CKD studies.)*	**IV/C & Ia/A**
◆ Multi-drug regimens are nearly universally required to achieve BP target, and should include either an ACE inhibitor or ARB when tolerated.	**IIa/B**
◆ Other useful agents in an effective multi-drug regimen include diuretics, β-blockers and calcium channel blockers.	**IV/C**
◆ RAS is considered a coronary disease equivalent and hyperlipidemia should be aggressively managed with a target LDL of <70mg/dL. *(No direct evidence in RAS [IV/C], but Ia/A evidence from CAD studies.)*	**IV/C & Ia/A**
◆ Smoking cessation is an important aspect of aggressive medical management of RAS.	**III/B**
◆ Treatment with at least 75mg/day of aspirin has not been directly studied in RAS, but is extrapolated from more general CAD studies as RAS is considered a CAD equivalent by most experts. *(No direct evidence in RAS [IV/C], but Ia/A evidence from CAD studies.)*	**IV/C & Ia/A**
◆ Diabetic control targeting HgB A1c <7.0% should be achieved in diabetic patients with RAS. *(No direct evidence in RAS [IV/C], but Ia/A evidence from DM studies.)*	**IV/C & Ia/A**

References

1. van Jaarsveld BC, *et al.* The effect of balloon angioplasty on hypertension in atherosclerotic renal-artery stenosis. Dutch Renal Artery Stenosis Intervention Cooperative Study Group. *N Engl J Med* 2000; 342(14): 1007-14.
2. Simon G. What is critical renal artery stenosis? Implications for treatment. *Am J Hypertens* 2000; 13(11): 1189-93.
3. Davidson RA, Barri Y, Wilcox CS. Predictors of cure of hypertension in fibromuscular renovascular disease. *Am J Kidney Dis* 1996; 28(3): 334-8.
4. Kalra PA, *et al.* Atherosclerotic renovascular disease in United States patients aged 67 years or older: risk factors, revascularization, and prognosis. *Kidney Int* 2005; 68(1): 293-301.
5. Balk E, *et al.* Effectiveness of management strategies for renal artery stenosis: a systematic review. *Ann Intern Med* 2006; 145(12): 901-12.
6. Romero JC, *et al.* New insights into the pathophysiology of renovascular hypertension. *Mayo Clin Proc* 1997; 72(3): 251-60.
7. Ploth DW. Angiotensin-dependent renal mechanisms in two-kidney, one-clip renal vascular hypertension. *Am J Physiol* 1983; 245(2): F131-41.
8. Tullis MJ, *et al.* Clinical evidence of contralateral renal parenchymal injury in patients with unilateral atherosclerotic renal artery stenosis. *Ann Vasc Surg* 1998; 12(2): 122-7.
9. Barri YM, *et al.* Prediction of cure of hypertension in atherosclerotic renal artery stenosis. *South Med J* 1996; 89(7): 679-83.
10. National Institutes of Health, N.I.o.D.a.D.a.K.D., U.S. Renal Data System, USRDS 2008 Annual Data Report: Atlas of Chronic Kidney Disease and End-Stage Renal Disease in the United States. Bethesda, MD, 2008.
11. Pearce JD, *et al.* Progression of atherosclerotic renovascular disease: a prospective population-based study. *J Vasc Surg* 2006; 44(5): 955-62; discussion 962-3.
12. Edwards MS, *et al.* Renovascular disease and the risk of adverse coronary events in the elderly: a prospective, population-based study. *Arch Intern Med* 2005; 165(2): 207-13.
13. Mui KW, *et al.* Incidental renal artery stenosis is an independent predictor of mortality in patients with peripheral vascular disease. *J Am Soc Nephrol* 2006; 17(7): 2069-74.
14. Conlon PJ, *et al.* Severity of renal vascular disease predicts mortality in patients undergoing coronary angiography. *Kidney Int* 2001; 60(4): 1490-7.
15. Brunner HR, *et al.* Hypertension of renal origin: evidence for two different mechanisms. *Science* 1971; 174(16): 1344-6.
16. Gavras H, *et al.* Reciprocation of renin dependency with sodium volume dependency in renal hypertension. *Science* 1975; 188(4195): 1316-7.
17. Textor SC. Pathophysiology of renovascular hypertension. *Urol Clin North Am* 1984; 11(3): 373-81.
18. Hughes JS, *et al.* Duration of blood pressure elevation in accurately predicting surgical cure of renovascular hypertension. *Am Heart J* 1981; 101(4): 408-13.
19. Grim CE, *et al.* Balloon dilatation for renal artery stenosis causing hypertension: criteria, concerns, and cautions. *Ann Intern Med* 1980; 92(1): 117-9.
20. Plouin PF, *et al.* Blood pressure outcome of angioplasty in atherosclerotic renal artery stenosis: a randomized trial. Essai Multicentrique Medicaments vs Angioplastie (EMMA) Study Group. *Hypertension* 1998; 31(3): 823-9.
21. Webster J, *et al.* Randomised comparison of percutaneous angioplasty vs continued medical therapy for hypertensive patients with atheromatous renal artery stenosis. Scottish and Newcastle Renal Artery Stenosis Collaborative Group. *J Hum Hypertens* 1998; 12(5): 329-35.
22. Miyamori I, *et al.* Effects of converting enzyme inhibition on split renal function in renovascular hypertension. *Hypertension* 1986; 8(5): 415-21.
23. Chobanian AV, *et al.* Seventh report of the Joint National Committee on Prevention, Detection, Evaluation, and Treatment of High Blood Pressure. *Hypertension* 2003; 42(6): 1206-52.
24. Caps MT, *et al.* Risk of atrophy in kidneys with atherosclerotic renal artery stenosis. *Kidney Int* 1998; 53(3): 735-42.
25. Wenzel UO, *et al.* Adverse effect of the calcium channel blocker nitrendipine on nephrosclerosis in rats with renovascular hypertension. *Hypertension* 1992; 20(2): 233-41.

26. Hackam DG, *et al.* Role of renin-angiotensin system blockade in atherosclerotic renal artery stenosis and renovascular hypertension. *Hypertension* 2007; 50(6): 998-1003.
27. Jackson B, *et al.* Pharmacologic nephrectomy with chronic angiotensin converting enzyme inhibitor treatment in renovascular hypertension in the rat. *J Lab Clin Med* 1990; 115(1): 21-7.
28. van de Ven PJ, *et al.* Angiotensin converting enzyme inhibitor-induced renal dysfunction in atherosclerotic renovascular disease. *Kidney Int* 1998; 53(4): 986-93.
29. Michel JB, *et al.* Myocardial effect of converting enzyme inhibition in hypertensive and normotensive rats. *Am J Med* 1988; 84(3A): 12-21.
30. Matsubara BB, *et al.* The effect of non-antihypertensive doses of angiotensin converting enzyme inhibitor on myocardial necrosis and hypertrophy in young rats with renovascular hypertension. *Int J Exp Pathol* 1999; 80(2): 97-104.
31. Jalil JE, *et al.* Coronary vascular remodeling and myocardial fibrosis in the rat with renovascular hypertension. Response to captopril. *Am J Hypertens* 1991; 4(1 Pt 1): 51-5.
32. Losito A, *et al.* Long-term follow-up of atherosclerotic renovascular disease. Beneficial effect of ACE inhibition. *Nephrol Dial Transplant* 2005; 20(8): 1604-9.
33. Demeilliers B, Jover B, Mimran A. Contrasting renal effects of chronic administrations of enalapril and losartan on one-kidney, one clip hypertensive rats. *J Hypertens* 1998; 16(7): 1023-9.
34. Carmines PK, Navar LG. Disparate effects of Ca channel blockade on afferent and efferent arteriolar responses to ANG II. *Am J Physiol* 1989; 256(6 Pt 2): F1015-20.
35. Ribstein J, Mourad G, Mimran A. Contrasting acute effects of captopril and nifedipine on renal function in renovascular hypertension. *Am J Hypertens* 1988; 1(3 Pt 1): 239-44.
36. Miyamori I, *et al.* Comparative effects of captopril and nifedipine on split renal function in renovascular hypertension. *Am J Hypertens* 1988; 1(4 Pt 1): 359-63.
37. Stone NJ, Bilek S, Rosenbaum S. Recent National Cholesterol Education Program Adult Treatment Panel III update: adjustments and options. *Am J Cardiol* 2005; 96(4A): 53E-9.
38. Ray KK, *et al.* Early and late benefits of high-dose atorvastatin in patients with acute coronary syndromes: results from the PROVE IT-TIMI 22 trial. *J Am Coll Cardiol* 2005; 46(8): 1405-10.
39. Nissen SE, *et al.* Effect of very high-intensity statin therapy on regression of coronary atherosclerosis: the ASTEROID trial. *JAMA* 2006; 295(13): 1556-65.
40. Chade AR, *et al.* Simvastatin promotes angiogenesis and prevents microvascular remodeling in chronic renal ischemia. *Faseb J* 2006; 20(10): 1706-8.
41. Chade AR, *et al.* Simvastatin abates development of renal fibrosis in experimental renovascular disease. *J Hypertens* 2008; 26(8): 1651-60.
42. Khong TK, *et al.* Regression of atherosclerotic renal artery stenosis with aggressive lipid lowering therapy. *J Hum Hypertens* 2001; 15(6): 431-3.
43. Baggio B, *et al.* Atherosclerotic risk factors and renal function in the elderly: the role of hyperfibrinogenaemia and smoking. Results from the Italian Longitudinal Study on Ageing (ILSA). *Nephrol Dial Transplant* 2005; 20(1): 114-23.
44. Collaborative meta-analysis of randomised trials of antiplatelet therapy for prevention of death, myocardial infarction, and stroke in high risk patients. *BMJ* 2002; 324(7329): 71-86.
45. Hennekens CH, Dyken ML, Fuster V. Aspirin as a therapeutic agent in cardiovascular disease: a statement for healthcare professionals from the American Heart Association. *Circulation* 1997; 96(8): 2751-3.
46. Intensive blood-glucose control with sulphonylureas or insulin compared with conventional treatment and risk of complications in patients with type 2 diabetes (UKPDS 33). UK Prospective Diabetes Study (UKPDS) Group. *Lancet* 1998; 352(9131): 837-53.
47. Stratton IM, *et al.* Association of glycaemia with macrovascular and microvascular complications of type 2 diabetes (UKPDS 35): prospective observational study. *BMJ* 2000; 321(7258): 405-12.
48. Gerstein HC, *et al.* Effects of intensive glucose lowering in type 2 diabetes. *N Engl J Med* 2008; 358(24): 2545-59.
49. Skyler JS, *et al.* Intensive glycemic control and the prevention of cardiovascular events: implications of the ACCORD, ADVANCE, and VA diabetes trials: a position statement of the American Diabetes Association and a scientific statement of the American College of Cardiology Foundation and the American Heart Association. *Circulation* 2009; 119(2): 351-7.

Chapter 5

Optimal regimen-based pharmacotherapy of hypertension in patients with concomitant conditions

C. Venkata S. Ram MD MACP FACC
Clinical Professor of Internal Medicine
Texas Blood Pressure Institute
Dallas Nephrology Associates
University of Texas Southwestern Medical Center
Dallas, Texas, USA

Introduction

Systemic hypertension remains a major risk factor for premature global morbidity and mortality; it is also the most prevalent risk factor for systemic vascular disease. Hypertension is the most common reason for Americans to see a healthcare provider. In spite of national and international awareness and dissemination of scientific information, hypertension control rates are dismally low [1, 2]. A majority of hypertension patients have a blood pressure (BP) level above the treatment goal (<140/90mm Hg). Hence, uncontrolled hypertension can be considered as a rampant but a treatable risk factor. Due to increasing life expectancy of the aging population, we can expect to see a growing prevalence of hypertension in the community. With advancing degree of hypertension, it becomes difficult to achieve the target blood pressure goal. Therefore, it is important to initiate appropriate therapy as early as possible to control and contain the pandemic of hypertension.

System hypertension is a disorder of circulatory homeostasis resulting from a complex interaction of various humoral, non-humoral, and local vasoconstrictor mechanisms. The sympathetic nervous system (SNS), the renin-angiotensin-aldosterone system (RAAS), and the kidney are major sources of vasoactive and sodium/fluid balance aberrations resulting in an elevated blood pressure level. Despite elegant studies and rigorous scientific investigations, no single theory can explain the pathogenesis of hypertension. Multiple mechanisms interdigitate with each other to raise the level of blood pressure; genetic factors play an important role in the blood pressure disorders.

Treatment principles

Whereas specific therapeutic avenues to treat hypertension in patients with comorbid conditions will be discussed below, certain general principles should be followed in clinical practice. The decision to treat hypertension should not only take blood pressure levels into account, but also the presence of other cardiovascular risk factors, associated comorbid conditions, and the extent of target organ damage (TOD). The risk stratification guidelines are provided by the Joint National Committee (JNC) [1, 2] and also by WHO/ISH [3]. A number of lifestyle modifications have been shown to lower blood pressure and to reduce the prevalence of hypertension and should be recommended for all patients with hypertension. Appropriate body weight, increasing physical fitness, moderation of alcohol intake, increasing potassium consumption, increased consumption of fruits and vegetables, and a reduction of sodium intake and saturated fat – all have been shown to reduce the blood pressure to a variable degree. The effectiveness of lifestyle changes is highly variable depending on the patient's adherence and other influences, but for most, a modest reduction is achieved through hygienic measures. Since even slight reductions in blood pressure reduce the risk of cardiovascular disease (CVD), lifestyle modifications are recommended for all patients with hypertension. In addition to reducing the prevalence of hypertension, lifestyle modifications are also beneficial to improve the management of diabetes, hyperlipidemia, and obesity which often co-exist with hypertension; non-pharmacological therapy while rendering no side effects may actually enhance the sense of well-being of patients. In contrast to a drug treatment strategy which has to be individualized, lifestyle modifications reduce blood pressure levels across the whole population.

In uncomplicated hypertension differences between antihypertensive drug classes tend to be small relative to the general benefits of overall blood pressure reduction. Most patients with hypertension require multiple antihypertensive drugs to achieve the blood pressure goal; so, it is useful to apply effective combinations of drugs instead of seeking superiority of one class over others. In patients with comorbid conditions or 'complicated' hypertension, certain classes of antihypertensive drugs may be advantageous evidenced by randomized clinical trials (RCTs).

Optimizing pharmacotherapy in hypertensive patients with concomitant conditions

Hypertension with diabetes

Systemic hypertension accentuates cardiovascular and renal morbidity and mortality in patients with diabetes mellitus (DM) [4, 5] **(IIa/B)**. Hypertension and DM are two of the most commonly seen disorders in clinical practice. The prevalence of hypertension in DM is twice that observed in the general population. Hypertension and diabetes interact with each other adversely and synergistically in increasing the cardiovascular complication rates and premature mortality [6]. An overwhelming number of patients with diabetes develop CVD. Systemic hypertension in diabetic patients exaggerates the development of diabetic retinopathy, nephropathy, coronary artery disease (CAD), stroke, and congestive heart failure

(CHF). Diabetes and hypertension together account for the majority of patients who develop chronic kidney disease (CKD) and end-stage renal disease (ESRD).

Several studies have demonstrated that effective blood pressure control in patients with diabetes provides important therapeutic benefits. The JNC 7 and other guideline committees have recommended a blood pressure goal of <130/80mmHg for hypertensive patients with concomitant diabetes (Table 1). It is unclear whether the same therapeutic goal is applicable to those patients who have insulin resistance without overt DM. Suffice it to understand that hypertension should be treated aggressively in patients with impaired glucose metabolism. As mentioned above, non-pharmacological treatment should be implemented prior to or along with initiation of drug therapy for hypertension.

Table 1. Goals of therapy.
• Reduce CVD and renal morbidity and mortality
• Treat to BP <140/90mmHg or BP <130/80mmHg in patients with diabetes or chronic kidney disease
• Achieve SBP goal especially in a person ≥50 years of age

Recommended antihypertensive drugs

Judged from the results of different RCTs, the JNC 7 suggested that for hypertensive patients with DM, RAAS blockers, β-blockers (BBs), calcium channel blockers (CCBs) or diuretics can be considered as initial therapy.

Angiotensin receptor blockers (ARBs) have been widely advocated as desirable antihypertensive drugs in DM, particularly type 2 DM based on positive outcomes from RCTs. ARBs block the actions of angiotensin II at the vascular level by inhibiting its vasoconstrictive and other actions. The general mechanisms and hemodynamic results of ARBs are similar except for the differences in their duration of action. A number of studies utilizing either short- or long-acting ARBs have demonstrated their usefulness in patients with diabetes by delaying the progression of CKD/ESRD or by a reduction of proteinuria, microalbuminuria, or both [7] **(Ib/A)**. ARBs are very well tolerated and are indicated to treat hypertension in patients with diabetes. Patients receiving ARBs should be monitored periodically or closely (depending on renal function) for potassium, BUN, and creatinine levels. Angiotensin-converting enzyme inhibitors (ACE-Is) have become the cornerstone of antihypertensive drug therapy in patients with DM. ACE-Is, as the name implies, block the ACE and thus, attenuate the generation of angiotensin II. Like ARBs, the general mechanism of action and hemodynamic effects of all ACE-Is are similar; there may be some differences in their duration of action and pharmacokinetic properties. Several studies have convincingly proven the benefits of ACE-Is in DM, particularly in those with type 1 DM [8]. In the Captopril Prevention Project (CAPPP) trial, diabetic patients who were on an ACE-I experienced lesser morbidity and mortality [9] **(Ib/A)**. Subsequent studies in DM with or without hypertension have confirmed the usefulness of ACE-Is in reducing proteinuria and in arresting the progression of CKD/ESRD [10, 11]. Unless contraindicated or not tolerated ACE-Is should be included in the optimal therapeutic regimen for patients with diabetes. Furthermore, studies have shown that ACE-Is are superior to CCBs in the management of hypertension in patients with diabetes. Despite their equal effects on blood pressure, ACE-Is are preferred over CCBs in patients with diabetes.

β-blockers (BBs) have a therapeutic role in providing protection against CVD in patients with diabetes [12, 13]. Various cardiovascular actions of BBs make them an attractive option to treat hypertension in patients with diabetes. Concerns with traditional BBs (side effects, tolerability, effects on metabolic parameters) are less likely to be manifested with the new generation of vasodilating BBs such as carvedilol and nebivolol. BBs differ in their cardio-selectivity, lipophilicity, degree and nature of adrenergic blockade, duration of action, and effects on glucose and lipid parameters. The positive clinical outcomes from BBs in diabetic hypertensives were established many years ago in the United Kingdom Prospective Diabetes Study (UKPDS) [14, 15]. However, older BBs (propranolol, atenolol, and metoprolol) may exert adverse effects on glucose and lipid parameters; newer (vasodilating) BBs by virtue of their unique actions at the tissue level exert favorable or neutral effects on glucose and lipid metabolism. In comparison with metoprolol, carvedilol has been shown to reduce proteinuria in diabetic patients [16] **(Ib/A)**. Despite their desirable pharmacological and metabolic actions, outcome studies are needed to judge the ultimate place of newer BBs in the modern hypertension treatment. Guidelines from the American College of Clinical Endocrinology favor the use of metabolically advantageous BBs (like carvedilol or nebivolol) over the conventional BBs. As stated above, we do not have any outcome studies or RCTs with the vasodilating BBs.

Although calcium channel blockers (CCBs) are effective drugs to control hypertension, their role as initial or monotherapy is limited because of negative outcomes with dihydropyridine (DHP) CCBs in this subset of the patient population. CCBs effectively lower the blood pressure in hypertensive patients with diabetes but certain studies such as the Fosinopril versus Amlodipine Cardiovascular Events Trial (FACET) [17] and Appropriate Blood Pressure Control in Diabetes (ABCD) [11] trial have shown that RAAS blockers are superior to CCBs. Hence, DHP CCBs are not recommended as initial therapy for hypertension in diabetes but they are certainly utilized as adjunctive therapy for blood pressure control on the background of RAAS blockade. The non-DHP CCBs like diltiazem and verapamil have less adverse effects compared to DHPs in diabetes, but outcome trials are lacking. DHP CCBs, although not contraindicated in diabetes, may worsen proteinuria, a prognostic factor.

Thiazide diuretics which have been routinely recommended by the guideline committees for the general treatment of hypertension also have a role in the long-term blood pressure control in diabetic patients. From a pharmacological point of view, thiazide diuretics may have an adverse effect on glucose metabolism, insulin resistance, and on lipids but in the large outcome trials such as the Systolic Hypertension in the Elderly Program (SHEP), diuretics were shown to be beneficial in the diabetic cohort. In the SHEP, low-dose chlorthalidone therapy was shown to reduce mortality from CVD in the diabetic cohort. In another large outcome study, Antihypertensive and Lipid-Lowering Treatment to Prevent Heart Attack Trial (ALLHAT), the diabetic cohort (36% of the entire study group) benefited from chlorthalidone therapy to a similar degree as CCBs or ACE-Is [18, 19] **(Ib/A)**; the diuretic group experienced a significantly lower level of systolic blood pressure. The beneficial effects of diuretics compared to CCBs and ACE-Is were particularly favorable in the prevention of CHF. Glycemic control was negatively impacted by chlorthalidone but the clinical outcomes were comparable to lisinopril or amlodipine. While it is recommended that glycemic control be followed closely, diuretics remain an integral component of a multi-drug regimen for BP control in diabetic subjects.

The role of α-adrenergic blockers in the treatment of hypertension has been called into question by the ALLHAT study, because of unsatisfactory patient outcomes. Based on this study and other observations, α-adrenergic blockers are not desirable as first-line drugs for diabetic patients. The centrally acting α-agonists, such as clonidine, have metabolically neutral actions on glucose and hence may be used as an add-on treatment to achieve the blood pressure goal in diabetics. Ongoing research with endothelin antagonists and direct renin inhibitors is warranted to evaluate their precise role in the diabetic population.

The majority of hypertensive patients with diabetes require multiple drugs to achieve and maintain the blood pressure goal; thus, the advantages and disadvantages of individual drug classes should be judged on the basis of overall blood pressure control and assessment of outcome trials. In addition to the blood pressure goal, careful attention should be given to assess the impact of therapy on kidney function and the cardiovascular system. Tight blood pressure control while reducing proteinuria should be dual objectives in the chronic management of hypertension in patients with diabetes, insulin resistance, and metabolic syndrome.

Hypertension in chronic kidney disease (CKD)

Systemic hypertension, diabetes, and proteinuria are critical factors in the development of chronic kidney disease (CKD) which may lead to end-stage renal disease (ESRD) [20-22] **(IV/C)**. Once CKD/ESRD is established, there is a high likelihood of developing CVD. Hence, there is a link between hypertension and CVD via the occurrence and progression of CKD. More than 80% of patients with CKD have hypertension. Not only does hypertension contribute to the development of CKD, the complications and manifestations of hypertension are aggravated by CKD. The normal circadian rhythm of blood pressure regulation is lost in CKD resulting in the lack of nocturnal dip in the blood pressure level which portends poor prognosis. A number of studies have shown the aggressive control of hypertension in both diabetic and non-diabetic nephropathy slows the progression of proteinuria and CKD, and delays the culmination to ESRD. A number of factors/markers may explain the adverse relationship between hypotension and CKD. A decrease in the glomerular filtration rate (GFR) is an early sign of CKD; progression of CKD is more likely in hypertensive individuals who present with diminished GFR. Many patients with hypertension also have hyperlipidemia which may further accentuate CKD; hyperlipidemia correlates with structural changes in the kidney in hypertensive nephrosclerosis. Another factor in the development of hypertensive CKD is tobacco consumption [23, 24].

It is well established that hypertension and CKD together are powerful risk factors for CVD. Patients with hypertension and CKD have a high risk for coronary artery disease (CAD), myocardial infarction (MI), and congestive heart failure (CHF). Therefore, optimal management of hypertension in patients with CKD should embrace concomitant aggressive treatment of diabetes, hyperlipidemia, obesity, and abstinence from tobacco; all the components of metabolic syndrome should be addressed in the evaluation and management of hypertension in patients with CKD.

Recommended antihypertensive drugs

The National Kidney Foundation and other guidelines recommend a therapeutic goal of blood pressure <130/80mm Hg for all hypertensive patients with CKD. And in order to

Table 2. Summary of recommendations on hypertension and antihypertensive agents in CKD.
Reproduced from the National Kidney Foundation. Am J Kidney Dis 2004; 43: S1-290.

Type of kidney disease	Blood pressure target (mm Hg)		Preferred agents for CKD, with or without hypertension		Other agents to reduce CVD risk and reach blood pressure target	
Diabetic kidney disease	<130/80	B	Ace inhibitor or ARB	A (A)	Diuretic preferred then BB or CCB	A
Non-diabetic kidney disease with spot urine total protein-to-creatinine ratio ≥200mg/g	<130/80	A	Ace inhibitor or ARB	A (C)	Diuretic preferred then BB or CCB	A
Non-diabetic kidney disease with spot urine total protein-to-creatinine ratio <200mg/g	<130/80	B	None preferred		Diuretic preferred then ACE inhibitor, ARB, BB or CCB	A
Kidney disease in the transplant recipient	<130/80	B	None preferred		CCB, diuretic, BB ACE inhibitor, ARB	B

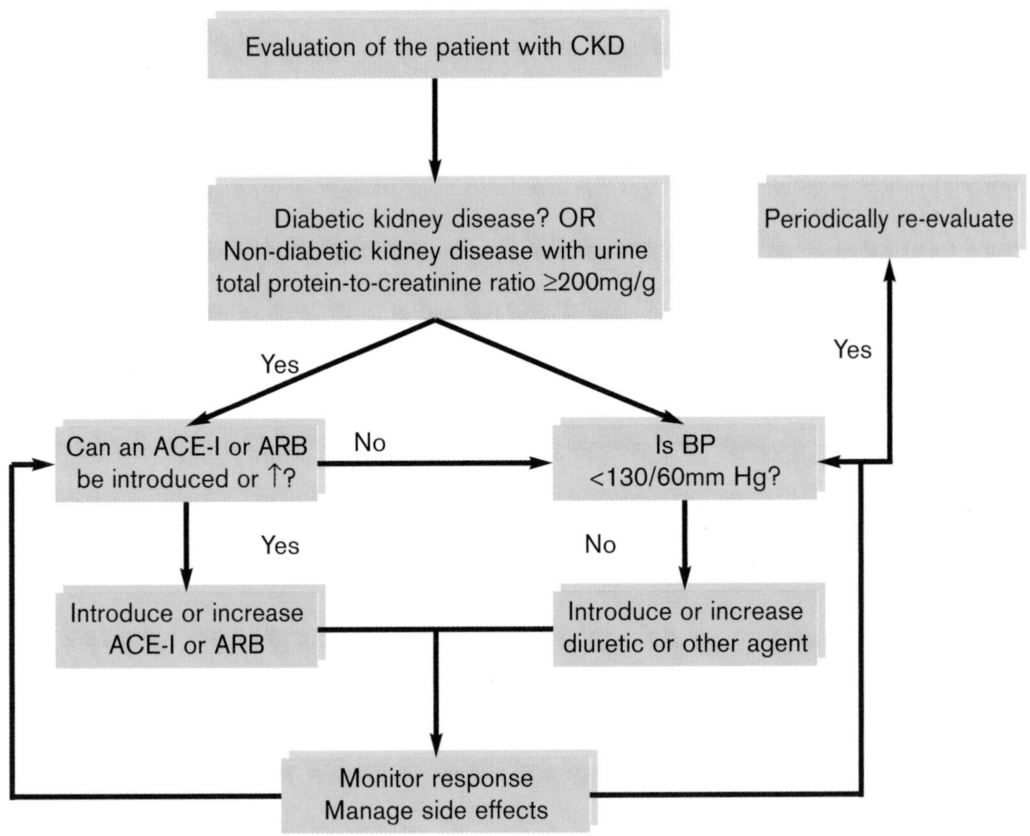

Figure 1. Algorithm for the evaluation and management of hypertension and use of antihypertensive agents in CKD. *Reproduced from the National Kidney Foundation. Am J Kidney Dis 2004; 43: S1-290.*

prevent progression of CKD and its conversion to ESRD, the blood pressure goal should be pursued and maintained. Two key considerations are to lower the blood pressure and to block the RAAS to preserve kidney function (Table 2 and Figure 1). All patients with hypertension and CKD should be advised to follow lifestyle modifications: aerobic exercise, smoking cessation, limiting alcohol, and sodium intake, and ideal body weight. Without implementation of and adherence to non-pharmacological approaches, it is extremely difficult to achieve success with drug therapy.

Achieving blood pressure goal levels in patients with CKD is not only useful for renal protection, but also for cardiovascular protection. Unless contraindicated or not tolerated, drugs blocking the RAAS should be an essential component of the treatment plan. Studies have shown that both ACE-Is and ARBs exert significant renoprotection and cardiovascular protection in diabetic and non-diabetic, hypertensive patients with CKD [25-27] **(Ib/A & IV/C).**

Inappropriate or sustained activation of RAAS contributes to the glomerular hyperfiltration and structure changes in the kidney. Therefore, RAAS blockade may provide functional benefits in the preservation of GFR. Recent studies have confirmed ARBs are not only helpful in CKD, but are superior to DHP CCBs for the prevention of TOD. In studies such as the Reduction of Endpoints in NIDDM with A-II Antagonist Losartan (RENAAL) trial, Irbesartan Diabetic Nephropathy Trial (IDNT), and Irbesartan Renal Micro-Albuminuria (IRMA) trial, the advantages of ARBs in patients with CKD have been firmly established. Of course, all patients with CKD receiving RAAS blockers should be closely monitored not only for blood pressure, but also for renal function, and potassium level (risk of hyperkalemia). Whereas RAAS blockers play an important role in the management of hypertension in CKD, an appropriate diuretic (usually a loop diuretic) should also be integrated into the treatment plan [28]. To reach the therapeutic goal, additional classes of drugs (BBs, direct vasodilators, CCBs, and central α-agonists, etc.) are often required. In the absence of hyperkalemia, an aldosterone antagonist can also be added with usual precautions and monitoring (hyperkalemia) [29]. While RAAS blockers, diuretics, and other antihypertensive drugs are used to treat hypertension in patients with CKD, one should not hesitate to use hydralazine or minoxidil for patients with uncontrolled or refractory hypertension. The objective for hypertension control in patients with CKD is to achieve and maintain the goal blood pressure level which is only possible through close follow-up and aggressive application of therapeutic options.

Hypertension and hyperlipidemia

In patients with metabolic syndrome and hypertension, there is a clustering of multiple additional risk factors such as hyperlipidemia [2, 30]. The combined presence of hypertension and hyperlipidemia augments the cardiovascular risk and promotes excessive morbidity and mortality. It is therefore essential that in patients with hypertension, concurrent management of hyperlipidemia should also be implemented if indicated. Achieving the blood pressure goals but leaving hyperlipidemia unattended exposes the patient to residual risk. The JNC and other guideline committees recommend the determination of lipids and appropriate treatment in patients with hypertension.

Recommended antihypertensive drugs

There is a generalized consensus that both hypertension and hyperlipidemia be concurrently treated to achieve goal levels of blood pressure and lipids. In this context, it should be noted that certain antihypertensive drugs may exert an unfavorable effect on lipid levels; the consequences of antihypertensive drugs on lipid levels is highly variable and unpredictable. Whereas thiazide diuretics (including chlorthalidone) may cause mild increases in total cholesterol and triglyceride concentrations, they have been shown to reduce cardiovascular mortality because of their blood pressure lowering effects which are of considerable importance. BBs often used as a component of combination therapy may raise serum triglyceride levels. These may be subtle (not clinically proven) differences among the BBs on their propensity to alter the lipid levels. It appears that the 'vasodilating' BBs such as carvedilol and nebivolol are less likely to induce lipid abnormalities in the long run; whether this effect provides an additional advantage has not been established. α-blockers (such as doxazosin) may improve lipid metabolism but studies such as ALLHAT failed to show an outcome benefit. Other classes of drugs such as ACE-Is, ARBs, aldosterone antagonists, centrally acting α-agonists, and direct vasodilators have a neutral effect on lipids. Because hyperlipidemia is an independent and additional risk factor for CVD, lipids should be monitored in patients with hypertension and any adverse effect of antihypertensive drugs should be detected and corrected. In the Anglo-Scandinavian Cardiac Outcomes Trial (ASCOT), it was noted that concurrent treatment of hypertension and hyperlipidemia provided greater protection of TOD than treatment of hypertension alone [31, 32] **(Ib/B)**. On the basis of this study as well as on the pathobiology of vascular disease, it is critical to prevent and treat hyperlipidemia in patients with hypertension.

Hypertension and coronary artery disease (CAD)

Hypertension is a principal independent risk factor for CAD and its complications. There is a strong correlation between blood pressure level and manifestations of CAD. After the age of 50 years, systolic blood pressure becomes a more sensitive predictor of CAD than diastolic blood pressure. Nevertheless, both systolic and diastolic levels of blood pressure have a prognostic significance for overall mortality from CAD. Various humoral, physical, metabolic and local factors mediate the link between blood pressure and CAD. Aggressive treatment of hypertension to a goal is mandated for primary and secondary prevention of CAD. With careful and gradual treatment of hypertension, the so-called J-curve (myocardial hypoperfusion) is less likely to occur; however, precipitous and excessive lowering of blood pressure should be avoided to reduce the potential of the J-curve. It goes without saying that management and prevention of CAD requires attention to all the risk factors for CVD; hypertension is only one factor in the complex vascular biology of CAD.

Recommended antihypertensive drugs

Due to the multi-factorial etiology of CAD, non-pharmacological treatment measures should be implemented. The use of BBs in patients with CAD (particularly in the elderly) has become controversial. While the benefits of BBs in patients with CHF or left ventricular dysfunction are established, the precise role of these drugs in patients with CAD remains under scrutiny. The ASCOT was stopped prematurely due to the superiority of the amlodipine-based regimen over atenolol-based therapy in reducing cardiovascular events. In this study, atenolol-based therapy failed to reduce the central aortic pressure, raising questions about the central versus peripheral hemodynamic effects of antihypertensive drugs. BBs which have a heart rate lowering effect may be beneficial in patients with CAD.

In general, RAAS blockers tend to provide possible benefits in patients with CAD due to their pharmacological actions [33-35] **(Ia/A, Ib/A & IV/C)**. ACE-Is and ARBs, therefore, are suitable to treat hypertension in patients with CVD. Non-DHP CCBs, such as diltiazem or verapamil, although not widely used for hypertension, have beneficial effects on coronary blood flow [36]. In the ALLHAT, DHP CCB-based therapy was as good as ACE-I-based therapy for cardiovascular protection. For patients with CAD, the goal blood pressure should be <130/80mm Hg. The choice of drugs is controversial. Clinical trials support the benefits of RAAS blockers, CCBs, or thiazide diuretics in patients with CAD. In patients with a history of angina or myocardial infarction, a BB is an appropriate option (Table 3).

Table 3. Treatment of hypertension in the prevention and management of ischemic heart disease. Summary of the main recommendations. *Adapted from Rosendorff et al. Circulation. 2007; 115: 2761-8.*

Area of concern	BP target mm Hg	Lifestyle modification†	Specific drug indications	Comments
General CAD prevention	<140/90	Yes	Any effective antihypertensive drug or combination ‡	If SBP >160mm Hg or DBP >100mm Hg, then start with 2 drugs
High CAD risk *	<130/80	Yes	ACE-I or ARB or CCB or thiazide diuretic or combination	If SBP >160mm Hg or DBP >100mm Hg, then start with 2 drugs
Stable angina, UA/STEMI, STEMI	<130/80	Yes	β-blocker and ACE-I or ARB §	If β-blocker contraindicated, or if side effects occur, can substitute diltiazem or verapamil (but not if bradycardia or LVD is present) Can add dihydropyridine CCB (not diltiazem or verapamil) to β-blocker A thiazide diuretic can be added for BP control
LVD	<120/80	Yes	ACE-I or ARB and β-blocker and aldosterone antagonist ¥ and thiazide or loop diuretic and hydralazine/ isosorbide dinitrate	Contraindicated: verapamil, diltiazem, clonidine, moxonidine, α-blockers

UA = unstable angina; LVD = LV dysfunction; ACE-I = ACE inhibitor

Before making any management decisions, you are strongly urged to read the full text of the relevant section of the Scientific Statement

* Diabetes mellitus, chronic kidney disease, known CAD or CAD equivalent (carotid artery disease, peripheral arterial disease, abdominal aortic aneurism), or 10-year Framingham risk score ≥10%

† Weight loss if appropriate, healthy diet (including sodium restriction), exercise, smoking cessation, and alcohol moderation

‡ Evidence supports ACE-I (or ARB), CCB, or thiazide diuretic as first-line therapy

§ If anterior MI is present, if hypertension persists, if LV dysfunction or HF is present, or if the patient has diabetes mellitus

¥ If severe HF is present (New York Heart Association class III or IV, or LVEF <40% and clinical HF)

Hypertension and congestive heart failure (CHF)

Systemic hypertension is a major risk factor for CHF – either by a direct biophysical/mechanical effect on left ventricular function and structure or via decreasing coronary profusion. Most patients with left ventricular dysfunction or frank CHF have a history of hypertension. By causing systolic and diastolic dysfunction and CAD, hypertension has a complex pathophysiological etiological connection to CHF.

Recommended antihypertensive drugs

The therapeutic objectives in CHF are to relieve the symptoms and to reverse bio-mechanical hemodynamic abnormalities. Diuretics in combination with other drugs have a therapeutic benefit in CHF but excessive sodium and water losses may activate the SNS and RAAS. Drugs which block the RAAS [37-40] **(Ia/A, Ib/A & IV/C)** are extremely useful and indicated for patients with CHF. Various RCTs have clearly shown that morbidity and mortality in CHF is significantly curtailed by effective utilization of ACE-Is. The role of ARBs in CHF is not as clearly identified as ACE-Is. Clinical trials, however, have shown the benefits of combining ARBs with ACE-Is in subsets of patients with CHF. Aldosterone antagonists such as spironolactone and eplerenone have been shown to be extremely useful in patients with CHF receiving standard therapy [41, 42]. Although the trials have not specifically evaluated aldosterone antagonists in patients with CHF and hypertension, they may be useful in this setting based on the pathophysiology of aldosterone in CVD.

The role of BBs in the management of CHF is well established. By attenuating the negative consequences of SNS activation in CHF, BBs have been shown to decrease the morbidity and mortality in CHF [43-45]. Large RCTs utilizing metoprolol or carvedilol, or bisoprolol have demonstrated the usefulness of these BBs in patients with compensated CHF and/or LV dysfunction. Consequently, BBs are recommended for patients with CHF and/or LV dysfunction. The target blood pressure level for patients with CHF is not clear, but the evidence favors lowering the blood pressure close to 120/80mm Hg.

Hypertension and prevention of stroke

It is well known that systemic hypertension is the most correctible risk factor for stoke prevention. A substantial number of strokes is attributable to hypertension. Treatment of hypertension reduces the risk of stroke. In individuals older than 60 years, for each 10mm Hg reduction in systolic blood pressure, the risk of stroke is reduced by a third. Since the stroke risk increases with age, hypertension should be controlled vigorously in the elderly population. While there is some dispute about blood pressure management immediately after stroke, long-term control of hypertension prevents cerebrovascular disease. There is ample evidence to support the view that blood pressure control prevents not only the first but also recurrent stroke [46, 47] **(Ia/A, Ib/A & IV/C)**.

Recommended antihypertensive drugs

Recent studies such as PROGESS, MOSES, and PRoFESS [48-50] **(Ia/A)** have shed additional light on the management of hypertension to prevent stroke. For stroke prevention, the degree of achieved blood pressure level is more important than the choice of antihypertensive drugs. Both ACE-Is and ARBs have been shown to reduce stroke risk but whether the observed benefit is from their pharmacological actions or the blood pressure level is not clear; it is hard to separate one from the other. BBs are less likely to protect against stroke. Whether the newer vasodilating BBs are helpful for stroke prevention is not known. Despite their possible adverse effects, thiazide diuretics have been shown to be as effective as other classes of antihypertensive drugs. Similarly, CCBs have also been shown to be effective for stroke prevention in patients with hypertension

Conclusions

There is substantial evidence to demonstrate that high levels of blood pressure are associated with significant morbidity and mortality. Fortunately, there is compelling evidence also to suggest that proper blood pressure control reduces the complication rates in patients with hypertension. Hence, for all patients with hypertension, therapeutic goals should be achieved and maintained. While the degree of blood pressure reduction is more paramount than the type of antihypertensive drug class, certain comorbid conditions discussed in this chapter require special considerations. Evidence-based medicine and RCTs suggest the importance of specific preferred antihypertensive drugs in patients with co-existing medical conditions; therapy in such circumstances should take into consideration both the blood pressure goal as well as the type of antihypertensive drug. With careful consideration of comorbid conditions, patients with hypertension can benefit considerably by individualized, tailored therapy.

Key points	Evidence level
◆ Systemic hypertension is an important cause of premature and excessive morbidity and mortality.	Ia/A
◆ Uncontrolled hypertension puts the patient at a high risk for stroke, kidney disease, cardiovascular disease, disability and death.	Ia/A
◆ A steady increase in systemic arterial blood pressure leads to target organ damage.	Ia/A
◆ Fortunately hypertension can be easily detected and treated.	Ia/A
◆ Based upon comorbid conditions and other clinical considerations, antihypertensive drugs can be tailored to achieve the goal levels of blood pressure.	Ib/A
◆ Adherence to published guidelines on the management of hypertension reduces the disease burden and protects public health.	Ib/A

References

1. Chobanian AV, Bakris GL, Black HR, *et al.* The seventh report of the Joint National Committee on Prevention, Detection, Evaluation and Treatment of High Blood Pressure: The JNC 7 Report. *JAMA* 2003; 289: 2560-72.
2. Greenlund KJ, Croft JB, Mensah GA. Prevalence of heart disease and stroke risk factors in persons with prehypertension in the United States, 1999-2000. *Arch Intern Med* 2004; 164: 2113-8.
3. Guidelines Committee. 2003 European Society of Hypertension - European Society of Cardiology guidelines for the management of arterial hypertension. *J Hypertens* 2003; 21: 1011-53.
4. Bloomgarden ZT. Cardiovascular disease in type 2 diabetes. *Diabetes Care* 1999; 22: 1729-44.
5. Stamler J, Vaccaro O, Neaton JD, Wentworth D. Diabetes, other risks, and 12 yr cardiovascular mortality for men screened in the Multiple Risk Factor Intervention Trial. *Diabetes Care* 1993; 16: 434-44.
6. Lithall HO. Hyperinsulinemia, insulin resistance, and the treatment of hypertension. *Am J Hypertens* 1996; 9: 1508-45.
7. Brenner BM, Cooper ME, de ZeeuwD, KeaneW, Mitch WE, Parving HH, Remuzzi G, Snappin SH, Zhang Z, Shahinfar S, RENAAL Study Investigators. Effects of losartan on renal and cardiovascular outcomes in patients with type 2 diabetes and nephropathy. *N Engl J Med* 2001; 345: 861-9.
8. Lewis EJ, Hunsicker LG, Bain RP, Rohde RD. The effect of angiotensin-converting-enzyme inhibition on diabetic nephropathy. *N Engl J Med* 1993; 329-1456-62.
9. Hannson L, Lindlholm LH, Niskanen L, Lanke J, Hendner T, *et al.* Effect of angiotensin-converting-enzyme inhibition compared with conventional therapy on cardiovascular morbidity and mortality in hypertension: the Captopril Prevention Project (CAPPP) randomized trial. *Lancet* 1999; 353: 611-6.
10. Bakris GL, Weir MR, DeQuattro V, McMahon FG. Effects of an ACE inhibitor/calcium antagonist combination on proteinuria in diabetic nephropathy. *Kidney Int* 1998: 54(4): 1283-9.
11. Schrier RW, Estacio RO, Esler A, *et al.* Effects of aggressive blood pressure control in normotensive type 2 diabetic patients on albuminuria, retinopathy and strokes. *Kidney Int* 2002; 61: 1086-97.
12. Jacob S, Rett K, Henriksen EJ. Antihypertensive therapy and insulin sensitivity: do we have to redefine the role of ß-blocking agents? *Am J Hypertens* 1998; 11: 1256-65.
13. Jacob S, Balletshofer B, Henriksen EJ, *et al.* ß-blocking agents in patients with insulin resistance: effects of vasodilating ß-blockers. *Blood Press* 1999; 8: 261-8.
14. UK Prospective Diabetes Study Group. Tight blood pressure control and risk of macrovascular and microvascular complications in type 2 diabetes: UKPDS 38. *BMJ* 1998; 317: 703-13.
15. UK Prospective Diabetes Study Group. Intensive blood-glucose control with sulphonylureas or insulin compared with conventional treatment and risk of complications in patients with type 2 diabetes (UKPDS 33). *Lancet* 1998; 352: 837-53.
16. Bakris GL, Fonseca V, Katholi RE, *et al.* Metabolic effects of carvedilol versus metoprolol in patients with type 2 diabetes mellitus and hypertension: a randomized controlled trial. *JAMA* 2004; 292: 2227-36.
17. Tatti P, Pahor M, Byington RP, Di Mauro P, Guarisco R, Strollo G, Strollo F. Outcome results of the Fosinopril Versus Amlodipine Cardiovascular Events Randomized trial (FACET) in patients with hypertension and NIDDM. *Diabetes Care* 1998; 21: 597-603.
18. ALLHAT Collaborative Research Group. Major cardiovascular events in hypertension patients randomized to doxazosin vs chorthalidone: the Antihypertension and Lipid-lowering Treatment to Prevent Heart Attack Trial (ALLHAT). (Published correction appears in *JAMA* 2002; 288: 2976.) *JAMA* 2000; 283: 1967-75.
19. Wright JT Jr, Harris-Haywood S, Pressel S, Brazilay J, Baimbridge C, Bareis CJ, Baselie JN, Black HR, Dart R, Gupta AK, Hamilton BP, Einhorn PT, Haywood LJ, Jafri SZ, Louise GT, Whelton PK, Scott CL, Simmons DL, Stanford C, Davis BR. Clinical outcomes by race in hypertensive patients with and without the metabolic syndrome: Antihypertensive and Lipid-Lowering Treatment to Prevent Heart Attack Trial (ALLHAT). *Arch Intern Med* 2008; 168: 207-17.
20. Perry HM Jr, Miller JP, Fornoff JR, *et al.* Early predictors of 15-year end-stage renal disease in hypertensive patients. *Hypertension* 1995; 25: 587-94.
21. Ritz E, Ryehlik I, Locatelli F, Halimi S. End-stage renal failure type 2 diabetes: a medical catastrophe of worldwide dimensions. *Am J Kidney Dis* 1999; 34: 795-808.
22. Toto RD, Mitchell HC, Smith RD, *et al.* 'Strict' blood pressure control and progression of renal disease in hypertensive nephrosclerosis. *Kidney Int* 1995; 48: 851-9.

23. Ritz E, Ogata H, Orth SR. Smoking: a factor promoting onset and progression of diabetic nephropathy. *Diabet Med* 2000; 26: 54-63.
24. Regalado M, Yang S, Wesson DE. Cigarette smoking is associated with augmented progression of renal insufficiency in severe essential hypertension. *Am J Kidney Dis* 2000; 35: 667-94.
25. Lewis EJ, Hunsicker LG, Clark WR, *et al* (Collateral Study Group). Renoprotective effect of the angiotensin-receptor antagonist irbesartan in patients with nephropathy due to type 2 diabetes. *N Engl J Med* 2001; 345: 851-60.
26. Agoda LY, Appel L, Bakris GL, *et al* (African American Study of Kidney Disease and Hypertension Study Group). Effect of ramipril vs amlodipine on renal outcomes in hypertensive nephrosclerosis: a randomized controlled trial. *JAMA* 2001; 285: 2719-28.
27. Wright JT Jr, Bakris G, Greene T, *et al* (African American Study of Kidney Disease and Hypertension Study Group). Effect of blood pressure lowering and antihypertensive drug class on progression of hypertensive kidney disease: results from the AASK trial. *JAMA* 2002; 288: 2421-31.
28. Douglas JG, Bakris GL, Epstein M, *et al.* Management of high blood pressure in African Americans: consensus statement of the Hypertension in African Americans Working Group of the International Society on Hypertension in Blacks. *Arch Intern Med* 2003; 163: 525-41.
29. Sato A, Hayashi K, Naruse M, Saruta T. Effectiveness of aldosterone blockade in patients with diabetic nephropathy. *Hypertension* 2003; 41: 640-68.
30. Expert Panel on Detection, Evaluation and Treatment of High Blood Cholesterol in Adults. Executive summary of the Third Report of the National Cholesterol Education Program (NCEP) Expert Panel on Detection, Evaluation, and Treatment of High Blood Cholesterol in Adults (Adult Treatment Panel III). *JAMA* 2001, 285: 1486-2497.
31. Sever PS, Dahlof B, Poulter NR, *et al.* Rationale, design, methods and baseline demography of participants of the Anglo-Scandinavian Cardiac Outcomes Trial. ASCOT investigators. *J Hypertens* 2001; 19: 1139-47.
32. Sever PS, Dahlof B, Poulter NR, *et al.* ASCOT investigators. Prevention of coronary and stroke events with atorvastatin in hypertensive patients who have average or lower-than-average cholesterol concentrations, in the Anglo-Scandinavian Cardiac Outcomes Trials - Lipid Lowering Arm (ASCOT-LLA): a multicentre randomized controlled trial. *Lancet* 2003; 361: 1149-58.
33. Braunwald E, Domanski MJ, Fowler SE, Geller NOL, Gersh BJ, Hsia J, Pfeffer MA, Rice MM, Rosenberg YD, Rouleau JL. PEACE Trial Investigators. Angiotensin-converting-enzyme inhibition in stable coronary artery disease. *N Engl Med* 2004; 351: 2058-68.
34. The Acute Infarction Ramipril Efficacy (AIRE) Study Investigators. Effect of ramipril on mortality and morbidity of survivors of acute myocardial infarction with clinical evidence of heart failure. *Lancet* 1993; 342: 821-8.
35. Longobardi G. Ferrara N, Furgi G, Abete P, Rengo F. Improvement of myocardial blood flow to ischemic regions by angiotensin-converting enzyme inhibition. *J Am Coll Cardiol* 2000; 35: 1437-8.
36. Hansson L, Hedner T, Lund-Johansen P, Kjeldsen SE, Lindbolm LH, Syvertsen JO, Lanke J, de Faire U, Duhlof B, Karlberg BE. Randomised trial of effects of calcium antagonists compared with diuretics and ß-blockers on cardiovascular morbidity and mortality in hypertension: the Nordic Diltiasem (NORDIL) study, *Lancet* 2000; 356: 359-65.
37. Pfeffer MA, Swedberg K, Granger CB, Held P, McMurray JJ, Michelson EL, Olofsson B, Ostergren J, Yusuf S, Pocock S. CHARM Investigators and Committees. Effects of candesartan on mortality and morbidity in patients with chronic heart failure: the CHARM - overall programme. *Lancet* 2003; 362: 759-66.
38. The SOLVD Investigators. Effect of enalapril on mortality and the development of heart failure in asymptomatic patients with reduced left ventricular ejection fractions (published correction appears in *N Engl J Med* 1992; 327: 685-91).
39. The SOLVD Investigators. Effect of enalapril on survival in patients with reduced left ventricular ejection fractions and congestive heart failure. *N Engl J Med* 1991; 325: 293-302.
40. Kostis JB. The effect of enalapril on mortal and morbid events in patients with hypertension and left ventricular dysfunction. *Am J Hypertens* 1995; 8: 909-14.
41. Pitt B, White H, Nicolau , Martinez P, Gheorghiade M, Aschermann M, van Veldhuisen DJ, Zannad F, Krum H, Mukherjee R, Vincent J; EPHESUS Investigators. Eplerenone reduces mortality 30 days after randomization following acute myocardial infarction in patients with left ventricular systolic dysfunction and heart failure. *J Am Coll Cardiol* 2005; 46: 425-31.

42. Pitt B, Zannad F, Remme WJ, Cody R, Catnigne A, Perez A, Puleosky J, Wittes J; Randomized Aldosterone Evaluation Study Investigators. The effect of spironolactone on mortality in patients with severe heart failure. *N Engl J Med* 1999; 341: 707-17.
43. Poole-Wilson PA, Swedberg K, Cleland JG, DiLenardo A, Hanrath P. Komajda M, Lubsen J, Cutlger B, Metra M, Remroe WJ. Torp-Pederson C, Scherbag A, Skenc A; Carvedilol or Metoprolol European Trial Investigators. Comparison of carvedilol and metoprolol on clinical outcomes in patients with chronic heart failure in the Carvedilol or Metoprolol European Trial (COMET): randomized controlled trial. *Lancet* 2003; 362: 7-13.
44. Packer M, Fowler MB, Recker EB, Coats AJ, Katus HA, Krum H. Mohaesi P, Rouleau JL. Tendera M. Staiger C, Holeslaw TL, Amann-Zalan I, Demets DL; Carvedilol Prospective Randomized Cumulative Survival (COPERNICUS) Study Group. Effect of carvedilol on the morbidity of patients with severe chronic heart failure: results of the Carvedilol Prospective Randomized Cumulative Survival (COPERNICUS) Study. *Circulation* 2002; 106: 2194-9.
45. MERIT-HF Study Group. Effect of metoprolol CR/XL in chronic heart failure: Metoprolol CR/XL. Randomized Intervention Trial in Congestive Heart Failure (MERIT-HF). *Lancet* 1999; 353: 2001-7.
46. Aiyagari V, Gorlick PB. Management of blood pressure for acute and recurrent stroke. *Stroke* 2009; 40: 2251-6.
47. Laws CM, Bennet DA, Feigin VL, Roger A. Blood pressure and stroke; an overview of published reviews. *Stroke* 2004; 35: 1024.
48. PROGRESS Collaborate Group. Randomised trial of a perindopril-based blood-pressure-lowering regimen among 6105 individuals with previous stroke or transient ischaemic attack. *Lancet* 2001; 358: 1033-41.
49. Schruder J, Loders S, Katsehewsk A, Hammersen F, Plate K, Berger J, Zidek W, Dominiak P, Diener HC; MOSES Study Group morbidity and mortality after stroke. Eprosartan Compared with Nitrendipine for secondary prevention; principal results of a prospective randomized controlled study (MOSES). *Stroke* 2005; 36: 1218-26.
50. Yusuf S, Diener HC, Sacco RL, Cotton D, Ounpuu S, Lawton WA, Palesch Y, Martin RH, Albers GW, Bath P, Bornstein N, Chan BP, Chen ST, Cunha L, Dablof B, De Keyser J, Donnan GA, Estol C, Gorlick P, Gu V, Hermansson K, Hilbrich L, Kaste M, Lu C, Machng T, Pais P, Roberts R, Skvortsova V, Teal P, Toni D, VanderMaelen C, Voigt T, Weber M, Yoon BW; PRoFess Study Group. Telmisartan to prevent recurrent stroke and cardiovascular events. *N Engl J Med* 2008; 359: 1225-37.

Chapter 6

The optimal management of patients with resistant hypertension due to aldosterone excess

Eduardo Pimenta MD, Clinical Research Fellow
Endocrine Hypertension Research Centre and Clinical Centre of Research Excellence in Cardiovascular Disease and Metabolic Disorders
University of Queensland School of Medicine, Princess Alexandra Hospital
Brisbane, Australia

David A. Calhoun MD, Professor of Medicine
Vascular Biology and Hypertension Program
University of Alabama at Birmingham, Birmingham, Alabama, USA

Introduction

Resistant hypertension is defined as blood pressure (BP) that remains above goal in spite of the use of three antihypertensive medications of different classes in effective doses, ideally including a diuretic [1]. Patients with controlled blood pressure but needing four or more medications should also be considered to have resistant hypertension [2]. Resistant hypertension is defined accordingly in order to identify patients with reversible causes of hypertension or patients that may benefit from diagnostic and therapeutic considerations [2]. The goal blood pressure is less than 140/90mm Hg for general hypertensive patients and less than 130/80mm Hg in patients with diabetes and chronic kidney disease (glomerular filtration rate <60mL/min/1.73m^2; serum creatinine >1.5mg/dL in men or >1.3mg/dL in women; albuminuria >300mg/24-hr or >200mg/g creatinine) [1] **(Ia/A)**.

Although the awareness and control of hypertension have increased, only 37% of hypertensive patients in the United States achieve the conservative goal of <140/90mmHg [3], emphasizing the widespread persistence of poorly controlled hypertension. While the prevalence of resistant hypertension as currently defined is unknown, clinical studies suggest that it is a common clinical problem **(Ib/A)**. For example, in the Antihypertensive and Lipid-Lowering Treatment to Prevent Heart Attack Trial (ALLHAT) [4], 34.4% of subjects never achieved blood pressure control in spite of intensive therapy including 27.3% of patients receiving three or more medications after 5 years of follow-up. In The International Verapamil-Trandolapril Study (INVEST) [5], 51% of patients were on three or more antihypertensive drugs after 24 months. While uncontrolled hypertension is not synonymous with resistant hypertension (the former would include patients with poorly controlled hypertension secondary to poor adherence and/or undertreatment), these clinical studies indicate that difficult to control hypertension remains a common medical problem.

Factors that predispose to antihypertensive treatment resistance include older age, obesity, physical inactivity, chronic kidney disease, diabetes, African American race and high dietary salt intake. Use of exogenous substances such as alcohol, sympathomimetic agents, oral contraceptives and especially non-steroidal anti-inflammatory agents (NSAIDs) can interfere with treatment **(Ia/A)**. Lastly, secondary causes of hypertension are more common in patients presenting with resistant hypertension (Table 1) **(III/B)**.

Table 1. Secondary causes of resistant hypertension.
• Hyperaldosteronism
• Obstructive sleep apnea
• Chronic kidney disease
• Renal artery stenosis
• Pheochromocytoma
• Central nervous system tumors
• Coarctation of the aorta
• Thyroid diseases

Hyperaldosteronism

Primary aldosteronism (PA) was first described by Jerome Conn in 1955 [6]. The index case was a young women presenting with resistant hypertension, hypokalemia, and a metabolic alkalosis. She was subsequently found to have an aldosterone-producing adenoma (APA), which when surgically resected, effectively cured her of the syndrome. However, the modern syndrome of hyperaldosteronism differs from the classical description of PA. Hypokalemia and adrenal tumors are no longer required for the diagnosis of hyperaldosteronism. Other forms of PA are now recognized and should also be investigated (Table 2). Screenings done during Dr. Conn's lifetime suggested that PA was an uncommon cause of hypertension, with an estimated prevalence of 1-2% of general hypertensive patients. In the early 1990s, however, investigators in Brisbane, Australia, reported [7] a surprisingly high prevalence of PA of approximately 12% among 52 hypertensive subjects responding to a newspaper

Table 2. Causes of primary aldosteronism.
◆ Aldosterone-producing adenoma
◆ Bilateral or idiopathic hyperplasia
◆ Unilateral hyperplasia
◆ Aldosterone-producing adrenocortical carcinoma
◆ Familial hyperaldosteronism: o type I or glucocorticoid-remediable aldosteronism o type II

advertisement for participation in an antihypertensive drug trial. A follow-up study [8] of 199 subjects referred to the hypertension clinic in Brisbane confirmed the high occurrence of PA, with an estimated prevalence of at least 9.5% and perhaps as high as 13%.

Since these reports, multiple studies have confirmed that PA is much more common than had been demonstrated historically with a prevalence among general hypertensive patients of approximately 10% **(IIb/B)**. In one of the more compelling and clinically informative studies [9], Mosso *et al* screened over 600 hypertensive patients for PA. The severity of the untreated hypertension based on JNC VI stages (Stage 1 140-159/90-99, Stage 2 160-179/100-109, Stage 3 ≥180/110mm Hg) was known for each subject. The investigators were therefore able to relate the prevalence of PA to the severity of the underlying hypertension. The overall prevalence of PA was 6.1%. The prevalence, however, increased progressively with increasing severity of hypertension. In subjects with Stage 1 hypertension, the PA prevalence was only 2%, which was not different from normotensive controls; in subjects with Stage 2 hypertension the PA prevalence was 8%; and in subjects with Stage 3 hypertension, the prevalence was 13%. The results are clinically relevant in demonstrating that the likelihood of PA increases with increasing severity of hypertension such that patients with mild hypertension are at low risk while patients with severe hypertension are at a high risk of having PA.

PA is particularly common in subjects with resistant hypertension with a prevalence of approximately 20% **(IIb/B)**. In an evaluation of patients referred to the University of Alabama at Birmingham hypertension clinic [10], we found that 18 of 88 (20%) of consecutively evaluated patients with resistant hypertension were diagnosed with PA based on a suppressed plasma renin activity (PRA) (<1.0ng/mL/hr) and a high 24-hr urinary aldosterone excretion (>12µg/24-hr) during high dietary sodium intake (>200mEq/24-hr). The prevalence of PA was similar in African American and white patients. A prevalence of PA of approximately 20% in patients with resistant hypertension has been a consistent observation of prospective studies done at different clinics worldwide. In a study conducted in Seattle, Washington [11], PA was diagnosed in 17% of patients with difficult to control hypertension. Similarly, investigators in Oslo, Norway [12], have confirmed PA in 23% of patients with resistant hypertension. Investigators in Prague, Czech Republic, have reported [13] a prevalence of PA of 19% in patients referred to a university hypertension clinic for moderate to severe hypertension.

Prognosis

In animal studies, aldosterone excess in combination with high dietary salt intake has been shown to promote target-organ deterioration independent of increases in blood pressure [14-16] **(III/B)**. This target-organ decline is characterized by perivascular inflammation and necrosis progressing to diffuse fibrosis. These pro-inflammatory and profibrotic effects of aldosterone observed experimentally are consistent with observational studies of patients with PA indicating an increased likelihood of left ventricular hypertrophy [17], chronic kidney disease [18], and endothelial dysfunction [19], each of which independently predicts increased cardiovascular risk.

Cross-sectional comparisons of patients with PA and hypertensive control patients indicate that the former are at increased risk of having cardiovascular disease **(III/B)**. In a recent analysis [20], compared to control patients matched for severity and duration of hypertension, patients confirmed to have PA were more than four times as likely to have had a stroke, 6.5 times as likely to have had a prior myocardial infarction, and more than 12 times as likely to have developed atrial fibrillation. Although prospective evaluations are lacking, observational studies do suggest that patients with evidence of aldosterone excess are at increased risk of cardiovascular complications compared to patients with primary hypertension.

Diagnosis

Given the particularly high association between hyperaldosteronism and treatment resistance, all patients with resistant hypertension, even those who are normokalemic, should be evaluated for all forms of PA **(III/B)**. Although originally described as an essential characteristic of the syndrome, Conn later recognized [21] that hypokalemia was more often a late manifestation of the syndrome that was generally preceded by the development of hypertension. The recent prospective assessments determining the prevalence of PA seem to confirm such a progression in finding that hypertensive patients diagnosed with PA usually have normal serum potassium levels **(III/B)**. In our experience [22] 50% of patients with hyperaldosteronism and resistant hypertension have normal potassium levels or have never needed potassium supplementation. While patients who present with hypokalemia (especially spontaneously occurring hypokalemia, but also including hypokalemia that develops with thiazide diuretic use) are at increased risk of having PA, the absence of hypokalemia does not exclude the presence of PA.

Screening

As opposed to assessing plasma aldosterone levels or PRA independently, measurement of the plasma aldosterone/plasma renin activity ratio (ARR) has been shown to have sufficient sensitivity to serve as an effective screening test for PA **(IIb/B)**. Although the exact test characteristics of the ARR vary between studies, its negative predictive value has been generally good such that a low ARR (<20 when plasma aldosterone is measured in ng/dL and PRA is measured in ng/mL/hr) reliably excludes PA. The specificity of ARR is low such that a high ratio (>20-30) is suggestive but not diagnostic of PA. The lower specificity of the ARR likely reflects a high prevalence of low-renin hypertension, particularly among patients with resistant hypertension. Accordingly, a high ARR is suspicious for PA, but the diagnosis must be confirmed with suppression testing.

Use of the ARR to screen for PA is best done after withdrawal of antihypertensive medications and correction of low potassium levels **(IIb/B)**. Angiotensin-converting enzyme (ACE) inhibitors, angiotensin receptor blockers (ARBs), and diuretics tend to increase PRA, while β-blockers have the opposite effect, tending to suppress PRA. ACE inhibitors and ARBs may suppress plasma aldosterone levels, particularly with initial use. However, as the effects of these medications on the ARR would tend to result in a falsely low ratio, a high ratio in the context of ongoing medication is even more sensitive for aldosterone excess. (The exception being potassium-sparing diuretics, particularly mineralocorticoid receptor antagonists such as spironolactone or eplerenone, that must be withdrawn for 4-6 weeks before screening as they falsely elevate both PRA and plasma aldosterone.)

Alpha antagonists and non-dihydropiridine calcium channel blockers likely have the least effect on the ARR **(III/B)**. However, as it is often not possible to withdraw antihypertensive treatment from patients with resistant hypertension, it is more pragmatic to first check the ARR without withdrawing medications as a high ratio in this setting is still suspicious for PA [23]. A low ratio in the setting of ongoing medication use loses sensitivity and is less reliable in excluding PA.

The higher the ARR, the more likely the patient has PA (Table 3). However, the ARR is very dependent on the PRA, so that if the PRA is extremely low, it can result in a falsely positive ratio. This risk can be reduced by using a minimum PRA value of 0.5ng/mL/hr to calculate the ARR such that a plasma aldosterone of at least 10ng/dL is needed to have a ratio of 20 or greater. The risk of a falsely positive ratio can be further reduced by requiring a minimum plasma aldosterone level of 15ng/dL, but this will reduce the sensitivity of the ratio, resulting in more falsely negative screenings (Table 3).

Confirmation

Confirmation of PA requires demonstration of lack of suppression of aldosterone secretion with volume expansion **(IIb/B)**. Current guidelines for detection and diagnosis of PA

Table 3. Test characteristics of various levels of the plasma aldosterone/plasma renin activity ratio (ARR) to identify primary aldosteronism in patients being treated for resistant hypertension. ***Adapted from Nishizaka MK, et al. Am J Hypertens 2005; 18: 805-12.***

Cut-off	Sensitivity (%)	Specificity (%)	+PV (%)	-PV (%)
ARR>20	78	83	56	93
ARR>50	10	99	86	80
ARR>20 and PAC>15	57	88	57	88

+PV = positive predictive value; -PV = negative predictive value; PAC = plasma aldosterone concentration

Table 4. Confirmatory tests for primary aldosteronism.

- Oral sodium loading test
- Saline infusion test
- Fludrocortisone suppression test
- Captopril challenge test

recommend that patients with a positive ARR undergo testing to confirm or exclude the diagnosis of PA [24]. Four different confirmatory tests are recommended (Table 4).

Historically, the gold standard to confirm the diagnosis of PA has been the fludrocortisone suppression test **(III/B)**. Patients receive oral dietary salt loading (sufficient to maintain a urinary sodium excretion rate of at least 3mmol/kg of body weight) with concomitant administration of fludrocortisone (0.1mg orally every 6 hours) for 4 days. Upright PAC >6ng/dl on day 4 at 10am confirms PA, provided the PRA is <1.0ng/ml/h and the plasma cortisol concentration is lower than the value obtained at 7am to exclude confounding ACTH stimulation [24]. Such an approach, however, produces extreme fluid retention and potassium wasting such that hospitalization is required to monitor for excessive fluid overload and to avoid severe hypokalemia.

Alternatively, failure to suppress plasma aldosterone to <5-10ng/dL after infusion of 2L of normal saline over 4 hours confirms the diagnosis of PA **(IIb/B)**. Failure of captopril 25mg given orally to suppress plasma aldosterone to <12ng/dL after 2 hours has been suggested to reliably indicate PA, but there has been much less experience with this method of suppression testing **(IV/C)**.

Demonstration of increased 24-hr urinary excretion of aldosterone in spite of dietary salt loading for 3 days can also be used to confirm the diagnosis of PA [24, 25] **(IIb/B)**. Such an approach is generally safe and can be done on an out-patient basis. A urinary aldosterone ≥12g/24-hr in sodium replete patients (>200mmol/24-hr) is considered positive for PA. If the sodium intake is <200mmol/24-hr, the 24-hr urinary assessment is repeated after 3 days of dietary salt supplementation sufficient to increase sodium intake >200mmol/24-hr.

CT imaging

After confirmation of biochemical PA, thin-cut abdominal CT imaging is recommended in an attempt to identify adrenal tumors that are potentially APAs. The specificity of CT imaging to identify APAs is poor, therefore, screening for APAs with CT imaging without having confirmed biochemical PA is not recommended **(III/B)**. Presence of an adrenal tumor(s) suggestive of an APA increases the likelihood that the patient will benefit from adrenalectomy. The absence of a visible tumor on CT imaging does not exclude the possibility of a micro-adenoma as a possible source of the excess aldosterone.

Adrenal vein sampling

Even in the setting of confirmed biochemical PA, CT imaging has a poor specificity for identifying APAs. In a recent retrospective analysis [26] of cases of confirmed PA, concordance between CT imaging and adrenal vein sampling (AVS) was observed in only 54% of patients such that 45% of patients would have received inappropriate therapy (either incorrectly excluded from having surgery, having non-indicated surgery, or having the wrong adrenal gland removed) if CT imaging alone had been used to guide therapy.

AVS confirms or excludes lateralization of aldosterone excretion consistent with a unilateral APA **(IIb/B)**. Although generally safe, it is technically difficult, particularly in terms of reliably sampling the right adrenal vein. According to a review [27] of 47 reports, the success rate for cannulating the right adrenal vein in 384 patients was 74%. With experience, the success rate increased to 90-96% [28, 29]. It is sometimes suggested [25] that young patients (<40 years) with confirmed PA and a unilateral tumor on CT imaging can be reliably referred for surgery without confirmation of lateralization (i.e. AVS). Likewise, because of increased cancer potential, resection of very large tumors (>2-3cm) is also often recommended regardless of AVS results **(IV/C)**. These recommendations, however, are based largely on anecdote such that opinions as to when AVS is needed or not needed prior to surgery can vary widely between experts. In equivocal cases, referral to an institution experienced with AVS and adrenalectomy is recommended.

Treatment

Adrenalectomy

Resection of unilateral APAs generally corrects the hyperaldosteronism, particularly the associated potassium wasting **(IIb/B)**. The blood pressure response to adrenalectomy is variable, with young patients more likely to have complete resolution of hypertension and older patients less likely, particularly if there is a lengthy history of poorly controlled hypertension [30]. Unless there is a contraindication, adrenalectomy should be done laparoscopically to minimize the recovery time.

Medical treatment

Treatment of the patient with resistant hypertension includes removal of contributing factors, appropriate treatment of secondary causes, and use of effective multi-drug regimens **(III/B)**. Interfering substances should be withdrawn or down-titrated as possible. Multidisciplinary teams, including nurses, pharmacists, nutritionists, and fitness trainers can improve treatment results [31]. Non-pharmacologic therapies such as weight loss, exercise, dietary salt reduction, and moderation of alcohol intake should be encouraged as appropriate for all patients **(III/B)**.

Patients with resistant hypertension seem to be exquisitely sensitive to salt intake. A cross-over prospective study [32] compared blood pressure levels in 12 patients with resistant hypertension during a low- and high-salt diet. Plasma aldosterone concentration was moderately elevated in those patients. Systolic and diastolic 24-hr ambulatory blood pressure decreased by 20.3 and 9.3mmHg, respectively, from a high- to low-salt diet. This effect occurred secondary both to intravascular fluid retention and impairment of vascular function.

A triple combination of an ACE inhibitor or an angiotensin receptor blocker, calcium channel blocker, and a thiazide diuretic is generally very effective and well tolerated. Patients with resistant hypertension often have occult volume retention and effective diuretic therapy is essential for blood pressure control [33, 34]. Long-acting thiazide diuretics are effective in most patients with resistant hypertension. Loop diuretics are preferable in patients with CKD if the creatinine clearance is <30mL/min. Furosemide is relatively short-acting and if used should be prescribed at least twice-daily.

Mineralocorticoid receptor antagonists promote significant additional blood pressure reduction independent of aldosterone/renin levels in patients with resistant hypertension [22, 35-38] **(IIb/B)**. In a prospective assessment, spironolactone 25-50mg daily produced a mean reduction of 24.1mm Hg in systolic blood pressure (SBP) and 10.6mm Hg in diastolic blood pressure (DBP) (Figure 1) [39]. In a study [22] done at the University of Alabama at Birmingham, the effect of spironolactone in patients with uncontrolled blood pressure on an average of four medications, including an ACE inhibitor or ARB, and a diuretic, was prospectively assessed. After 6 months of follow-up, office SBP was reduced by 25mm Hg and DBP by 12mm Hg. Blood pressure reductions were similar in patients with and without PA and the blood

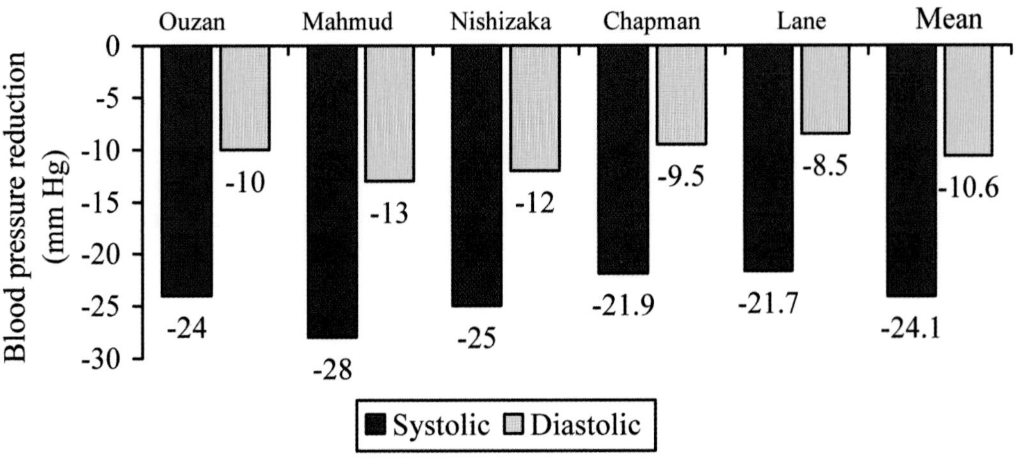

Figure 1. Spironolactone-induced blood pressure reductions observed in studies of patients with resistant hypertension. *Reproduced from Pimenta E, Calhoun DA [39].*

pressure response to spironolactone was not predicted by baseline PAC or PRA or by 24-hr urinary aldosterone excretion. The benefit was also similar in African American and white subjects.

Lane *et al* reported [37] the effect of spironolactone (25-50mg) in 133 patients with resistant hypertension. Spironolactone was associated with a fall in SBP of 21.7mm Hg and DBP of 8.5mm Hg. Data from the Anglo-Scandinavian Cardiac Outcomes Trial – Blood Pressure Lowering Arm (ASCOT) [38] also demonstrated a significant blood pressure lowering effect of spironolactone when prescribed as fourth-line therapy. SBP and DBP were reduced by 21.9 and 9.5mm Hg, respectively, in 1411 participants.

Generally, we use spironolactone in combination with a thiazide diuretic to maximize the antihypertensive benefit and to minimize the risk of hyperkalemia **(IV/C)**. Spironolactone is generally well tolerated, with breast tenderness occurring in about 10% of men with the 25mg dose. Occurrence of breast tenderness with or without gynecomastia increases sharply with higher doses. The more selective mineralocorticoid receptor antagonist, eplerenone, with a lower affinity for progesterone and androgen receptors, is better tolerated than spironolactone. It has been shown [40] to effectively reduce blood pressure in general hypertensive patients with a low incidence of breast tenderness, gynecomastia, sexual dysfunction, and menstrual irregularities. Eplerenone has also been shown to provide substantial add-on benefit when added to the existing regimen of patients with resistant hypertension. In a prospective study, 52 patients with resistant hypertension (SBP >140mm

Hg or DBP >90mm Hg on maximal doses of ≥3 antihypertensive agents, including a loop or thiazide diuretic) received eplerenone (50-100mg daily). After 12 weeks of treatment, 24-hr systolic and diastolic blood pressure decreased by 17.6 and 12.2mm Hg, respectively [41]. As with spironolactone, hyperkalemia can occur with eplerenone, necessitating monitoring.

In our experience, spironolactone-associated hyperkalemia is uncommon in patients with normal renal function even when added to an ACE inhibitor or ARB, but it can occur, necessitating close monitoring. The risk of hyperkalemia is increased in older patients, in patients with CKD or diabetes, and in patients receiving ACE inhibitors or ARBs and/or NSAIDs. In these higher-risk patients, spironolactone can be started at 12.5mg daily (requires splitting of 25mg tablet). Serum potassium and creatinine levels should be monitored in patients treated with mineralocorticoid receptor antagonists. Potassium supplementation or salt substitutes that contain potassium should be discontinued or reduced in patients who are started on mineralocorticoid receptor antagonists.

Amiloride, in blocking the epithelial sodium channel, acts as an indirect mineralocorticoid receptor antagonist. It has been documented to be effective in treating aldosterone-related hypertension, particularly in patients with resistant hypertension, but there is less experience using it to specifically treat PA [11, 42] **(IV/C)**. It is well tolerated without any of the sex-hormone-related adverse effects of spironolactone. Like direct mineralocorticoid receptor antagonists, there is a risk of hyperkalemia.

Evolving perspectives

Controversy exists as to whether or not to pursue confirmation of PA in patients with a high ARR as opposed to simply beginning a MR antagonist. The argument for the latter approach is that even with confirmation of PA the majority of patients will not be surgical candidates and, therefore, will simply end up being treated medically [43]. The counter argument is that in treating all patients with a high ARR without having excluded PA, those patients with aldosterone-producing tumors, although a minority will never be identified and, therefore, must endure lifelong medical therapy when they might have been more effectively or even cured of their hypertension with adrenalectomy.

Recent studies have demonstrated that treatment with an MR antagonist is as effective as adrenalectomy for preventing target organ damage and cardiovascular disease. A prospective study [44] followed 54 patients with PA (either APA or hyperplasia) for 6.4 years (Figure 2). They were treated with adrenaletomy (those with APA) or aldosterone antagonists (including 5 patients with APA). Both treatments effectively reduced left ventricular hypertrophy independent of blood pressure. However, left ventricular hypertrophy decreased more rapidly in those patients treated with adrenalectomy compared to those treated with aldosterone antagonists. In a separate study [45], the same authors compared cardiovascular outcomes (acute myocardial infarction, stroke, myocardial revascularization and arrhythmias) in the same population. There was no difference in the incidence of combined endpoints between patients treated with adrenalectomy or aldosterone antagonists after an average follow-up of 7.4 years despite similar blood pressure reduction.

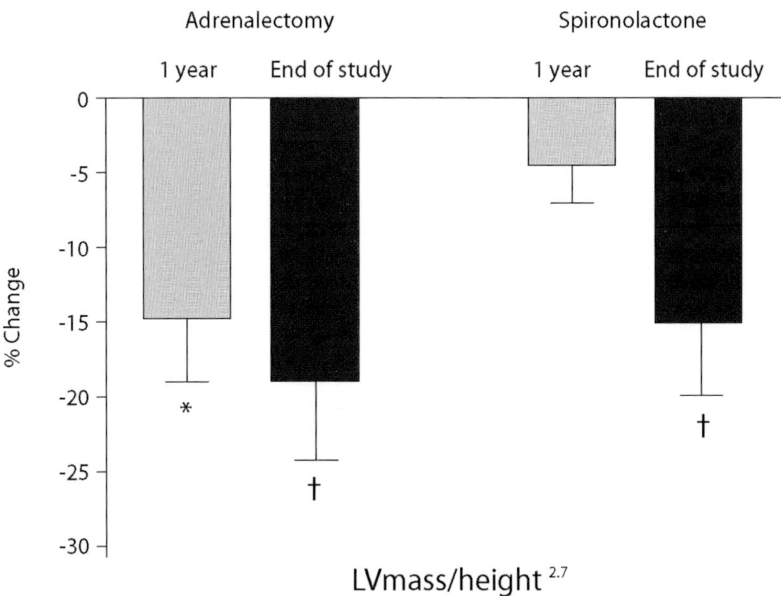

Figure 2. Percentage changes of left ventricular mass index (LVMI) during short- and long-term follow-up in patients with primary aldosteronism who were treated with adrenalectomy (n=24) or spironolactone (n=30). Short-term and long-term follow-up measurements were done after 1 year and an average of 6.4 years, respectively. * P_0.05 vs. baseline; † P_0.01 vs. baseline. *Reproduced with permission from Catena C, et al* [44].

Conclusions

The evidence suggests that:

- resistant hypertension, defined as uncontrolled blood pressure in spite of the use of at least three antihypertensive medications, is an increasingly common problem;
- for reasons that are unclear, PA is particularly common in subjects with resistant hypertension with a prevalence of approximately 20%;
- mineralocorticoid receptor antagonists are an effective therapeutic option for the treatment of resistant hypertension even in the absence of demonstrable aldosterone excess.

Key points	Evidence level
◆ Hypokalemia and adrenal tumors are no longer required for the diagnosis of PA.	III/B
◆ Patients with PA are at increased risk of having cardiovascular disease.	III/B
◆ All patients with resistant hypertension, even those who are normokalemic, should be evaluated for PA.	III/B
◆ The plasma aldosterone/plasma renin activity ratio (ARR) has been shown to have sufficient sensitivity to serve as an effective screening test for PA.	IIb/B
◆ Confirmation of PA requires demonstration of lack of suppression of aldosterone secretion with volume expansion.	IIb/B
◆ Screening for APA with CT imaging without having confirmed biochemical PA is not recommended.	III/B
◆ AVS is the gold standard for diagnosis of unilateral forms of PA.	IIb/B
◆ Laparoscopic unilateral adrenalectomy is recommended for patients with APA.	IIb/B
◆ Mineralocorticoid receptor antagonists are recommended for treatment of patients with resistant hypertension with or without aldosterone excess.	IIb/B

References

1. Chobanian AV, Bakris GL, Black HR, *et al.* Seventh Report of the Joint National Committee on Prevention, Detection, Evaluation, and Treatment of High Blood Pressure. *Hypertension* 2003; 42: 1206-52.
2. Calhoun DA, Jones D, Textor S, *et al.* Resistant hypertension: diagnosis, evaluation, and treatment: a scientific statement from the American Heart Association Professional Education Committee of the Council for High Blood Pressure Research. *Hypertension* 2008; 51: 1403-19.
3. Ong KL, Cheung BMY, Man YB, Lau CP, Lam KS. Prevalence, awareness, treatment, and control of hypertension among United States adults 1999-2004. *Hypertension* 2007; 49: 69-75.
4. Cushman WC, Ford CE, Cutler JA, *et al.* Success and predictors of blood pressure control in diverse North American settings: the Antihypertensive and Lipid-Lowering Treatment to Prevent Heart Attack Trial (ALLHAT). *J Clin Hypertens* 2002; 4: 393-404.
5. Pepine CJ, Handberg EM, Cooper-DeHoff RM, *et al.* A calcium antagonist vs a non-calcium antagonist hypertension treatment strategy for patients with coronary artery disease - The International Verapamil-Trandolapril Study (INVEST): a randomized controlled trial. *JAMA* 2003; 290: 2805-16.
6. Conn JW. Presidential address. I. Painting background. II. Primary aldosteronism, a new clinical syndrome. *J Lab Clin Med* 1955; 45: 3-17.
7. Gordon RD, Ziesak MD, Tunny TJ, Stowasser M, Klemm SA. Evidence that primary aldosteronism may not be uncommon: 12% incidence among antihypertensive drug trial volunteers. *Clin Exp Pharmacol Physiol* 1993; 20: 296-8.
8. Gordon RD, Stowasser M, Tunny TJ, Klemm SA, Rutherford JC. High incidence of primary aldosteronism in 199 patients referred with hypertension. *Clin Exp Pharmacol Physiol* 1994; 21: 315-8.
9. Mosso L, Carvajal C, González A, *et al.* Primary aldosteronism and hypertensive disease. *Hypertension* 2003; 42: 161-5.

10. Calhoun DA, Nishizaka MK, Zaman MA, Thakkar RB, Weissmann P. Hyperaldosteronism among black and white subjects with resistant hypertension. *Hypertension* 2002; 40: 892-6.
11. Gallay BJ, Ahmad S, Xu L, Toivola B, Davidson RC. Screening for primary aldosteronism without discontinuing hypertensive medications: plasma aldosterone-renin ratio. *Am J Kidney Dis* 2001; 37: 669-705.
12. Eide IK, Torjesen PA, Drolsum A, Babovic A, Lilledahl NP. Low-renin status in therapy-resistant hypertension: a clue to efficient treatment. *J Hypertens* 2004; 22: 2217-26.
13. Strauch B, Zelinka T, Hampf M, Bernhardt R, Widimsky J Jr. Prevalence of primary hyperaldosteronism in moderate to severe hypertension in the Central Europe region. *J Hum Hypertens* 2003; 17: 349-52.
14. Rocha R, Rudolph AE, Frierdich GE, *et al.* Aldosterone induces a vascular inflammatory phenotype in the rat heart. *Am J Physiol Heart Circ Physiol* 2002; 283: H1802-10.
15. Brilla CG, Weber KT. Mineralocorticoid excess, dietary sodium, and myocardial fibrosis. *J Lab Clin Med* 1992; 120: 893-901.
16. Sato A, Saruta T. Aldosterone-induced organ damage: plasma aldosterone level and inappropriate salt status. *Hypertens Res* 2004; 27: 303-10.
17. Rossi GP, Sacchetto A, Visentin P, *et al.* Changes in left ventricular anatomy and function in hypertension and primary aldosteronism. *Hypertension* 1996; 27: 1039-45.
18. Fox CS, Larson MG, Hwang S-J, *et al.* Cross-sectional relations of serum aldosterone and urine sodium excretion to urinary albumin excretion in a community-based sample. *Kidney Int* 2006; 69: 2064-9.
19. Nishizaka MK, Zaman MA, Green SA, Renfroe KY, Calhoun DA. Impaired endothelium-dependent flow-mediated vasodilation in hypertensive subjects with hyperaldosteronism. *Circulation* 2004; 109: 2857-61.
20. Milliez P, Girerd X, Plouin PF, Blacher J, Safar ME, Mourad JJ. Evidence for an increased rate of cardiovascular events in patients with primary aldosteronism. *J Am Coll Cardiol* 2005; 45: 1243-8.
21. Conn JW. The evolution of primary aldosteronism. *Harvey Lect* 1968; 62: 257-91.
22. Nishizaka MK, Zaman MA, Calhoun DA. Efficacy of low-dose spironolactone in subjects with resistant hypertension. *Am J Hypertens* 2003; 16: 925-30.
23. Pimenta E, Calhoun DA. Primary aldosteronism: diagnosis and treatment. *J Clin Hypertens* 2006; 8: 887-93.
24. Funder JW, Carey RM, Fardella C, *et al.* Case detection, diagnosis, and treatment of patients with primary aldosteronism: an endocrine society clinical practice guideline. *J Clin Endocrinol Metab* 2008; 93: 3266-81.
25. Mattsson C, Young Jr WF. Primary aldosteronism: diagnostic and treatment strategies. *Nat Clin Pract Nephrol* 2006; 2: 198-208.
26. Nwariaku FE, Miller BS, Auchus R, *et al.* Primary hyperaldosteronism: effect of adrenal vein sampling on surgical outcome. *Arch Surg* 2006; 141: 497-503.
27. Young Jr WF, Klee GG. Primary aldosteronism. Diagnostic evaluation. *Endocrinol Metab Clin North Am* 1988; 17: 367-95.
28. Young WF, Stanson AW, Thompson GB, Grant CS, Farley DR, van Heerden JA. Role for adrenal venous sampling in primary aldosteronism. *Surgery* 2004; 136: 1227-35.
29. Stowasser M, Gordon RD. Familial hyperaldosteronism. *J Steroid Biochem Mol Biol* 2001; 78: 215-29.
30. Sawka AM, Young WF, Thompson GB, *et al.* Primary aldosteronism: factors associated with normalization of blood pressure after surgery. *Ann Intern Med* 2001; 135: 258-61.
31. Goessens BM, Visseren FL, Olijhoek JK, Eikelboom BC, van der Graaf Y. Multidisciplinary vascular screening program modestly improves treatment of vascular risk factors. *Cardiovasc Drugs Ther* 2005; 19: 429-35.
32. Pimenta E, Gaddam KK, Husain S, Aban I, Oparil S, Calhoun DA. High dietary salt ingestion increases blood pressure secondary to increases in intravascular volume and vascular resistance in patients with resistance hypertension. *Hypertension* 2008; 52: e97 (abstract).
33. Garg JP, Elliott WJ, Folker A, Izhar M, Black HR, RUSH University Hypertension Service. Resistant hypertension revisited: a comparison of two university-based cohorts. *Am J Hypertens* 2005; 18: 619-26.
34. Ventura HO, Taler SJ, Strobeck JE. Hypertension as a hemodynamic disease: the role of impedance cardiography in diagnostic, prognostic, and therapeutic decision making. *Am J Hypertens* 2005; 18: 26S-43.
35. Ouzan J, Perault C, Lincoff AM, Carré E, Mertes M. The role of spironolactone in the treatment of patients with refractory hypertension. *Am J Hypertens* 2002; 15: 333-9.
36. Mahmud A, Mahgoub M, Hall M, Feely J. Does aldosterone-to-renin ratio predict the anti-hypertensive effect of the aldosterone antagonist spironolactone? *Am J Hypertens* 2005; 18: 1631-5.
37. Lane DA, Shah S, Beevers DG. Low-dose spironolactone in the management of resistant hypertension: a surveillance study. *J Hypertens* 2007; 25: 891-94.

38. Chapman N, Dobson J, Wilson S, *et al.* Effect of spironolactone on blood pressure in subjects with resistant hypertension. *Hypertension* 2007; 49: 839-45.
39. Pimenta E, Calhoun DA. Resistant hypertension and aldosteronism. *Curr Hyp Rep* 2007; 9: 353-9.
40. Flack JM, Oparil S, Pratt JH, *et al.* Efficacy and tolerability of eplerenone and losartan in hypertensive black and white patients. *J Am Coll Cardiol* 2003; 41: 1148-55.
41. Calhoun DA, White WB. Effectiveness of the selective aldosterone blocker, eplerenone, in patients with resistant hypertension. *J Am Soc Hypertens* 2008; 2: 462-8.
42. Saha C, Eckert GJ, Ambrosius WT, *et al.* Improvement in blood pressure with inhibition of the epitelial sodium channel in blacks with hypertension. *Hypertension* 2005; 46: 481-7.
43. Kaplan NM. Is there an unrecognized epidemic of primary aldosteronism? *Con Hypertension* 2007; 50: 454-8.
44. Catena C, Colussi G, Lapenna R, *et al.* Long-term cardiac effects of adrenalectomy or mineralocorticoid antagonists in patients with primary aldosteronism. *Hypertension* 2007; 50: 911-8.
45. Catena C, Colussi G, Nadalini E, *et al.* Cardiovascular outcomes in patients with primary aldosteronism after treatment. *Arch Intern Med* 2008; 168: 80-5.

Chapter 7

Should pre-hypertension be treated?

Joseph L. Izzo, Jr. MD
Professor of Medicine and Pharmacology
State University of New York at Buffalo
New York, USA

Introduction

The term 'pre-hypertension' arose in 2003 from the Seventh Report of the Joint National Committee on the Prevention, Detection, Evaluation, and Treatment of High Blood Pressure (JNC 7) [1] to describe individuals whose blood pressures (BP) fall within the range of 120-139/80-89mmHg. Although not formally studied and still debated today, it appears the concept has had a significant impact on medical practice. In the United States, pre-hypertension replaces older terms such as 'borderline hypertension' and 'high normal blood pressure', although variants of these categories persist in the literature and in other countries.

Rationale for the term pre-hypertension

The critical scientific underpinning of the concept of pre-hypertension is the linear increase in systolic blood pressure (SBP) that occurs with advancing age in industrialized societies (about 0.5mmHg per year) [2]. From this trend, it can be appreciated that there is a 'residual risk' of developing hypertension at any age; the chance that a normotensive middle-aged individual will eventually be classified as having hypertension (BP >140/90mmHg) within 20 years exceeds 90% [3]. In this context, pre-hypertension is a scientifically accurate and clinically useful descriptive term that underscores the age-related progression of hypertension.

The primary intention of introducing the term pre-hypertension was to alert the large number of individuals with blood pressures above 'normal' but below the traditional threshold of hypertension (about 1/4 of the United States population) that they were at increased risk for cardiovascular, cerebrovascular, and renal diseases [1]. Epidemiological support for this statement includes a report from the Framingham Heart Study that individuals with 'high normal' blood pressures (130-139/85-89mmHg) had 12-year rates of ischemic heart disease that were roughly double those of optimal blood pressure [4]. Subsequently, a worldwide meta-analysis in almost a million people corroborated that the log-linear relationship between elevated blood pressure and cardiovascular disease mortality extended down to levels at least as low as 115/75mmHg [5]. Based on these findings, the JNC 7 Executive Committee felt strongly that the public health benefits of alerting the public to the dangers of 'borderline' blood pressure elevations outweighed any negative risks of labeling these individuals as having an abnormal medical condition.

It was clear from the beginning that there would be substantial scientific and practical concerns attached to any attempt to define a highly heterogeneous population by a blood pressure range alone. Most obvious is that the concept of 'pre'-hypertension immediately breaks down when it is (mis)applied to individuals with blood pressures in the range of 120-139/80-89mm Hg who are receiving treatment or those 'post-hypertensives' with complications of hypertension, particularly heart failure. Another problematic issue that limits the value of blood pressure categorization is the amount of blood pressure variability within individuals. The 20mmHg 'slices' that currently define the JNC 7 stages of hypertension are actually quite narrow given the observed patterns of variation in many patients. Normal circadian rhythms can be sufficiently large that a given patient may fall within two or more categories (e.g. pre-hypertension and Stage 1 hypertension) within the same visit. In addition, there can be dramatic effects of meals, timing of medications, exercise conditioning, emotional state, and intercurrent diseases that confound accurate classification. Since the release of JNC 7, the loudest protests have arisen from individuals who have felt that the label 'pre-hypertension' is too alarmist in nature and inappropriately labels a large healthy population with a non-disease. It is true that half the U.S. population has pre-hypertension or hypertension, so the potential impact is great. It should also be noted that these and other implications were debated at length by the JNC 7 Executive Committee, which actually field-tested the term pre-hypertension; all groups tested, including lay persons and health professionals, favored pre-hypertension over 'high normal blood pressure' or 'borderline hypertension'.

Pathophysiology of pre-hypertension

Ultimately, if the blood pressure is elevated, there must be excessive flow or impedance; in hypertension, both flow and impedance tend to be inappropriately high, irrespective of the etiology of hypertension. Much of the literature has implied erroneously that increased vascular resistance is the principal hemodynamic abnormality in essential hypertension but even casual inspection of available data demonstrates clearly that there is almost complete overlap between normal and hypertensive individuals with respect to resting cardiac output and systemic vascular resistance [6-7]. It also appears that with aging, there is a transition from high flow ('hyperkinetic hypertension') to high resistance [8-9]. The problem of disproportionately high cardiac output is particularly apparent in younger, obese, pre-hypertensive, pre-diabetic individuals said to have the 'metabolic syndrome' [7].

If both flow and resistance are inappropriately high in hypertension, what underlying physioregulatory mechanisms are at the root of the problem? As time passes, a variety of interactions can be expected to occur and an integrated model for the progression of hypertension is presented in Figure 1. The most comprehensive explanation is that hypertension is at least partially the result of an underlying tendency toward overactivity of the sympathetic nervous and renin-angiotensin systems, coupled with exaggerated renal salt and water retention. Pre-hypertension is closely associated with abdominal (truncal, visceral) obesity [10], the major cause of insulin resistance and hyperlipidemia. The hyperdynamic circulation in obese individuals has also been associated with insulin

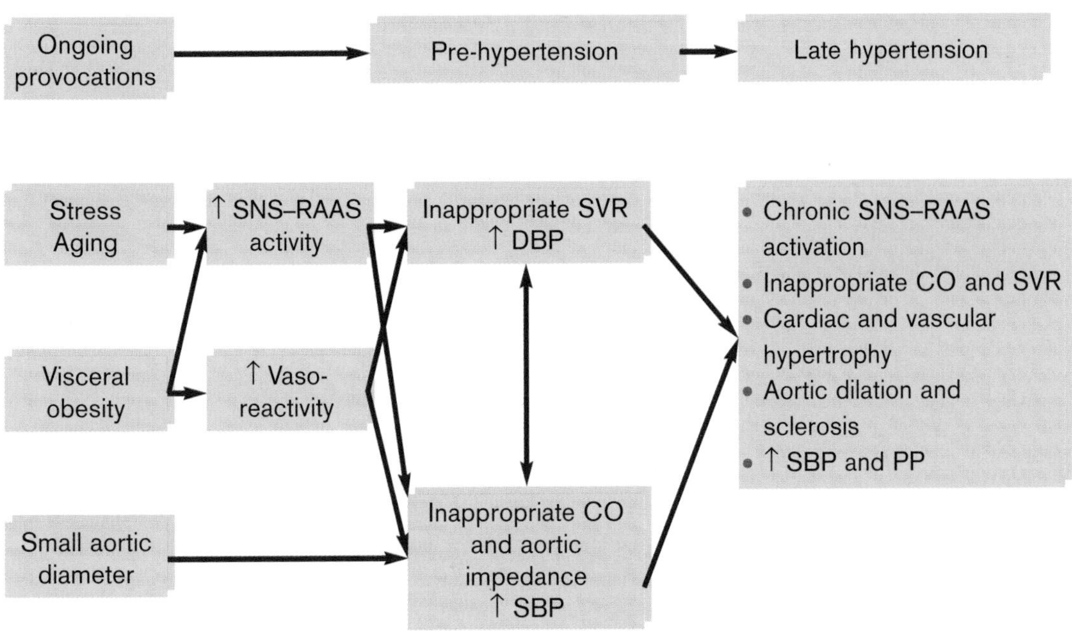

Figure 1. Integrated pathophysiology of essential hypertension. Pre-hypertension is characterized by excessive activation of a number of physiologic systems (see text). *Adapted from Izzo JL Jnr. Curr Hypertens Rep 2007; 9: 264-6.*

resistance in the offspring [11]. Other closely related phenomena, including 'endothelial dysfunction', may be present but exaggerated vasoreactivity is not required for the development of sustained hypertension and in fact there is virtually no correlation between degree of BP reactivity and baseline BP [7].

The concept of excessive neurohumoral activation in essential hypertension has been accepted for decades but remains hard to prove in large clinical populations. The largest cross-sectional physiologic profiles come from the Tecumseh Study [10] and the Strong Heart study [12]. There is also indirect evidence from the TRial Of Prevention of HYpertension (TROPHY), in which obese pre-hypertensive individuals were randomized to receive either placebo or candesartan therapy for 2 years, followed in each case by placebo for an additional 2 years [13]. Candesartan caused an immediate decrease in blood pressure (about 10/4mmHg compared to pretreatment values) that persisted for the full 2 years of ARB therapy. Upon cessation of the angiotensin blocker, however, blood pressures in those treated with ARB immediately returned to their prior baseline values and remained there for the duration of the subsequent 2-year placebo follow-up. This pattern indicates strongly that inappropriate activation of the renin-angiotensin system occurs in pre-hypertension. Because the renin-angiotensin and sympathetic nervous systems are intimately inter-related in a low-grade positive feedback process, it can be inferred directly that there is excess neurohumoral activation in pre-hypertension. Viewed from the perspective of the usual degree of age-related blood pressure increase, TROPHY also demonstrates that the rate of rise of blood pressure with age can be slowed by neurohumoral blockade and that pre-hypertension is predominantly a functional, not structural disorder. One important caveat: in younger, predominantly obese people, diastolic prehypertension is usually due to inappropriately high systemic vascular resistance, whereas systolic prehypertension in older people is usually due to increased arterial stiffness or narrow aortic diameters [14].

Treatment of pre-hypertension

According to JNC 7, anyone with BP values >120/80mmHg should sustain an optimal lifestyle by practicing weight control, maintaining adequate physical activity, following a modified Mediterranean diet, restricting dietary salt, and avoiding tobacco or excessive alcohol consumption. There is relatively little hard outcome evidence to support the treatment of prehypertension with lifestyle or pharmacologic therapies, yet both approaches have been shown to lower blood pressure in this population and may be beneficial for delaying the onset of Stage 1 hypertension (BP >140/90mmHg). A summary with evidence levels is presented in Table 1.

Weight loss

The correlation of hypertension and abdominal obesity, with increased waist circumference and increased intra-abdominal fat stores, is extremely strong. A meta-analysis of 25 studies in which the mean SBP ranged from 111 to 171mmHg revealed that a weight loss of 5.1kg was associated with a mean reduction in blood pressure of 4.4/3.6mmHg (about 1mmHg SBP for each kg of weight loss) [15]. There is a trend for greater antihypertensive effect in those with the greatest degree of weight loss, higher blood pressure prior to weight loss, and in those taking concomitant antihypertensive drugs [16]. The Trial Of Hypertension Prevention (TOHP) found that sustained weight loss reduced the onset of hypertension by about 20%[16-17]. This finding can best be interpreted as a slower increase in SBP with age but weight loss did not fully abolish the age-related increase in SBP in TOHP participants. In general, the effects of weight loss are not limited by age, race or gender. From a practical point of view, it is reasonable to propose that weight loss is the cornerstone of treatment for obese pre-hypertensive individuals.

Physical activity

Most data relating to exercise and blood pressure have been small cross-sectional studies or trials in which higher levels of physical activity are typically associated with lower blood pressure levels [18]. In a meta-analysis of 72 trials, 105 study groups, and 3936 participants, physical training reduced daytime ambulatory blood pressure by 3.3/3.5mm Hg ($p<0.01$), with the greatest reductions observed in hypertensives (6.9/4.9mmHg) [19]. The thorniest issue, whether the potential antihypertensive effects of chronic exercise are independent of weight reduction, has never been answered unequivocally; when weight loss does not occur, the effects of exercise on blood pressure are often quite small [20]. Nevertheless, JNC 7 recommended regular physical activity as part of an overall non-pharmacologic lifestyle-improvement activity [1]. The American College of Sports Medicine has gone further, stating unequivocally that physical exercise lowers blood pressure in normotensive and hypertensive individuals and it has recommended at least 30 minutes daily of moderate physical activity [21]. The mechanisms by which physical activity may lower blood pressure include reduced systemic vascular resistance, sympathetic nervous activity, and plasma renin activity [19].

Dietary composition

The Dietary Approaches to Stop Hypertension (DASH) studies have provided quantitative information about modifications in diet and dietary salt content and their effects on blood pressure. Entry criteria in DASH were SBP <160 and DBP 80-95mmHg but because the initial mean blood pressure for the participants was about 131/84mmHg, the study was essentially conducted in pre-hypertensives to identify whether the DASH diet (an isocaloric diet designed to maintain current weight that was rich in fruits, vegetables, whole grains, and low-fat meats) could lower blood pressure when compared to a standard American diet (rich in saturated fats and refined carbohydrates and low in fiber). In this parallel-arm, short-term (8 weeks) trial, the experimental group received all foods in the form of 'box lunches'. The main result was that the DASH diet lowered clinic blood pressure by about 11/6mmHg [22] and 24-hour mean ambulatory blood pressure by 3.2/1.9mmHg compared to controls [23]. Recurring criticisms about the applicability of DASH are that it was very short and that all foods were provided by the investigators, so the participants' role in dietary modification was somewhat passive. The specific mechanisms by which diet reduces blood pressure are not fully known, but weight reduction decreases sympathetic nervous [24] and therefore renin-angiotensin activity. Weight loss also ameliorates insulin resistance and hyperlipidemia and therefore remains attractive as a component of lifestyle modification.

Dietary salt intake

The role of salt restriction in blood pressure-lowering is a complex topic that requires knowledge of the degree of 'salt-sensitivity' in the individual. Nevertheless, the DASH-salt studies have given important insight into the question: how much does sodium restriction lower blood pressure? Results indicate that DASH participants on the low-sodium diet (about 2.3g sodium daily) had BP values about 7/4mmHg lower than those on the DASH diet without salt restriction [25]. Secondary analyses revealed that the effects of the DASH diet were most pronounced in those with higher initial BP levels or isolated systolic hypertension [26], but the diet was also effective in women and African Americans and exerted a positive effect on 24-hour ambulatory BP values as well [23].

Table 1. Summary of therapeutic recommendations.

Modality	Recommendation	Evidence grade
Weight control	Achievement and maintenance of ideal body weight	III/B
Physical activity	Regular physical activity as part of an overall weight maintenance program to maintain ideal body weight	III/B
Dietary composition	Adherence to a DASH-style (reduced-fat, modified Mediterranean) diet	Ib/A
Dietary sodium intake	Adherence to moderate salt restriction (less than 2.3g of sodium daily)	III/B
Alcohol and tobacco	Moderation in alcohol use and avoidance of tobacco products (benefits not directly related to BP)	IV/C
Drug therapy	ARB therapy may be considered to lower BP in all men and in women without child-bearing potential if there is elevated risk for cardiovascular disease (e.g. microalbuminuria, insulin resistance, dyslipidemia, or early renal impairment)	IV/C

Other lifestyle measures

The impact of cigarette smoking, alcohol consumption, dietary divalent cation content, omega-3 fatty acid supplementation, and other lifestyle or nutritional measures on blood pressure appear to be less striking [1]. Cigarettes raise blood pressure acutely and are likely to contribute to increased 24-hour blood pressures but do not always affect clinic or overnight blood pressure. Alcohol is a vasodilator that is usually cardioprotective but when taken chronically in excess, may contribute to weight gain and blood pressure elevation. JNC 7 recommended avoidance of tobacco use and moderation in alcohol intake.

Drug therapy: angiotensin receptor blockade

The randomized, placebo-controlled TROPHY study is instructive not only for its insights into pathophysiology but also into the potential value of drug therapy in pre-hypertension [13]. The prevalence of hypertension (BP exceeding 140/90mmHg) after 2 years of active therapy with 16mg candesartan daily and again after 2 additional years of placebo was about 66% less at 2 years and 16% less at 4 years. The Randomized Olmesartan And Diabetes MicroAlbuminuria Prevention (ROADMAP) study [27] recently found that early ARB therapy in pre-hypertensive diabetics (mean pre-treatment BP 136/81mmHg) reduces the occurrence of microalbuminuria, a biomarker for diabetic nephropathy and vascular disease (ASN Abstracts). There is no outcome study in pre-hypertension but since hypertension is an accepted surrogate for CVD morbidity and mortality, it is likely that CVD benefits are possible with early ARB therapy. Proof of this statement will not be immediately forthcoming, however, because the overall CVD event rate is relatively low in pre-hypertension, necessitating very long, large, and expensive clinical trials.

Ultimately, the value of drug therapy must be established. It is not sufficient to study only up-front costs but establishing true long-term value is extremely difficult. It is not fully possible to extrapolate TROPHY results to the entire population because of the small numbers of blacks included and the unclear value of ARB therapy in African Americans or other important subgroups such as those older individuals with systolic pre-hypertension due to increased arterial stiffness. In these subgroups, diuretics or other agents may be preferable as first-line therapy. Another major concern is that women of child-bearing potential should not take ACE inhibitors or ARBs due to potential fetal abnormalities. Given the further enhancement of risk by common coexisting conditions, it is not unreasonable to propose that pre-hypertensive individuals (men or women without child-bearing potential) who also have the metabolic syndrome (any three or more of: SBP >130mmHg, waist circumference >40" for men or 30" for women, HDL-cholesterol <40 for men or <50mg/dL for women, triglycerides >150mg/dL, or fasting glucose >100mg/dL) or those with microalbuminuria are potential candidates for ARB therapy, not only because of the theoretical benefits and proven efficacy of these agents in pre-hypertension and microalbuminuria, but because of their exceptionally benign adverse effect profile, at least in men. With the advent of generic ARBs, a much stronger case can be made for ARB-based disease prevention.

Conclusions

Systolic blood pressure increases steadily with age and weight gain in industrialized societies. In middle age, an individual's blood pressure tends to pass through an intermediate stage of systolic or diastolic 'pre-hypertension' characterized by truncal obesity and excessive neurohumoral stimulation. Non-pharmacologic therapy (diet, exercise, sodium restriction, reduced dietary fat and carbohydrate content, moderation of alcohol intake, avoidance of tobacco) is generally recommended for pre-hypertension despite relatively thin evidence for clinical effectiveness. Major challenges to the treatment of pre-hypertension include absence of clinical symptoms, the extremely long latent period (decades) before target organ disease becomes clinically apparent, psychological barriers to lifestyle modification, and practical issues such as time constraints and the relatively high cost of healthier diets. In high-risk pre-hypertensives such as those with metabolic syndrome, angiotensin receptor blocker therapy could be beneficial, although the number-needed-to-treat is probably too high to justify universal use.

Key points	Evidence level
◆ About a quarter of the US population has pre-hypertension (BP 120-139/80-89 mmHg).	
◆ The concept of pre-hypertension is based on the linear increase in SBP that occurs with advancing age in industrialized societies (about 0.5mmHg per year) and the 'residual risk' of developing hypertension at any age.	
◆ The underlying pathophysiology of pre-hypertension is usually related to obesity and inappropriately high sympathetic nervous activity, renin-angiotensin activity, salt-sensitivity, cardiac output, and systemic vascular resistance.	
◆ Achievement and maintenance of ideal body weight is recommended for all pre-hypertensives.	III/B
◆ Regular physical activity should be included as part of an overall weight maintenance program to maintain ideal body weight.	III/B
◆ Adherence to a DASH-style (reduced-fat, modified Mediterranean) diet with reduced sodium content is appropriate for all pre-hypertensives.	Ib/A
◆ Adherence to moderate salt restriction (less than 2.3g of sodium daily) is a useful adjunct for blood pressure control.	III/B
◆ Moderation in alcohol use and avoidance of tobacco products (based on benefits not directly related to blood pressure) should be advocated.	IV/C
◆ ARB therapy may be considered to lower blood pressure in all men and in women without child-bearing potential if there is sufficiently elevated risk for cardiovascular disease, including concomitant micro-albuminuria, insulin resistance, dyslipidemia, or early renal impairment.	IV/C

References

1. Chobanian AV, Bakris GL, Black HR, *et al.* The Seventh Report of the Joint National Committee on Prevention, Detection, Evaluation, and Treatment of High Blood Pressure: the JNC 7 report. *JAMA* 2003; 289: 2560-72.
2. Burt VL, Whelton P, Roccella EJ, *et al.* Prevalence of hypertension in the US adult population: Results from the Third National Health and Nutrition Examination Survey, 1988-1991. *Hypertension* 1995; 25: 305-13.
3. Vasan RS, Beiser A, Seshadri S, *et al.* Residual lifetime risk for developing hypertension in middle-aged women and men: The Framingham Heart Study. *JAMA* 2002; 287: 1003-10.
4. Lloyd-Jones DM, Evans JC, Larson MG, O'Donnell CJ, Wilson PW, Levy D. Cross-classification of JNC VI blood pressure stages and risk groups in the Framingham Heart Study. *Arch Int Med* 1999; 159: 2206-12.
5. Lewington S, Clarke R, Qizilbash N, Peto R, Collins R. Age-specific relevance of usual blood pressure to vascular mortality: a meta-analysis of individual data for one million adults in 61 prospective studies. *Lancet* 2002; 360: 1903-13.
6. Julius S, Conway J. Hemodynamic studies in patients with borderline blood pressure elevation. *Circulation* 1968; 38: 282-8.
7. Julius S, Mejia A, Jones K, *et al.* 'White coat' versus 'sustained' borderline hypertensions in Tecumseh Michigan. *Hypertension* 1990; 16: 617-23.
8. Julius S. Transition from high cardiac output to elevated vascular resistance in hypertension. *Am Heart J* 1988; 116(2 part 2): 600-6.
9. Lund-Johansen P. Twenty-year follow-up of hemodynamics in essential hypertension during rest and exercise. *Hypertension* 1991; 18.
10. Julius S, Krause L, Schork NJ, *et al.* Hyperkinetic borderline hypertension in Tecumseh, Michigan. *J Hypertension* 1991; 9: 77-84.
11. Palatini P, Vriz O, Nesbitt S, *et al.* Parental hyperdynamic circulation predicts insulin resistance in offspring: The Tecumseh offspring study. *Hypertension* 1999; 33: 769-74.
12. Drukteinis JS, Roman MJ, Fabsitz RR, *et al.* Cardiac and systemic hemodynamic characteristics of hypertension and prehypertension in adolescents and young adults: the Strong Heart Study. *Circulation* 2007; 115: 221-7.
13. Julius S, Nesbitt SD, Egan BM, *et al.* Feasibility of treating prehypertension with an angiotensin-receptor blocker. *New Engl J Med* 2006; 354: 1685-97.
14. Mitchell GF, Lacourciere Y, Ouellet JP, *et al.* Determinants of elevated pulse pressure in middle-aged and older subjects with uncomplicated systolic hypertension: the role of proximal aortic diameter and the aortic pressure-flow relationship. *Circulation* 2003; 108: 1592-8.
15. Neter JE, Stam BE, Kok FJ, Grobbee DE, Geleijnse JM. Influence of weight reduction on blood pressure: a meta-analysis of randomized controlled trials. *Hypertension* 2003; 42: 878-84.
16. Stevens VJ, Obarzanek E, Cook NR, *et al.* Long-term weight loss and changes in blood pressure: results of the Trials of Hypertension Prevention, phase II. *Ann Int Med* 2001; 134: 1-11.
17. Stevens VJ, Corrigan SA, Obarzanek E, *et al.* Weight loss intervention in phase 1 of the Trials of Hypertension Prevention. The TOHP Collaborative Research Group. *Arch Int Med* 1993; 153: 849-58.
18. Gidding SS, Barton BA, Dorgan JA, *et al.* Higher self-reported physical activity is associated with lower systolic blood pressure: the Dietary Intervention Study in Childhood (DISC). *Pediatrics* 2006; 118: 2388-93.
19. Cornelissen VA, Fagard RH. Effects of endurance training on blood pressure, blood pressure-regulating mechanisms, and cardiovascular risk factors. *Hypertension* 2005; 46: 667-75.
20. Stewart KJ, Bacher AC, Turner KL, *et al.* Effect of exercise on blood pressure in older persons: a randomized controlled trial. *Arch Int Med* 2005; 165: 756-62.
21. Pescatello LS, Franklin BA, Fagard R, *et al.* American College of Sports Medicine position stand. Exercise and hypertension. *Medicine & Science in Sports & Exercise* 2004; 36: 533-53.
22. Appel LJ, Moore TJ, Obarzanek E, *et al.* A clinical trial of the effects of dietary patterns on blood pressure. DASH Collaborative Research Group. *New Engl J Med* 1997; 336: 1117-24.
23. Moore TJ, Vollmer WM, Appel LJ, *et al.* Effect of dietary patterns on ambulatory blood pressure: results from the Dietary Approaches to Stop Hypertension (DASH) Trial. DASH Collaborative Research Group. *Hypertension* 1999; 34: 472-7.

24. Straznicky NE, Lambert EA, Lambert GW, Masuo K, Esler MD, Nestel PJ. Effects of dietary weight loss on sympathetic activity and cardiac risk factors associated with the metabolic syndrome. *J Clin Endocrinol Metab* 2005; 90: 5998-6005.
25. Sacks FM, Svetkey LP, Vollmer WM, *et al.* Effects on blood pressure of reduced dietary sodium and the Dietary Approaches to Stop Hypertension (DASH) diet. DASH-Sodium Collaborative Research Group. *New Engl J Med* 2001; 344: 3-10.
26. Moore TJ, Conlin PR, Ard J, Svetkey LP. DASH (Dietary Approaches to Stop Hypertension) diet is effective treatment for stage 1 isolated systolic hypertension. *Hypertension* 2001; 38: 155-8.
27. Haller H, Viberti GC, Mimran A, Remuzzi G, Rabelink AJ, Ritz E, Rump LC, Ruilope LM, Katayama S, Ito S, Izzo JL Jr, Januszewicz A. Preventing microalbuminuria in patients with diabetes: rationale and design of the Randomized Olmesartan And Diabetes MicroAlbuminuria Prevention (ROADMAP) study. *J Hypertension* 2006; 24: 403.

Chapter 8

What are optimal treatment goals for older patients with isolated systolic hypertension?

Raymond R. Townsend MD
Director of the Hypertension Program
Department of Medicine
University of Pennsylvania
Philadelphia, USA

Introduction

This chapter's intriguing title presents three immediate semantic difficulties. These are, simply, what is 'optimal', what is 'older' and what is 'hypertension'. So that the reader starts from a similar premise as the author, let us begin by defining these terms and acknowledging their limitations when appropriate. The a priori notion in this chapter is that the word 'goal' refers to benefit (defined as protection from target organ damage or better survival) since the goal of any treatment is a benefit that exceeds any risk(s) associated with the treatment. The assignment then is to define two aspects of the 'goal', namely treatment threshold and treatment goal blood pressure. The first task is to determine that level of systolic blood pressure where treating it has been shown to produce a benefit (threshold). The second task is determining to what level the systolic blood pressure was reduced to in order to accomplish a benefit (target).

Optimal is easy to define. With unexpected brevity, the Oxford English Dictionary portrays it as: "Best, most favourable, esp. under a particular set of circumstances" [1]. Older is more difficult. Moving from a superlative like 'optimal', to a comparative like 'older' represents a conundrum as it has to be defined with respect to a range or a reference group. Since this chapter (as is thematic in this book) seeks an evidence-based approach it would be appropriate to define 'older' or 'elderly' based on evidence. In this regard evidence is scant, and often arbitrary. Older age will, therefore, be defined as >60 years of age since one of the first elderly trials used that as criteria [2], and most of the trials we will consider also used that criteria. The special scenario of an age >80 years carries the additional modifier of 'very' so that it is said to characterize the 'very elderly'. We will assume that 'elderly' and 'older age' are interchangeable terms in a discussion focused on blood pressure.

Hypertension is the most difficult of the three terms and is the least well defined, despite the ability to measure blood pressure for more than 100 years. A logical definition of hypertension would be that level of blood pressure where the risks in reducing it with drug therapy outweigh the risks of leaving it untreated [3] **(IV/C)**. Such a definition is vague and without definitive trial evidence to support it. Thus, we will use the JNC 7 definition of 'hypertension' as >140mm Hg systolic or >90mm Hg diastolic. Since this chapter is focused on the subgroup of isolated systolic hypertension, using JNC 7 terminology then would refer to people with an untreated systolic blood pressure of >140mm Hg and a diastolic blood pressure of <90mm Hg [4] **(IV/B)**. A caveat is in order, though, because if you skip ahead to Table 2 you will notice that I have violated this definition and included trials enrolling subjects up to a diastolic of 95mm Hg. This arose from a difference in the definition of diastolic 'hypertension' which for years was set at 95mm Hg in Europe [5], though it is now set at 90mm Hg in the 2007 guidelines [6].

So we begin this chapter with a reformulation of the titular question as follows: "What are the best or most favourable goals of treating people who are at least 55 years of age if not older whose systolic blood pressure is more than 139mm Hg and whose diastolic blood pressure is less than 90mm Hg?". An examination of evidence supporting the role of isolated systolic hypertension in target organ damage will be covered next. The term 'target organ damage' indicates stroke or transient ischemic attack, heart failure, heart attack or a reperfusion intervention, chronic kidney disease and peripheral arterial disease as defined in JNC 7 [4]. After that a discussion of mechanisms contributing to isolated systolic hypertension will be undertaken followed at the end by a review of evidence that supports treating it.

Epidemiology and impact of isolated systolic hypertension

Isolated systolic hypertension is the most common form of blood pressure encountered in people aged 60 or higher [7] **(III/B)**. As shown in Framingham data, the untreated systolic pressure rises continuously across the age range with every decade having a higher mean systolic pressure than the previous one, and a lower mean systolic pressure than the next one as shown in Figure 1 [7]. Moreover, systolic blood pressure elevations (>140mm Hg) remain relatively common, even among drug-treated hypertensives [8]. The latest data from the Health and Nutrition Examination Survey (NHANES) show a substantial increase in the prevalence of hypertension when spanning the years of 1988 to 2004 [9] **(III/B)**. The populations most likely to have elevations in systolic blood pressure are women, particularly when over 70 years of age, non-Hispanic blacks and Mexican Americans, and those with diabetes and chronic kidney disease [9]. The latter group, i.e. those with CKD, is worthy of emphasis since the prevalence rate of people with a systolic BP of >150mm Hg (19.8% of 88,559 people) in the Kidney Early Evaluation Program (KEEP) is more than twice that of NHANES (8.7% of 20,095) [10]. Our experience with NHANES data indicates that isolated systolic hypertension is less commonly found as BMI increases, particularly in men [11] **(III/B)**.

The first report of an impact of increased systolic pressure (150mm Hg) when diastolic pressure was 90mm Hg or less was presented in the 1959 Build and Blood Pressure study,

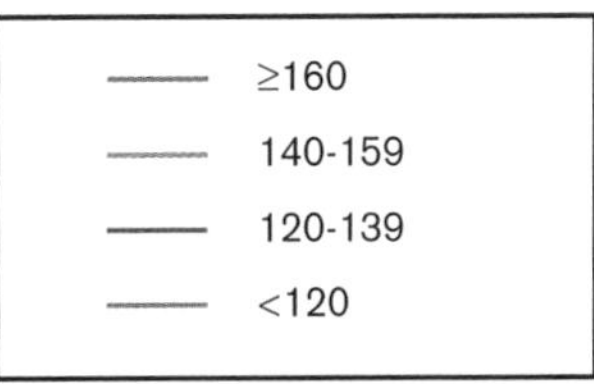

n=2036

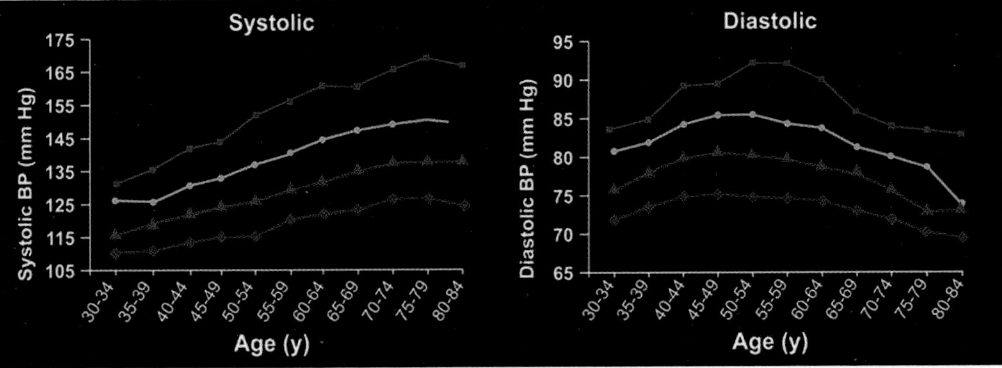

Figure 1. Framingham Heart Study data showing the continual increase in systolic blood pressure across decades of life, but peaking of diastolic blood pressure in the 6th decade of life with decline thereafter. *Adapted from Franklin SS, et al* [7].

an actuarial database using data gathered by life insurance companies [12] **(IIb/B)**. They noted that in men less than 60 years of age with this profile they have about double the mortality. In the report prepared by the Canada Life Insurance Medical Officer's Association, using this data they noted that "...an elevation of systolic pressure of 15mm Hg above average systolic or 10mm Hg above average diastolic was associated with an extra mortality of at least 25%" [13] **(IV/B)**.

The coronary heart disease consequences of an increase in systolic blood pressure were noted in the Framingham study in 1971 [14] **(III/B)**. In this report of 5127 men and women, the investigators stated that "The current practice of assessing the importance of blood pressure at all ages largely on the basis of diastolic pressure and the commonly held view concerning the innocuous nature of an elevated level of systolic pressure in the elderly requires reevaluation". Nonetheless it would be another 20 years before the Systolic Hypertension in the Elderly trial was published [15] **(Ib/A)**. The impact of isolated systolic hypertension is principally noted in higher stroke and heart failure rates [16-18] **(Ia/A)**. In the review of NHANES 2003-2004 data by Wong *et al*, the extraordinary burden of systolic pressure was evident in those who already manifest target organ damage wherein the prevalence of hypertension (and it was predominantly systolic blood pressure driving these results) was 2-3 times more common than in those without target organ damage [19] **(III/B)**. In the Hypertension Detection and Follow-up Program, each one mm Hg elevation in systolic blood pressure above 160mm Hg had an associated 1% increase in mortality during an 8-year time period [20] **(Ib/A)**.

Mechanisms relating systolic pressure to target organ damage

The systolic blood pressure as typically measured in the brachial artery is the result of several processes acting in concert. The increase in systolic pressure occurs by way of a change in the mechanical properties of large vessels. The net effect is a decrease in arterial compliance which both increases the systolic pressure necessary to accommodate the cardiac stroke volume, and also produces a decrease in diastolic blood pressure [21]. Stiffer arteries conduct the pulse wave at a higher velocity, and this increase in pulse wave velocity accelerates the return of the reflected pressure wave to the heart where the arrival in late systole instead of early diastole places an added systolic pressure load on the left ventricle [22]. Aging is a major determinant of stiffening of blood vessels because it promotes changes in collagen, and other aspects of the extracellular vessel wall matrix that enhance cross-linking of collagen causing an alteration in the anatomy and functional properties of the vasculature that reduces compliance [23]. Arterial wall elastin also decreases with age, resulting in thin elastic laminae and fragmented, poorly demarcated media. In animal models the change in the ratio of elastin to collagen in vessel wall favors more stiffness as collagen accumulates and elastin is depleted or damaged [24]. Other processes important in systolic hypertension are salt intake, activation of the sympathetic nervous system and processes which promote vascular calcification such as inflammatory states, diabetes and chronic kidney disease [25, 26] **(III/B)**.

It is important to note that isolated systolic hypertension does have a differential diagnosis associated with it. Although most cases are due to the effects of aging and intercurrent comorbidities (like hypertension, diabetes and dyslipidemias lumped under the rubric of 'atherosclerosis'), there are a few potentially curable secondary causes of isolated systolic hypertension. These include aortic valve insufficiency, arteriovenous fistulae, thyrotoxicosis, Paget's disease of bone, beriberi, and severe anemia, which are generally evident by history or on physical exam and easily corroborated with appropriate laboratory studies and imaging [26]. In addition, the possible presence of 'pseudohypertension' in which the rigidity of arterial vessels from processes like medial calcification produces a falsely elevated systolic pressure reading because of difficulty collapsing the vessel wall with a sphygmomanometer cuff [27]. It is thought to be more common when patients have severe systolic pressure elevations but lack signs of target organ damage.

Evidence supporting the treatment of isolated systolic hypertension

Non-drug measures

Customarily one begins a discussion of hypertension treatment with a review of non-drug therapy and we will respect that convention. Two non-drug therapies that reduce systolic blood pressure in isolated systolic hypertension include restriction of salt intake and an increase in physical activity.

Table 1 provides the evidence for both of these approaches. As is evident, the data are far from overwhelming, but they are encouraging and almost surprising in that relatively modest changes in sodium intake produce changes in systolic pressure that are in the range of about 10mm Hg. Even if not used as stand alone therapy, such a recommendation if successfully carried out is likely to enhance the effectiveness of medication-based approaches. This chapter's charge was isolated systolic hypertension, and the reader is reminded that there is a plethora of lifestyle measure effectiveness available with respect to pre-hypertension (systolic pressures of 120-139mm Hg, for example as in the DASH and PREMIER diet

Table 1. Effects of diet/sodium reduction (upper section) and exercise (lower section) on systolic BP.

Author / Year	N	BP	Mean age	Sodium mmol Δ	Duration	SBP/DBP Δ in mmHg
Diet/sodium reduction						
Moore 2001 [50]	72	146/85	55	No change**	8 weeks	12/3
Gates 2004 [51]	12 (6M/6F)	148/84	64	135->54mmol/d	4 weeks	12/6*
He 2006 [52]	24	166/86	63	175->87mmol/d	1 month	10/1
Exercise regimen						
Ferrier 2001 [33]	10	154/77	64	Stationary bicycle 3x/week for 40 minutes	8 weeks	'No change'
Staffileno 2003 [53]	18 PMP women	'Hypertensive'	'PMP'	10 minutes; 3x/day; 5 days/wk	8 weeks	8/5
Westhof 2007 [54]	54	>140/≤90†	≥60	Treadmill (lactate)	12 weeks	8/5

BP = Blood pressure; SBP = systolic blood pressure; DBP = diastolic blood pressure; Δ = change beginning -> end; mmol/d = millimoles (milliequivalents) per day; ** this was a DASH diet comparing that diet with typical control diets; * data reported at week 2 (of 4); † = using ambulatory blood pressure monitoring studies [28, 29] **(Ib/A)**) and typical high blood pressure where there is no prescription for a diastolic pressure less than 90mm Hg and a systolic pressure of at least 140mm Hg [30-32].

Exercise is also useful in the patient with isolated systolic hypertension. The lower portion of Table 1 shows the benefits accrued by what amounts to about 30 minutes of a brisk activity done three to five times a week. The third study in the exercise group (Ferrier 2001 [33]) was designed to investigate aspects of arterial compliance and function. It is presented for completeness sake, but the small number of subjects and the lack of specific details about systolic and diastolic blood pressure changes warrant caution in using it as the definitive study in the overall context of exercise and isolated systolic hypertension.

One caution to bear in mind is the occasional exaggerated systolic blood pressure response to exercise. There is no evidence of which I am aware to guide us in how to manage these people, so what we recommend is that if an older person with systolic hypertension is willing to engage in some regular exercise we encourage them to purchase a home blood pressure monitor and start with minimal activity preferably on a treadmill or an exercise bicycle where they can control the intensity and check their blood pressure before and immediately after a period of exercise. We arbitrarily recommend 'concern' when the systolic pressure exceeds 180mm Hg, but there is a lot of room for individualization until more information is available to guide better our efforts in encouraging patients in this aspect of blood pressure care.

Drug therapies

Of historical note, until 1991 there were virtually no randomized trials of antihypertensive drug therapy published whose enrollment included those with a diastolic blood pressure <90mm Hg. With the publication of the Systolic Hypertension in the Elderly Program (SHEP) in 1991 [15] **(Ib/A)**, the first trial-based evidence was produced demonstrating cardiovascular benefit (principally in stroke reduction, the primary outcome measure of SHEP). Prior to that time a common clinical teaching was that the systolic blood pressure in an older person is ordinarily 100 + [their age in years] so in an 80-year-old a systolic pressure of about 180mm Hg was considered acceptable. What is still missing in this critical area of blood pressure care is trial-based evidence for treating systolic pressures of 140-159mm Hg when diastolic pressures are <90mm Hg. The Hypertension in the Very Elderly Trial (HYVET) has brought us closer to this goal but there is still much to be done **(Ib/A)**.

One of the more useful purposes of a meta-analysis is that it collects in one place all studies relevant to the question pursued. In this regard, an excellent meta-analysis of evidence supporting drug treatment of isolated systolic hypertension was published in 2000 whose findings remain supported by interval trials completed since the time the meta-analysis appeared [34] **(Ia/A)**. The findings of this meta-analysis are the main supporting data for much of the treatment-related statements in the final Key Points table. The absolute benefit treating isolated systolic hypertension with drug therapy is greater in men, in people aged 70 or older and in people with previous target organ damage or wider pulse pressure. Treatment prevented stroke more effectively than coronary events. Interestingly, in this meta-analysis there was little correlation between untreated systolic hypertension and coronary artery disease outcomes. Based on this finding the authors urged some caution interpreting their results in this area because the poor correlation between coronary events and systolic blood pressure in untreated patients may indicate that the coronary protection from drug treatment may have been underestimated [35]. What follows next in this final section is not so much a detailed review of every trial of isolated systolic hypertension, but more a milestone-related narrative that summarizes how we got from no evidence on treating this relatively common blood pressure circumstance culminating in an assessment of the next steps necessarily to definitively answer the question that forms this chapter's title. Table 2 contains, in summary

Table 2. Randomized clinical trials of systolic hypertension.

Trial name & year	SBP criteria mm Hg	Duration	Age (mean)	# Randomized: active/comparator	Baseline BP	SBP on active treatment	SBP on comparator treatment	Significant outcome benefits
SHEP 1991	160-219	4.5 yrs	(72)	2365/2371	170/77	143	155	✓Stroke ✓CAD
STONE 1996	160-220	2.5 yrs	60-79 (66)	912/764	168/96-100	147	156	✓Stroke
Syst-Eur 1997	160-219 /<95	2 yrs	>60 (70)	2398/2297	174/85	151	161	✓Stroke ✓Major CVE
Syst-China 2000	160-219 /<95	3 yrs	>60	1253/1142	171/86	151	160	Marginally significant stroke and CVE benefits
HYVET 2008	≥160	1.8 yrs	≥80	1933/1912	173/91	143	155	✓Death ✓Heart failure
JATOS 2008	≥160	2 years	65-85	2212/2206 (more vs less aggressive BP control)	171/89	136	146	No difference in more vs less aggressive Rx groups

SHEP = Systolic Hypertension in the Elderly Program [15]; STONE = Shanghai Trial of Nifedipine in the Elderly [39] (note enrollment allowed diastolic values >95mm Hg); Syst-Eur = Systolic Hypertension in Europeans [37]; Syst-China = Systolic Hypertension in Chinese [38]; HYVET = Hypertension in the Very Elderly Trial [43]; JATOS = JApanese Trial to assess Optimal Systolic blood pressure in elderly hypertensive patients [49]; CAD = coronary artery disease; CVE = cardiovascular endoints; Rx = treatment

format, the main trials that form the evidence base for the recommendations in the Key Points table. Figure 2 gives a sense of the time period involved.

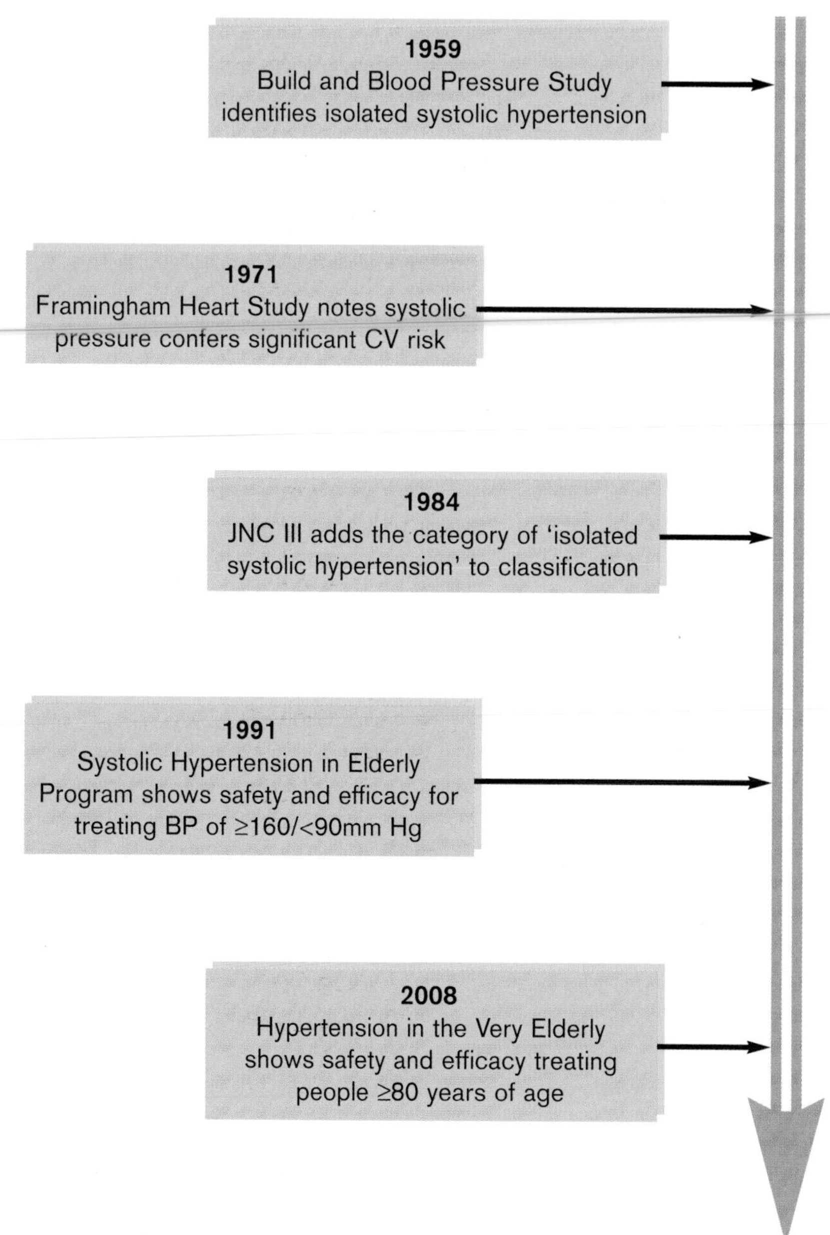

Figure 2. Timeline showing milestones in isolated systolic hypertension.

The blood pressure care world in 1991 was guided by the fourth report of the Joint National Committee (released in 1988) [36] **(IV/A)**, which classified high blood pressure based on the diastolic blood pressure value. At that time there was no guidance on what to do when diastolic blood pressure was <90mm Hg. The SHEP trial specifically enrolled subjects at least 60 years of age, where most isolated systolic hypertension is found, and randomized 2365 to active treatment and 2371 to placebo for 4.5 years [15]. The average age of participants in SHEP was 72 years and the blood pressure levels at enrollment were 170/77mm Hg. The drug treatment was chlorthalidone as a first-line agent, followed by the addition of atenolol after one step-up from 12.5 to 25mg of the diuretic. The principal finding of SHEP was a 12mm Hg greater reduction in systolic pressure in the drug treatment group (143mm Hg on average) compared with the placebo group (155mm Hg on average). This was associated with a 36% reduction in fatal and non-fatal stroke (the primary endpoint of SHEP) and a 27% reduction in fatal and non-fatal coronary heart disease. SHEP findings were confirmed by a similar placebo-controlled trial in Europe that based therapy on the calcium channel blocker, nitrendipine, as a first step and enalapril as a second step [37] **(Ib/A)**, and two trials in Asia which based therapy either on nitrendipine [38] **(Ib/A)** or on nifedipine [39] **(IIb/B)**. All four of these trials capped enrollment age at an upper limit of 75-79 years.

The data from these trials left two unanswered questions. These were:

- what about people over the age of 80 years?
- what about people with a systolic pressure of 140-159mm Hg?

An attempt to answer the first question appeared as a meta-analysis from the INDANA (based on the acronym INdividual Data ANalysis of Antihypertensive intervention trials) group in 1999 [40] **(Ia/B)**. Addressing the issue of benefit to treating people over the age of 80 they reviewed trial results on 1670 people and found that there was a suggestion that treatment reduced stroke but increased (by about 6%) the risk of death from all causes. The latter finding was not statistically significant but raised concern regarding the risk/benefit issue when treating the very elderly. On this background the Hypertension in the Very Elderly (PILOT) Trial was in progress supported initially by the British Heart Foundation and subsequently performed in 10 European centers [41] **(Ib/A)**. The findings of this pilot trial were published in 2003 [42]. They demonstrated that in 1283 patients older than 80 years of age who were enrolled with a blood pressure of 160-219/90-109mm Hg (so it is not a study of isolated systolic hypertension, but hang on...), treatment with the diuretic, bendroflumethiazide (one-third), or an angiotensin-converting enzyme (ACE) inhibitor (one-third) compared with no treatment and a target blood pressure of 150/80mm Hg showed findings very similar to the INDANA meta-analysis, i.e. prevention of stroke (19 strokes prevented for treating a 1000 patients for a year), but at the cost of 20 extra non-stroke deaths. Building upon the basic design of the HYVET pilot, the main HYVET trial began enrollment in 2000.

The main HYVET trial enrolled 3845 participants from around the world and specified age >80 years and systolic pressure (off any antihypertensive medications) of 160-199mm Hg [43] **(Ib/A)**. To be fair, this again is not a trial of isolated systolic hypertension, but the average blood pressure of 173/91mm Hg at the close of enrollment suggests that many of the participants had a diastolic blood pressure value of <90mm Hg. Treatment in HYVET was randomly assigned as either a diuretic (indapamide) or placebo. The second-line agent was the ACE inhibitor, perindopril, vs more placebo. The main HYVET trial was concluded prematurely after a mean follow-up of 1.8 years when the Safety Monitoring Board decided that the benefit of active drug treatment on the outcome of death from all causes was better than that noted in the placebo group. As with SHEP systolic blood pressure in those assigned to active drug therapy was 15mm Hg lower compared with the placebo group. What HYVET added was the assurance of safety in this population, an improvement in death rate, a nearly significant improvement in stroke incidence (p=0.06; but the trial was terminated early) and benefit in both heart failure and any cardiovascular endpoint. The other contribution of HYVET is the provision of data supporting the safety and feasibility of achieving a systolic blood pressure <150mm Hg as a treatment endpoint in elderly people.

The most recent meta-analysis on the value of treating high blood pressure that specifically considered older people (>65 years in this case) tabulated data from 31 trials and more than 190,000 participants and showed that older people benefit well from virtually all available antihypertensive agents proportionate to the magnitude of blood pressure reduction [44] **(Ia/A)**. Moreover, older patients experience this benefit without an increased risk from the treatment, a concern that was voiced in the literature [45] and was in the background and outcome of studies such as SHEP and the INDANA meta-analysis.

Although the outcomes of greatest interest in hypertension trials tend to be death, non-fatal heart attack and heart failure and non-fatal stroke, in the elderly an additional outcome is worthy of mention. This outcome is cognition. At present I think the things we can say about this outcome are the following:

- hypertension in middle-age years seems to engender more cognitive function impairment in older-age years [46] **(III/B)**;
- some trials suggest that treating hypertension in the elderly preserves cognitive function [47] **(IIa/B)**, while others do not think that the clinical trials show this benefit [48] **(IIb/B)**.

Conclusions

In summary, the answer as of Spring 2009 to the question posed, irrespective of how one defines 'older', is that a systolic blood pressure treated to <150-160mm Hg is the optimal treatment goal. There are still no data to support initiating antihypertensive drug therapy in people with a diastolic blood pressure value of <90mm Hg when the systolic blood pressure is <160mm Hg. The only trial achieving a systolic blood pressure below 140mm Hg on drug treatment was JATOS [49] **(Ib/A)** and perhaps due either to the relatively few number of events or the relatively short duration (2 years) of the trial there was no difference in the primary endpoint of cardiovascular events and kidney disease in the more compared with the less aggressive treatment groups (Table 2). Stay tuned.

Key points	Evidence level
◆ Isolated systolic hypertension is the most common form of blood pressure elevation in people older than 55 years of age.	IIb/B
◆ Older patients experience more cardiovascular disease from higher blood pressure in a 5-year period compared with younger patients.	Ia/A
◆ High blood pressure can be safely treated in older patients without excess morbidity.	Ia/A
◆ An important mechanism of isolated systolic blood pressure elevation in older patients is stiffening of blood vessels.	IIa/B
◆ Treating 59 older patients with isolated systolic hypertension for 5 years prevents 1 death from any cause.	Ia/A
◆ Treating 79 older patients with isolated systolic hypertension for 5 years prevents 1 death from cardiovascular disease.	Ia/A
◆ Treating 26 older patients with isolated systolic hypertension for 5 years prevents 1 cardiovascular event (fatal or non-fatal).	Ia/A
◆ Treating 48 older patients with isolated systolic hypertension for 5 years prevents 1 stroke (fatal or non-fatal).	Ia/A
◆ Treating 64 older patients with isolated systolic hypertension for 5 years prevents 1 coronary event (fatal or non-fatal).	Ia/A
◆ Even people 80 years of age and older benefit from drug therapy for hypertension when the systolic pressure is ≥160mm Hg.	Ia/A

References

1. Oxford English Dictionary. Accessed on 5-15-2009: http://dictionary.oed.com/cgi/entry/00332956?single=1&query_type=word&queryword=optimal&first=1&max_to_show=10.
2. Amery A, Birkenhager W, Brixko P, Bulpitt C, Clement D, Deruyttere M, *et al.* Mortality and morbidity results from the European Working Party on High Blood Pressure in the Elderly trial. *Lancet* 1985; 1(8442): 1349-54.
3. Brett AS. Ethical issues in risk factor intervention. *Am J Med* 1984; 76(4): 557-61.
4. Chobanian AV, Bakris GL, Black HR, Cushman WC, Green LA, Izzo JL, Jr. *et al.* Seventh report of the Joint National Committee on Prevention, Detection, Evaluation, and Treatment of High Blood Pressure. *Hypertension* 2003; 42(6): 1206-52.
5. Summary of 1993 World Health Organisation-International Society of Hypertension guidelines for the management of mild hypertension. Subcommittee of WHO/ISH Mild Hypertension Liaison committee. *BMJ* 1993; 307(6918): 1541-6.
6. Mancia G, De Backer G, Dominiczak A, Cifkova R, Fagard R, Germano G *et al.* 2007 Guidelines for the Management of Arterial Hypertension: The Task Force for the Management of Arterial Hypertension of the European Society of Hypertension (ESH) and of the European Society of Cardiology (ESC). *J Hypertens* 2007; 25(6): 1105-87.
7. Franklin SS, Gustin W, Wong ND, Larson MG, Weber MA, Kannel WB, *et al.* Hemodynamic patterns of age-related changes in blood pressure. The Framingham Heart Study. *Circulation* 1997; 96(1): 308-15.
8. Hyman DJ, Pavlik VN. Characteristics of patients with uncontrolled hypertension in the United States. *Clinical Nephrology* 2001; 345(7): 479-86.

9. Ostchega Y, Dillon CF, Hughes JP, Carroll M, Yoon S. Trends in hypertension prevalence, awareness, treatment, and control in older U.S. adults: data from the National Health and Nutrition Examination Survey 1988 to 2004. *J Am Geriatr Soc* 2007; 55(7): 1056-65.
10. Kalaitzidis R, Li S, Wang C, Chen SC, McCullough PA, Bakris GL. Hypertension in early-stage kidney disease: an update from the Kidney Early Evaluation Program (KEEP). *Am J Kidney Dis* 2009; 53(4 Suppl 4): S22-31.
11. Chirinos JA, Franklin SS, Townsend RR, Raij L. Body mass index and hypertension hemodynamic subtypes in the adult US population. *Arch Intern Med* 2009; 169(6): 580-6.
12. Hutchinson JJ. Highlights of the new Build and Blood Pressure study. *Trans Assoc Life Insur Med Dir Am* 1959; 43: 34-42.
13. MORTALITY trends in relation to blood pressure and build. *Can Med Assoc J* 1960; 82: 1033.
14. Kannel WB, Gordon T, Schwartz MJ. Systolic versus diastolic blood pressure and risk of coronary heart disease. The Framingham study. *American Journal of Cardiology* 1971; 27(4): 335-46.
15. SHEP Coop Res Group. Prevention of stroke by antihypertensive drug treatment in older persons with isolated systolic hypertension. Final results of the Systolic Hypertension in the Elderly Program (SHEP). *JAMA* 1991; 265: 3255-64.
16. Kannel WB, Wolf PA, McGee DL, Dawber TR, McNamara P, Castelli WP. Systolic blood pressure, arterial rigidity, and risk of stroke. The Framingham study. *JAMA* 1981; 245(12): 1225-9.
17. Haider AW, Larson MG, Franklin SS, Levy D. Systolic blood pressure, diastolic blood pressure, and pulse pressure as predictors of risk for congestive heart failure in the Framingham Heart Study. *Ann Intern Med* 2003; 138(1): 10-6.
18. Gasowski J, Grodzicki T. Systolic swing of the pendulum: relation between hypertension and heart failure revisited. *Hypertension* 2009; 53(3): 452-3.
19. Wong ND, Lopez VA, L'Italien G, Chen R, Kline SE, Franklin SS. Inadequate control of hypertension in US adults with cardiovascular disease comorbidities in 2003-2004. *Arch Intern Med* 2007; 167(22): 2431-6.
20. Curb JD, Borhani NO, Entwisle G, Tung B, Kass E, Schnaper H, *et al.* Isolated systolic hypertension in 14 communities. *Am J Epidemiol* 1985; 121(3): 362-70.
21. O'Rourke MF, Staessen JA, Vlachopoulos C, Duprez D, Plante GE. Clinical applications of arterial stiffness; definitions and reference values. *Am J Hypertens* 2002; 15(5): 426-44.
22. Nichols WW, Denardo SJ, Wilkinson IB, McEniery CM, Cockcroft J, O'Rourke MF. Effects of arterial stiffness, pulse wave velocity, and wave reflections on the central aortic pressure waveform. *J Clin Hypertens* (Greenwich) 2008; 10(4): 295-303.
23. Lakatta EG. Cardiovascular regulatory mechanisms in advanced age. *Physiol Rev* 1993; 73(2): 413-67.
24. Harkness ML, Harkness RD, McDonald DA. The collagen and elastin content of the arterial wall in the dog. *Proc R Soc Lond B Biol Sci* 1957; 146(925): 541-51.
25. Stokes GS. Treatment of isolated systolic hypertension. *Curr Hypertens Rep* 2006; 8(5): 377-83.
26. Kocemba J, Kawecka-Jaszcz K, Gryglewska B, Grodzicki T. Isolated systolic hypertension: pathophysiology, consequences and therapeutic benefits. *J Hum Hypertens* 1998; 12(9): 621-6.
27. Messerli FH. Osler's maneuver, pseudohypertension, and true hypertension in the elderly. *Am J Med* 1986; 80(5): 906-10.
28. Funk KL, Elmer PJ, Stevens VJ, Harsha DW, Craddick SR, Lin PH, *et al.* PREMIER - a trial of lifestyle interventions for blood pressure control: intervention design and rationale. *Health Promot Pract* 2008; 9(3): 271-80.
29. Appel LJ, Moore TJ, Obarzanek E, Vollmer WM, Svetkey LP, Sacks FM, *et al.* A clinical trial of the effects of dietary patterns on blood pressure. DASH Collaborative Research Group. *Clinical Nephrology* 1997; 336(16): 1117-24.
30. Dolor RJ, Yancy WS, Jr., Owen WF, Matchar DB, Samsa GP, Pollak KI, *et al.* Hypertension Improvement Project (HIP): study protocol and implementation challenges. *Trials* 2009; 10:13.
31. Neaton JD, Grimm RH, Jr., Prineas RJ, Stamler J, Grandits GA, Elmer PJ, *et al.* Treatment of Mild Hypertension Study. Final results. Treatment of Mild Hypertension Study Research Group. *JAMA* 1993; 270(6): 713-24.
32. Dickinson HO, Mason JM, Nicolson DJ, Campbell F, Beyer FR, Cook JV, *et al.* Lifestyle interventions to reduce raised blood pressure: a systematic review of randomized controlled trials. *J Hypertens* 2006; 24(2): 215-33.
33. Ferrier KE, Waddell TK, Gatzka CD, Cameron JD, Dart AM, Kingwell BA. Aerobic exercise training does not modify large-artery compliance in isolated systolic hypertension. *Hypertension* 2001; 38(2): 222-6.

34. Staessen JA, Gasowski J, Wang JG, Thijs L, Den Hond E, Boissel JP, *et al.* Risks of untreated and treated isolated systolic hypertension in the elderly: meta-analysis of outcome trials. *Lancet* 2000; 355(9207): 865-72.
35. Lloyd-Jones DM, Evans JC, Larson MG, O'Donnell CJ, Levy D. Differential impact of systolic and diastolic blood pressure level on JNC-VI staging. Joint National Committee on Prevention, Detection, Evaluation, and Treatment of High Blood Pressure. *Hypertension* 1999; 34(3): 381-5.
36. The 1988 report of the Joint National Committee on Detection, Evaluation, and Treatment of High Blood Pressure. *Arch Intern Med* 1988; 148(5): 1023-38.
37. Staessen JA, Fagard R, Thijs L, Celis H, Arabidze GG, Birkenhager WH, *et al.* Randomised double-blind comparison of placebo and active treatment for older patients with isolated systolic hypertension. The Systolic Hypertension in Europe (Syst-Eur) Trial Investigators. *Lancet* 1997; 350(9080): 757-64.
38. Wang JG, Staessen JA, Gong L, Liu L. Chinese trial on isolated systolic hypertension in the elderly. Systolic Hypertension in China (Syst-China) Collaborative Group. *Arch Intern Med* 2000; 160(2): 211-20.
39. Gong L, Zhang W, Zhu Y, Zhu J, Kong D, Page V, *et al.* Shanghai Trial of Nifedipine in the Elderly (STONE). *J Hypertens* 1996; 14(10):1237-45.
40. Gueyffier F, Bulpitt C, Boissel JP, Schron E, Ekbom T, Fagard R, *et al.* Antihypertensive drugs in very old people: a subgroup meta-analysis of randomised controlled trials. INDANA Group. *Lancet* 1999; 353(9155): 793-6.
41. Bulpitt CJ, Fletcher AE, Amery A, Coope J, Evans JG, Lightowlers S, *et al.* The Hypertension in the Very Elderly Trial (HYVET). Rationale, methodology and comparison with previous trials. *Drugs Aging* 1994; 5(3): 171-83.
42. Bulpitt CJ, Beckett NS, Cooke J, Dumitrascu DL, Gil-Extremera B, Nachev C, *et al.* Results of the pilot study for the Hypertension in the Very Elderly Trial. *J Hypertens* 2003; 21(12): 2409-17.
43. Beckett NS, Peters R, Fletcher AE, Staessen JA, Liu L, Dumitrascu D, *et al.* Treatment of hypertension in patients 80 years of age or older. *N Engl J Med* 2008; 358(18): 1887-98.
44. Turnbull F, Neal B, Ninomiya T, Algert C, Arima H, Barzi F, *et al.* Effects of different regimens to lower blood pressure on major cardiovascular events in older and younger adults: meta-analysis of randomised trials. *BMJ* 2008; 336(7653): 1121-3.
45. Verhaeverbeke I, Mets T. Drug-induced orthostatic hypotension in the elderly: avoiding its onset. *Drug Saf* 1997; 17(2): 105-18.
46. Launer LJ, Masaki K, Petrovitch H, Foley D, Havlik RJ. The association between midlife blood pressure levels and late-life cognitive function. The Honolulu-Asia Aging Study. *JAMA* 1995; 274(23): 1846-51.
47. Amenta F, Mignini F, Rabbia F, Tomassoni D, Veglio F. Protective effect of anti-hypertensive treatment on cognitive function in essential hypertension: analysis of published clinical data. *J Neurol Sci* 2002; 203-4: 147-51.
48. McGuinness B, Todd S, Passmore AP, Bullock R. Systematic review: blood pressure lowering in patients without prior cerebrovascular disease for prevention of cognitive impairment and dementia. *J Neurol Neurosurg Psychiatry* 2008; 79(1): 4-5.
49. Principal results of the Japanese Trial to Assess Optimal Systolic Blood Pressure in Elderly Hypertensive Patients (JATOS). *Hypertens Res* 2008; 31(12): 2115-27.
50. Moore TJ, Conlin PR, Ard J, Svetkey LP. DASH (Dietary Approaches to Stop Hypertension) diet is effective treatment for stage 1 isolated systolic hypertension. *Hypertension* 2001; 38(2): 155-8.
51. Gates PE, Tanaka H, Hiatt WR, Seals DR. Dietary sodium restriction rapidly improves large elastic artery compliance in older adults with systolic hypertension. *Hypertension* 2004; 44(1): 35-41.
52. He FJ, Markandu ND, MacGregor GA. Modest salt reduction lowers blood pressure in isolated systolic hypertension and combined hypertension. *Hypertension* 2005; 46(1): 66-70.
53. Staffileno BA, Braun LT, Rosenson RS. The accumulative effects of physical activity in hypertensive post-menopausal women. *J Cardiovasc Risk* 2001; 8(5): 283-290.
54. Westhoff TH, Franke N, Schmidt S, Vallbracht-Israng K, Meissner R, Yildirim H, *et al.* Too old to benefit from sports? The cardiovascular effects of exercise training in elderly subjects treated for isolated systolic hypertension. *Kidney Blood Press Res* 2007; 30(4): 240-7.

Chapter 9

What is optimal treatment of hypertension in minority populations?

Radhika Kanthety MD MSHS, Research Coordinator, Division of Nephrology and Hypertension, University Hospitals Case Medical Center, Cleveland, Ohio, USA

Jackson T Wright Jr. MD PhD, Professor of Medicine, Case Western Reserve University, Cleveland, Ohio, USA; Program Director, William T. Dahms Clinical Research Unit, Clinical and Translational Science Collaborative; Director, Clinical Hypertension Program, Division of Nephrology and Hypertension, University Hospitals Case Medical Center, Cleveland, Ohio, USA

Mahboob Rahman MD MS, Associate Professor of Medicine, Case Western Reserve University, Cleveland, Ohio, USA; Staff Nephrologist, Division of Nephrology and Hypertension, University Hospitals Case Medical Center, Cleveland, Ohio, USA and the Louis Stokes Cleveland VA Medical Center, Cleveland, Ohio, USA

Introduction

There is increasing racial and ethnic diversity in the population in the United States with the representation of Hispanics, especially Mexican Americans, and Asians on the rise. The epidemiology and manifestations of hypertension vary among racial and ethnic groups influenced, in part, by sociocultural factors and access to health care [1]. According to the NHANES (National Health and Nutrition Examination Survey) data, 28.9% of US adults have hypertension [2]. The prevalence is highest in blacks (40.1%), while it is 27.4% in non-Hispanic whites, and 27.1% among Mexican Americans, respectively (Table 1). African Americans have one of the highest prevalence of hypertension with a higher degree of morbidity, mortality, and target organ damage compared to the other populations. The prevalence in Hispanics is similar to non-Hispanic whites, though the risk of complications like stroke is higher in Puerto Rican and Mexican-Americans. Persons of Southeast Asian descent are also at a higher risk of hypertension [3] **(IV/C)**.

Of individuals with hypertension, 71.8 % are aware of their condition; awareness rates are the lowest among Mexican Americans. Among treated individuals, the mean blood pressure is lower in whites and highest in blacks even though blacks as a group are more likely to receive treatment than whites. Mexican Americans are the least likely to receive treatment perhaps, due to lack of insurance, lower socio-economic status or lack of access to health care [2, 4].

Table 1. Prevalence, awareness, treatment and control in the US population.

	Age-standardized and age-specific prevalence of hypertension in the US adult population	Hypertension awareness, treatment, and control in the the US adult hypertensive population		
		Awareness	Treatment	Control
All	28.9%	71.8	61.4	35.1
Non-hispanic white	27.4	72.0	62.1	36.8
Non-hispanic black	40.1	75.8	65.1	33.4
Mexican - American	27.1	61.3	47.4	24.3

These data suggest striking differences in hypertension based on race and ethnicity. In this chapter, we will review the implications of these differences for treatment of hypertension in these populations. We compiled our data by searching on PubMed and the internet using terms such as management of hypertension in minorities; evidence-based management of hypertension; targeted search for hypertension by race/ethnicity: treatment in African Americans, Hispanics, and Asians.

Epidemiology

African Americans

African Americans in general show an earlier development of hypertension, and higher prevalence rates in younger age groups than in whites. Compared to whites they have more Stage 2 hypertension, and have more target organ damage in the heart manifested as left ventricular hypertrophy with diastolic dysfunction, which often tends to be out of proportion to the level of blood pressure [5]. They are more likely to have chronic kidney disease and end-stage renal disease than their Caucasian counterparts [6], and are more prone to sudden cardiac death and out-of-hospital mortality due to cardiovascular, cerebrovascular and coronary artery disease [7]. In a study on persons of African descent, the risk of being hypertensive in men aged 40 and above was higher in black men and women compared to their white counterparts after controlling for factors such as age, obesity, socio-economic status, smoking and alcohol use. The mean blood pressures were 147.4/84.4mm Hg in black men and 141.6/81.5mm Hg in white men, whereas the values in women were 143.6/79.6 and 138.0/75.8mm Hg, respectively [8] **(III/B)**.

Hispanic

The age-adjusted prevalence of hypertension in Hispanics in the US (about 29%) is similar to non-Hispanic whites; major factors for morbidity and mortality among them being obesity and diabetes mellitus [2, 9]. Hispanics are a diverse group spanning various races: blacks, whites and native Americans and they also vary by their country of origin; the majority of this group in the United States is of Mexican origin. In some studies, mean blood pressures among these groups were higher than whites and second only to blacks [10] **(IV/C)**. When seen by a healthcare provider, Hispanics are more likely than whites to receive treatment for hypertension; however, they were less likely to have therapy intensified or target blood pressure attained compared to whites [11] **(III/B)**.

Asians/South Asians

The risk of hypertension in Asians is similar to the general population with the exception of South Asians in whom the risk is higher [12]. South Asians are also a diverse group and the mean blood pressures differ based on the country of origin [13] **(Ia/A)**; mean blood pressures are lower in Pakistanis and Bangladeshis, and higher in Indians living in the United Kingdom [14] **(IIa/A)**. The age-adjusted rates of hypertension in South Asian men (odds ratio 1.9; 95% confidence interval 1.4, 2.4; $p<0.001$) were similar to black men and the rates in South Asian women were similar to white women [8] **(III/B)**. Stroke and heart disease are the leading cause of death among South Asians [13] **(Ia/A)**. Hypertension is thought to be responsible for 57% of all stroke deaths and 24% of all coronary heart disease deaths in India [15] **(Ia/A)**. South Asians are more prone to cardiometabolic syndrome manifesting as insulin resistance, truncal obesity and dyslipidemia likely increasing their risk of coronary artery disease and stroke [16]. This trend is consistent in South Asians living in the US [17] **(Ib/A)**. The age-adjusted prevalence of angina or myocardial infarction in Asian Indian men in the US was about three times higher than controls in the Framingham Offspring Study (7.2% vs. 2.5%; $p<0.0001$) [18]. The prevalence of hypertension in Asian Indians is higher in urban compared to rural populations [3, 19] **(IV/C)** [15] **(Ia/A)**.

Others

Pima Indians have a high incidence of diabetes, and the incidence of hypertension is 34% among diabetic compared to 24% in non-diabetic Pima Indians [20]. Native Hawaiians and Pacific Islanders have lower rates of hypertension compared to their Caucasian counterparts (21.2% vs. 24.9%) [21], but have a greater risk of coronary artery disease perhaps due to the increased prevalence of diabetes and obesity [22]. A study of the residents living on the Molokai island in Hawaii found that more than 60% of its native population was obese thus increasing the risk of hypertension and cardiovascular disease [23].

Goals of treatment

The goal of treatment of hypertension in most patients with hypertension is to achieve a target BP of <140/90mm Hg and lower risk of cardiovascular and renal morbidity and mortality. In patients with coexisting risk factors such as diabetes, cardiovascular disease or chronic kidney disease, the treatment target is BP <130/80mm Hg [24] **(IV/C)**. These goals are consistent regardless of race or ethnicity.

Lifestyle

Non-pharmacologic interventions such as exercise and dietary modifications are an important adjunct in the management of hypertension. These include intake of ≥5 fruits and vegetables/day, regular exercise >12 times/month, maintaining healthy weight (body mass index 18.5-29.9kg/m^2), moderate alcohol consumption (up to one drink/day for women, two/day for men) and not smoking [24-26] **(I/A, IV/C)**. Adherence to a healthy lifestyle is generally lower in minorities compared to the general population (Table 2) [27] **(III/B)**.

Table 2. Adherence to healthy lifestyle behaviors in US adults.

	BMI <30	Physical activity >12 times/month	Non-smoker	≥5 servings /day of fruits and vegetables
Non-hispanic white	64.6	45.2	75.2	25.4
Non-hispanic black	57.0	34.6	65.6	24.6
Hispanic	66.1	36.2	72.9	28.6

Dietary modification

Current guidelines recommend that dietary sodium intake should be reduced to 2300mg/day in the general population, and 1500mg/day in hypertensive patients, African Americans, middle aged and older adults [28] **(IV/C)**. Dietary salt restriction is particularly in the management of hypertension in African American patients. Modest reduction in salt intake (169+/-73 to 89+/-52mmol per 24 hours) in black patients with hypertension showed a 8/3mm Hg blood pressure lowering; importantly, urinary protein excretion was also reduced by 19.4% [29] **(Ib/A)**. In addition, lower sodium intake has shown to improve other markers of target organ damage such as pulse wave velocity, more so in blacks compared to whites and Asians [30] **(Ib/A)**. South Asians also have a high salt intake and therefore restriction of sodium intake is as important in the management of hypertension in this population [17] **(Ib/A)**.

Optimal intake of potassium should accompany low salt intake and this is achieved best by eating more fruits and vegetables [28]. In general, intake of potassium is lower in African Americans than other racial ethnic groups [31] **(III/B)**, and potassium supplementation lowers blood pressure more [32] **(Ia/A)**. Increasing the potassium intake to 4.7g per day preferably in the form of fruits and vegetables or oral supplements helps optimize the treatment goals [28, 33] **(IIa/B, Ib/A)**.

The Dietary Approaches to Stop Hypertension (DASH) trial is a useful adjunct in the treatment of hypertension. In the DASH study, participants were randomized to 8 weeks of a control diet; a diet rich in fruits and vegetables; or a combination diet rich in fruits, vegetables, and low-fat dairy foods, and reduced in saturated fat, total fat, and cholesterol. The combination diet lowered systolic blood pressure significantly more in African Americans (6.8mm Hg) than in whites (3.0mm Hg) [34] **(Ib/A)**. Combining salt restriction with the DASH diet provides incremental lowering of blood pressure in African Americans and in other racial ethnic groups [35].

Exercise and weight loss

Weight loss and regular physical exercise are well known to have beneficial effects on hypertension and cardiovascular health. Current guidelines recommend moderately intense physical activity for about 30 minutes on most days of the week in the form of walking, swimming, or other aerobic activity [24]. Regular aerobic exercise lowers blood pressure in most hypertensive patients; the reduction in systolic blood pressure in African American patients may be as high as 10mm of Hg [36] **(Ia/A)**. Achieving and maintaining ideal body weight overcomes an important barrier to blood pressure control. A meta-analysis of 25 clinical trials has shown that an average weight loss of 5.1Kg by energy restriction, increased physical activity or both resulted in 4.4/3.5mm Hg reduction in blood pressures. Systolic blood pressure reduction associated with weight loss was higher in African Americans (-4.67) and Asians (-8.77), compared to Caucasians (-3.19) [37] **(Ia/A)**.

Alcohol use

Excessive alcohol consumption can be associated with resistant hypertension [38]. To improve blood pressure control, alcohol consumption should be limited to one to two drinks in men and one drink or less in women [24] **(IV/C)**. Reduction of alcohol consumption is associated with an average reduction in systolic and diastolic blood pressures of 3.31mm Hg and 2.04mm Hg, respectively [39] **(Ia/A)**.

Stress

Differences in stress levels, and responses to stress have been thought to contribute to racial differences in hypertension. Men with high stress levels and a family history of hypertension had higher systolic and diastolic blood pressures ($p<0.05$) and a seven-fold increase in relative risk of changes in blood pressure ($p<0.001$) when compared to men under less stress even though they had a family history of hypertension [40] **(IIa/B)**. Higher levels of socio-economic stress in African Americans may contribute to increased sympathetic nervous system activity that increases peripheral vascular resistance, one of the causes of hypertension [41]. A study on the association between stress related to racial discrimination and hypertension in an African American population based in Atlanta found that while exposure to incidents of racial discrimination was not significantly associated with an increased likelihood of hypertension, the magnitude of stress generally derived from exposure was, however, a highly significant predictor. Respondents reporting 'moderate' and a 'high to very high' level of derived stress were more than twice as likely to be hypertensive when compared to those reporting 'no to low' derived stress (p value=0.02 and 0.01, respectively) [42] **(IIa/B)**. Several studies have shown that techniques to lower stress and promote relaxation can lower blood pressure in African Americans [43-45] **(Ib/A)**.

Pharmacology

African Americans

Diuretics are the cornerstone of antihypertensive drug therapy in most African American hypertensive patients. The Seventh Report of the Joint National Committee on Prevention, Detection, Evaluation, and Treatment of High Blood Pressure (JNC 7) recommends thiazide diuretics as first-line therapy for treatment of most patients with hypertension [24]. The International Society on Hypertension in Blacks (ISHIB) guidelines though, endorse the use of any of the first-line agents (diuretics, β-blockers, ACE inhibitors or angiotensin receptor blockers) as initial monotherapy [46]. When used as monotherapy, African Americans have a better response in terms of blood pressure reduction treatment with diuretics and calcium channel blockers than β-blockers and inhibitors of the renin angiotensin axis, though the difference is ameliorated by use of combination therapy [47-50] **(Ib/A)**. Diuretics also increase the effectiveness of ACE inhibitors, β-blockers and other classes of antihypertensive drugs when used in combination [48] **(Ib/A)**. It should be noted that though angioedema is a rare complication of ACE inhibitor use (1.97 cases per 1000 person years), it is more likely in African Americans (OR 3.88) than in other racial ethnic groups [51].

While several studies document a difference in blood pressure response between racial groups [52] **(Ia/A)**, it is important to appreciate that there is significant overlap in blood pressure response. This was best illustrated by a meta-analysis by Sehgal *et al* which showed that the mean difference between whites and blacks ranged from 0.6 to 3.0mm Hg reduction in diastolic blood pressure. However, the percentage of whites and blacks with similar drug-associated changes in diastolic blood pressure was 90% for diuretics and β-blockers, 95% for calcium channel blockers, and 81% for angiotensin-converting enzyme inhibitors, suggesting that the majority of whites and blacks have similar responses to commonly used antihypertensive drugs [53] **(Ia/A)**. Recognizing that many patients will need more than one drug to control blood pressure, ISHIB guidelines recommend that combination therapy be used in African Americans when the systolic pressures are 15mm Hg or higher and the diastolic BP is 10mm Hg or more than the desired goal **(IV/C)** [46].

The Antihypertensive and Lipid-Lowering treatment to prevent Heart Attack Trial (ALLHAT) [54] **(Ib/A)** was a large study of over 40,000 patients, about one third of whom were blacks, offering important insights into treatment of hypertension in African Americans. This study compared amlodipine and lisinopril with chlorthalidone as first-line therapy for hypertension. There was no significant difference between the treatment groups (chlorthalidone, amlodipine and lisinopril) for the primary cardiovascular outcome in either racial subgroup. However, there were important differences in pre-specified secondary outcomes. Amlodipine was associated with a higher risk of heart failure than chlorthalidone in both blacks and non-blacks (blacks: RR [relative risk], 1.46; 95% CI, 1.24-1.73; non-blacks: RR, 1.32; 95% CI, 1.17-1.49; p<.001 for each comparison) with no difference in treatment effects by race (p=0.38 for interaction). In black patients, lisinopril was less effective than chlorthalidone in lowering blood pressure, and preventing stroke, and combined CVD outcomes (p<.001, p=0.01, and p=0.04, respectively, for interactions) [55]. In blacks and non-blacks, respectively, the RR for stroke was 1.40 (95% CI, 1.17-1.68) and 1.00 (95% CI, 0.85-1.17) and for combined cardiovascular disease were 1.19 (95% CI, 1.09-1.30) and 1.06 (95% CI, 1.00-1.13). For heart failure, the RR was 1.30 (95% CI, 1.10-1.54) and 1.13 (95% CI, 1.00-1.28), with no significant interaction by race. Adjustment for differences in blood pressure did not significantly alter differences in outcome for lisinopril vs chlorthalidone in blacks, suggesting that the difference in blood pressure did not entirely explain the difference in risk of outcomes. These findings were consistent in patients with metabolic syndrome [56] **(Ib/A)**.

The African American Study of Kidney Disease and Hypertension (AASK) study [57] **(Ib/A)** has also provided important insights into the management of African American patients with hypertensive chronic kidney disease (CKD). This study demonstrated that given adequate resources and availability of medications, blood pressure control could be achieved and maintained in this patient population [58] **(Ib/A)**. Use of ramipril was associated with a 38% reduced risk of clinical endpoints (reduction in glomerular filtration rate [GFR] of more than 50% or 25ml/min per 1.73m^2, end-stage renal disease, or death), a 36% slower mean decline in GFR after 3 months (p=0.002), and less proteinuria (p<0.001) compared to amlodipine. Similarly, ramipril was associated with a 22% lower risk of clinical outcomes when compared with metoprolol. Participants assigned to the lower mean arterial pressure goal (92mm Hg or less n=540) had similar rates of decline of GFR and clinical outcomes compared to those assigned to usual blood pressure goals (mean arterial pressure goals, 102 to 107mm Hg n=554) [57] **(Ib/A)**. Long-term follow-up of AASK participants indicates that despite good blood pressure control and inhibition of the renin angiotensin axis, renal disease inexorably progresses in many African American patients with hypertensive CKD [59] **(Ib/A)**.

Adherence remains very important in achieving blood pressure control; this can be better achieved by simplifying the regimen, patient education, and considering the cost to the patient which can be reduced by using generics when applicable. Systematic interventions to improve the patient physician relationship, adherence and blood pressure control are being studied [60, 61] **(Ib/A)**.

In summary, thiazide diuretics are a reasonable first choice in most African American hypertensive patients. In patients with chronic kidney disease and hypertension, use of an ACE-I/ARB is recommended. Finally, in patients presenting with BP >15mm Hg above goal, initiation with combination therapy should be considered.

Hispanics

There are more limited data about antihypertensive drug therapy in Hispanic patients. Subgroup analysis of the Hispanic participants in ALLHAT showed that Hispanics had a response to antihypertensive medications similar to non-Hispanics in terms of blood pressure lowering and cardiovascular outcomes [62, 63] **(Ib/A)**. Subgroup analysis of Hispanics enrolled in the INternational VErapamil SR/Trandolapril STudy (INVEST) trial (5017 Hispanic and 4710 non-Hispanic whites) showed that Hispanic patients achieved better blood pressure control, and were at significantly lower risk of experiencing a non-fatal myocardial infarction, non-fatal stroke, or death (hazard ratio [HR] 0.87, 95% CI 0.78-0.97) compared to non-Hispanic patients [64, 65] **(Ib/A)**. Pending further studies, it seems reasonable to follow current guidelines for choice of drug therapy based on the presence of co-existent conditions in this patient population [24].

Asians

While there are limited data specifically evaluating blood pressure lowering and long-term outcomes in Asian, native American or Pacific Islander populations [66, 67], it is thought that response to antihypertensive drugs is similar in Asians and Caucasians/whites [68]. Retrospective studies suggest that East Asians are more likely to develop an ACE-I cough compared with other racial ethnic groups [69].

Conclusions

In summary, hypertension can be managed effectively in minorities like in other groups with a combination of dietary and lifestyle modifications, exercise and pharmacotherapy. Though there are limited data, efficacy and side effects of antihypertensive drug therapy may vary in some minority populations. The ultimate goal of treatment of hypertension remains the same – achieving and maintaining blood pressure goal to lower long-term risks of cardiovascular and renal outcomes.

Key points	Evidence level
◆ Goal blood pressure for most patients with hypertension is less than 140/90mm Hg (<130/80mm Hg in patients with diabetes and with chronic kidney disease) regardless of race/ethnicity.	I/A
◆ Lifestyle modification is an important adjunct in the management of hypertension.	I/A
◆ Thiazide diuretics are the preferred initial choice for most African American patients with essential hypertension.	I/A
◆ RAS inhibitors are preferred in hypertensive patients with chronic kidney disease.	I/A
◆ Combination therapy should be considered in patients presenting with BP >20/10mm Hg than goal.	IV/C

References

1. Rahman M, Wright JT, Jr. Treatment of hypertension in minorities. In: *Hypertension Primer.* Izzo JL, Jr., Sica D, Black HR, Eds. Philadelphia: Lippincott Williams and Wilkins, 2008.
2. Cutler JA, Sorlie PD, Wolz M, Thom T, Fields LE, Roccella EJ. Trends in hypertension prevalence, awareness, treatment, and control rates in United States adults between 1988-1994 and 1999-2004. *Hypertension* 2008; 52(5): 818-27.
3. Ferdinand KC. Hypertension in minority populations. *J Clin Hypertens* (Greenwich) 2006; 8(5): 365-8.
4. Giles T, Aranda JM, Jr., Suh DC, Choi IS, Preblick R, Rocha R, *et al.* Ethnic/racial variations in blood pressure awareness, treatment, and control. *J Clin Hypertens* (Greenwich) 2007; 9(5): 345-54.
5. Rahman M, Douglas JG, Wright JT, Jr. Pathophysiology and treatment implications of hypertension in the African-American population. *Endocrinol Metab Clin North Am* 1997; 26(1): 125-44.
6. Choi AI, Rodriguez RA, Bacchetti P, Bertenthal D, Hernandez GT, O'Hare AM. White/black racial differences in risk of end-stage renal disease and death. *Am J Med* 2009; 122(7): 672-8.
7. Smith SC, Jr., Clark LT, Cooper RS, Daniels SR, Kumanyika SK, Ofili E, *et al.* Discovering the full spectrum of cardiovascular disease: Minority Health Summit 2003: report of the Obesity, Metabolic Syndrome, and Hypertension Writing Group. *Circulation* 2005; 111(10): e134-9.
8. Primatesta P, Bost L, Poulter NR. Blood pressure levels and hypertension status among ethnic groups in England. *J Hum Hypertens* 2000; 14(2): 143-8.
9. McWilliams JM, Meara E, Zaslavsky AM, Ayanian JZ. Differences in control of cardiovascular disease and diabetes by race, ethnicity, and education: U.S. trends from 1999 to 2006 and effects of medicare coverage. *Ann Intern Med* 2009; 150(8): 505-15.
10. Havas S, Fujimoto W, Close N, McCarter R, Keller J, Sherwin R. The NHLBI workshop on Hypertension in Hispanic Americans, Native Americans, and Asian/Pacific Islander Americans. *Public Health Rep* 1996; 111(5): 451-8.
11. Hicks LS, Shaykevich S, Bates DW, Ayanian JZ. Determinants of racial/ethnic differences in blood pressure management among hypertensive patients. *BMC Cardiovasc Disord* 2005; 5(1): 16.
12. Mathavan A, Chockalingam A, Chockalingam S, Bilchik B, Saini V. Madurai Area Physicians Cardiovascular Health Evaluation Survey (MAPCHES) - an alarming status. *Can J Cardiol* 2009; 25(5): 303-8.
13. Agyemang C, Bhopal RS. Is the blood pressure of South Asian adults in the UK higher or lower than that in European white adults? A review of cross-sectional data. *J Hum Hypertens* 2002; 16(11): 739-51.
14. Bhopal R, Unwin N, White M, Yallop J, Walker L, Alberti KG, *et al.* Heterogeneity of coronary heart disease risk factors in Indian, Pakistani, Bangladeshi, and European origin populations: cross-sectional study. *BMJ* 1999; 319(7204): 215-20.
15. Gupta R. Trends in hypertension epidemiology in India. *J Hum Hypertens* 2004; 18(2): 73-8.
16. Eapen D, Kalra GL, Merchant N, Arora A, Khan BV. Metabolic syndrome and cardiovascular disease in South Asians. *Vasc Health Risk Manag* 2009; 5: 731-43.
17. Venkataraman R, Nanda NC, Baweja G, Parikh N, Bhatia V. Prevalence of diabetes mellitus and related conditions in Asian Indians living in the United States. *Am J Cardiol* 2004; 94(7): 977-80.
18. Enas EA, Garg A, Davidson MA, Nair VM, Huet BA, Yusuf S. Coronary heart disease and its risk factors in first-generation immigrant Asian Indians to the United States of America. *Indian Heart J* 1996; 48(4): 343-53.
19. Mardikar HM, Deo D, Deshpande NV, Mukherjee D. Current perspectives on hypertension in Asian Indians. *Current Hypertension Reviews* 2007; 3(4): 264-9.
20. de Court, Pettitt DJ, Knowler WC. Hypertension in Pima Indians: prevalence and predictors. *Public Health Rep* 1996; 111 Suppl 2: 40-3.
21. Barnes PM, Adams PF, Powell-Griner E. Health characteristics of the Asian adult population: United States, 2004-2006. *Adv Data* 2008; (394): 1-22.
22. Aluli NE, Jones KL, Reyes PW, Brady SK, Tsark JU, Howard BV. Diabetes and cardiovascular risk factors in Native Hawaiians. *Hawaii Med J* 2009; 68(7): 152-7.
23. Curb JD, Aluli NE, Kautz JA, Petrovitch H, Knutsen SF, Knutsen R, *et al.* Cardiovascular risk factor levels in ethnic Hawaiians. *Am J Public Health* 1991; 81(2): 164-7.
24. Chobanian AV, Bakris GL, Black HR, Cushman WC, Green LA, Izzo JL, Jr., *et al.* The Seventh Report of the Joint National Committee on Prevention, Detection, Evaluation, and Treatment of High Blood Pressure: the JNC 7 report. *JAMA* 2003; 289(19): 2560-72.

25. Khan NA, Hemmelgarn B, Herman RJ, Bell CM, Mahon JL, Leiter LA, *et al.* The 2009 Canadian Hypertension Education Program recommendations for the management of hypertension: Part 2 - therapy. *Can J Cardiol* 2009; 25(5): 287-98.
26. Williams B. The changing face of hypertension treatment: treatment strategies from the 2007 ESH/ESC hypertension guidelines. *J Hypertens* 2009; 27 Suppl 3: S19-26.
27. King DE, Mainous AG, III, Carnemolla M, Everett CJ. Adherence to healthy lifestyle habits in US adults, 1988-2006. *Am J Med* 2009; 122(6): 528-34.
28. Appel LJ, Giles TD, Black HR, Izzo JL, Jr., Materson BJ, Oparil S, *et al.* ASH Position Paper: dietary approaches to lower blood pressure. *J Clin Hypertens* (Greenwich) 2009; 11(7): 358-68.
29. Swift PA, Markandu ND, Sagnella GA, He FJ, MacGregor GA. Modest salt reduction reduces blood pressure and urine protein excretion in black hypertensives: a randomized control trial. *Hypertension* 2005; 46(2): 308-12.
30. He FJ, Marciniak M, Visagie E, Markandu ND, Anand V, Dalton RN, *et al.* Effect of modest salt reduction on blood pressure, urinary albumin, and pulse wave velocity in white, black, and Asian mild hypertensives. *Hypertension* 2009; 54(3): 482-8.
31. Ford ES. Race, education, and dietary cations: findings from the Third National Health And Nutrition Examination Survey. *Ethn Dis* 1998; 8(1): 10-20.
32. Whelton PK, He J, Cutler JA, Brancati FL, Appel LJ, Follmann D, *et al.* Effects of oral potassium on blood pressure. Meta-analysis of randomized controlled clinical trials. *JAMA* 1997; 277(20): 1624-32.
33. Appel LJ, Brands MW, Daniels SR, Karanja N, Elmer PJ, Sacks FM. Dietary approaches to prevent and treat hypertension: a scientific statement from the American Heart Association. *Hypertension* 2006; 47(2): 296-308.
34. Svetkey LP, Simons-Morton D, Vollmer WM, Appel LJ, Conlin PR, Ryan DH, *et al.* Effects of dietary patterns on blood pressure: subgroup analysis of the Dietary Approaches to Stop Hypertension (DASH) randomized clinical trial. *Arch Intern Med* 1999; 159(3): 285-93.
35. Sacks FM, Svetkey LP, Vollmer WM, Appel LJ, Bray GA, Harsha D, *et al.* Effects on blood pressure of reduced dietary sodium and the Dietary Approaches to Stop Hypertension (DASH) diet. DASH-Sodium Collaborative Research Group. *N Engl J Med* 2001; 344(1): 3-10.
36. Whelton SP, Chin A, Xin X, He J. Effect of aerobic exercise on blood pressure: a meta-analysis of randomized, controlled trials. *Ann Intern Med* 2002; 136(7): 493-503.
37. Neter JE, Stam BE, Kok FJ, Grobbee DE, Geleijnse JM. Influence of weight reduction on blood pressure: a meta-analysis of randomized controlled trials. *Hypertension* 2003; 42(5): 878-84.
38. Calhoun DA, Jones D, Textor S, Goff DC, Murphy TP, Toto RD, *et al.* Resistant hypertension: diagnosis, evaluation, and treatment: a scientific statement from the American Heart Association Professional Education Committee of the Council for High Blood Pressure Research. *Circulation* 2008; 117(25): e510-26.
39. Xin X, He J, Frontini MG, Ogden LG, Motsamai OI, Whelton PK. Effects of alcohol reduction on blood pressure: a meta-analysis of randomized controlled trials. *Hypertension* 2001; 38(5): 1112-7.
40. Light KC, Girdler SS, Sherwood A, Bragdon EE, Brownley KA, West SG, *et al.* High stress responsivity predicts later blood pressure only in combination with positive family history and high life stress. *Hypertension* 1999; 33(6): 1458-64.
41. Calhoun DA. Hypertension in blacks: socioeconomic stress and sympathetic nervous system activity. *Am J Med Sci* 1992; 304(5): 306-11.
42. Davis SK, Liu Y, Quarells RC, Din-Dzietharn R. Stress-related racial discrimination and hypertension likelihood in a population-based sample of African Americans: the Metro Atlanta Heart Disease Study. *Ethn Dis* 2005; 15(4): 585-93.
43. Alexander CN, Schneider RH, Staggers F, Sheppard W, Clayborne BM, Rainforth M, *et al.* Trial of stress reduction for hypertension in older African Americans. II. Sex and risk subgroup analysis. *Hypertension* 1996; 28(2): 228-37.
44. Kondwani KA, Lollis CM. Is there a role for stress management in reducing hypertension in African Americans? *Ethn Dis* 2001; 11(4): 788-92.
45. Schneider RH, Staggers F, Alxander CN, Sheppard W, Rainforth M, Kondwani K, *et al.* A randomised controlled trial of stress reduction for hypertension in older African Americans. *Hypertension* 1995; 26(5): 820-7.
46. Douglas JG, Bakris GL, Epstein M, Ferdinand KC, Ferrario C, Flack JM, *et al.* Management of high blood pressure in African Americans: consensus statement of the Hypertension in African Americans Working Group of the International Society on Hypertension in Blacks. *Arch Intern Med* 2003; 163(5): 525-41.

47. Racial differences in response to low-dose captopril are abolished by the addition of hydrochlorothiazide. *Br J Clin Pharmacol* 1982; 14 Suppl 2: 97S-101S.
48. Materson BJ, Reda DJ, Cushman WC, Massie BM, Freis ED, Kochar MS, *et al.* Single-drug therapy for hypertension in men. A comparison of six antihypertensive agents with placebo. The Department of Veterans Affairs Cooperative Study Group on Antihypertensive Agents. *N Engl J Med* 1993; 328(13): 914-21.
49. Seedat YK. Varying responses to hypotensive agents in different racial groups: black versus white differences. *J Hypertens* 1989; 7(7): 515-8.
50. Sica D. Optimizing hypertension and vascular health: focus on ethnicity. *Clin Cornerstone* 2004; 6(4): 28-38.
51. Miller DR, Oliveria SA, Berlowitz DR, Fincke BG, Stang P, Lillienfeld DE. Angioedema incidence in US veterans initiating angiotensin-converting enzyme inhibitors. *Hypertension* 2008; 51(6): 1624-30.
52. Brewster LM, van Montfrans GA, Kleijnen J. Systematic review: antihypertensive drug therapy in black patients. *Ann Intern Med* 2004; 141(8): 614-27.
53. Sehgal AR. Overlap between whites and blacks in response to antihypertensive drugs. *Hypertension* 2004; 43(3): 566-72.
54. Major outcomes in high-risk hypertensive patients randomized to angiotensin-converting enzyme inhibitor or calcium channel blocker vs diuretic: the Antihypertensive and Lipid-Lowering Treatment to Prevent Heart Attack Trial (ALLHAT). *JAMA* 2002; 288(23): 2981-97.
55. Wright JT, Jr., Dunn JK, Cutler JA, Davis BR, Cushman WC, Ford CE, *et al.* Outcomes in hypertensive black and nonblack patients treated with chlorthalidone, amlodipine, and lisinopril. *JAMA* 2005; 293(13): 1595-608.
56. Wright JT, Jr., Harris-Haywood S, Pressel S, Barzilay J, Baimbridge C, Bareis CJ, *et al.* Clinical outcomes by race in hypertensive patients with and without the metabolic syndrome: Antihypertensive and Lipid-Lowering Treatment to Prevent Heart Attack Trial (ALLHAT). *Arch Intern Med* 2008; 168(2): 207-17.
57. Wright JT, Jr., Bakris G, Greene T, Agodoa LY, Appel LJ, Charleston J, *et al.* Effect of blood pressure lowering and antihypertensive drug class on progression of hypertensive kidney disease: results from the AASK trial. *JAMA* 2002; 288(19): 2421-31.
58. Wright JT, Jr., Agodoa L, Contreras G, Greene T, Douglas JG, Lash J, *et al.* Successful blood pressure control in the African American Study of Kidney Disease and Hypertension. *Arch Intern Med* 2002; 162(14): 1636-43.
59. Appel LJ, Wright JT, Jr., Greene T, Kusek JW, Lewis JB, Wang X, *et al.* Long-term effects of renin-angiotensin system-blocking therapy and a low blood pressure goal on progression of hypertensive chronic kidney disease in African Americans. *Arch Intern Med* 2008; 168(8): 832-9.
60. Cooper LA, Roter DL, Bone LR, Larson SM, Miller ER, III, Barr MS, *et al.* A randomized controlled trial of interventions to enhance patient-physician partnership, patient adherence and high blood pressure control among ethnic minorities and poor persons: study protocol NCT00123045. *Implement Sci* 2009; 4: 7.
61. Dolor RJ, Yancy WS, Jr., Owen WF, Matchar DB, Samsa GP, Pollak KI, *et al.* Hypertension Improvement Project (HIP): study protocol and implementation challenges. *Trials* 2009; 10: 13.
62. Einhorn PT, Davis BR, Massie BM, Cushman WC, Piller LB, Simpson LM, *et al.* The Antihypertensive and Lipid-Lowering Treatment to Prevent Heart Attack Trial (ALLHAT) Heart Failure Validation Study: diagnosis and prognosis. *Am Heart J* 2007; 153(1): 42-53.
63. Margolis KL, Piller LB, Ford CE, Henriquez MA, Cushman WC, Einhorn PT, *et al.* Blood pressure control in Hispanics in the Antihypertensive and Lipid-Lowering Treatment to Prevent Heart Attack Trial. *Hypertension* 2007; 50(5): 854-61.
64. Cooper-DeHoff RM, Aranda JM, Jr., Gaxiola E, Cangiano JL, Garcia-Barreto D, Conti CR, *et al.* Blood pressure control and cardiovascular outcomes in high-risk Hispanic patients - findings from the International Verapamil SR/Trandolapril Study (INVEST). *Am Heart J* 2006; 151(5): 1072-9.
65. Cooper-DeHoff RM, Zhou Q, Gaxiola E, Cangiano JL, Garcia-Barreto D, Handberg E, *et al.* Influence of Hispanic ethnicity on blood pressure control and cardiovascular outcomes in women with CAD and hypertension: findings from INVEST. *J Womens Health* (Larchmt) 2007; 16(5): 632-40.
66. Liu Y, Jia J, Liu G, Li S, Lu C, Liu Y, *et al.* Pharmacokinetics and bioequivalence evaluation of two formulations of 10-mg amlodipine besylate: an open-label, single-dose, randomized, two-way crossover study in healthy Chinese male volunteers. *Clin Ther* 2009; 31(4): 777-83.
67. Chia YC, Yeoh ES, Ng CJ, Khoo EM, Chua CT. Efficacy and tolerability of lercanidipine in mild to moderate hypertension among Asians of different ethnic groups. *Singapore Med J* 2009; 50(5): 500-5.
68. Khan JM, Beevers DG. Management of hypertension in ethnic minorities. *Heart* 2005; 91(8): 1105-9.
69. Morimoto T, Gandhi TK, Fiskio JM, Seger AC, So JW, Cook EF, *et al.* An evaluation of risk factors for adverse drug events associated with angiotensin-converting enzyme inhibitors. *J Eval Clin Pract* 2004; 10(4): 499-509.

Chapter 10

Treatment of hypertension in patients with ischemic heart disease

R. Michael Benitez MD FACC
Associate Professor of Medicine
University of Maryland School of Medicine
Maryland, USA

Introduction

Hypertension is a major independent risk factor for the development of ischemic heart disease (IHD), and data from the Framingham Heart Study supports a multiplicative interrelationship with other major risk factors, such as diabetes, smoking, and hyperlipidemia. The mechanisms by which hypertension increases the risks of ischemic coronary events may include impairment of endothelial function, increased oxidative stress, increased endothelial lipid permeability, as well as hemodynamic stress. Randomized trials have demonstrated that lowering blood pressure (BP) can rapidly reduce cardiovascular risk [1], with a sustained drop of 10mm Hg leading up to a 40-50% reduction in risk. There are, however, a number of controversies regarding the use of antihypertensives in patients with IHD. Within this chapter, we will address the evidence regarding some of these issues, including:

- what should the target goals of treatment be in patients with chronic IHD?
- are specific antihypertensive agents preferable in patients with IHD?
- how do these apply to special IHD populations, such as:

    - patients with acute coronary syndromes?
    - patients with left ventricular dysfunction?

Treatment goal – ischemic heart disease

The goals of antihypertensive therapy in patients with IHD include the prevention of death, myocardial infarction, stroke, and reduction of the frequency and severity of angina. To date, however, few clinical trials have been specifically designed to demonstrate the optimal goal of antihypertensive therapy in patients with IHD. The Seventh Report of the Joint National Committee on Prevention, Detection, Evaluation, and Treatment of High Blood Pressure (JNC 7) [2] supports a goal of <140/90mm Hg, or <130/80mm Hg in patients with diabetes or chronic kidney disease. The European Society of Cardiology, in a task force statement on the management of stable angina [3], has suggested pharmacologic therapy for patients with established IHD at the level of 130/85mm Hg. The American Heart Association advocates the goal of 130/80mm Hg for all patients with IHD [4], or IHD 'equivalents' (carotid artery disease, peripheral arterial disease, or abdominal aortic aneurysm) with a 'Class IIa indication' – a classification that inherently recognizes conflicting evidence and divergence of opinion. In fact, data from a meta-analysis of prospective studies evaluating the age-specific relevance of 'usual' blood pressure to vascular mortality demonstrated that risk for fatal IHD is elevated at levels that many clinicians would consider 'normal' [5] **(Ia/A)**. In this robust study that included nearly 1 million adults, blood pressure was associated with ischemic death over a range from 115/75mm Hg to 185/115mm Hg, with a doubling of risk for each 20mm Hg of systolic pressure (Figure 1). Despite this type of large volume data, there has been continued concern about the possible deleterious effects of lowering diastolic blood pressure too aggressively, principally due to a theoretic reduction in coronary blood flow. Such a 'J'-type mortality curve (with respect to decrease in blood pressure) is predicated upon a reduction in diastolic coronary flow in patients with either fixed atherosclerotic disease (and loss of coronary blood flow reserve), or the reduction of a diastolic pressure gradient to below the auto-regulatory threshold of normal endothelium.

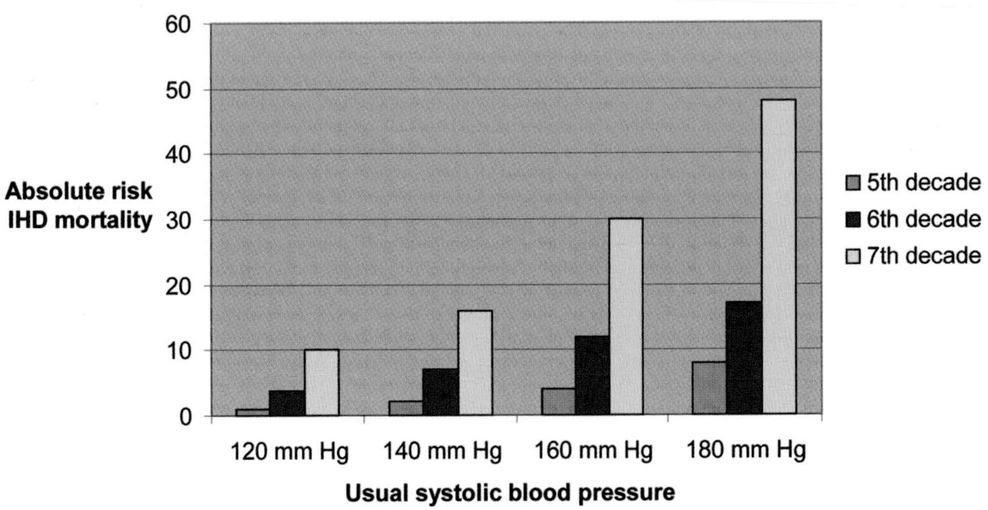

Figure 1. Ischemic heart disease (IHD) mortality as a function of age and systolic blood pressure. *Adapted from Lewington S, et al* [5].

The INVEST trial enrolled 22,000 patients with a history of hypertension and coronary artery disease [6] **(Ib/A)**. In this international trial of verapamil (plus trandolapril as needed) versus atenolol (plus HCTZ if needed), diastolic blood pressure <70mm Hg was associated with an increased risk of myocardial infarction. However, this group of subjects also tended to be older, with a higher incidence of prior MI, bypass, percutaneous coronary intervention, diabetes, heart failure and cancer. These confounding variables make conclusions difficult with respect to the effects of diastolic blood pressure. Within the Systolic Hypertension in the Elderly trial (SHEP), lowering diastolic blood pressure to <55-60mm Hg resulted in an increase in myocardial infarction and total cardiovascular events [7] **(Ib/A)**. In the Hypertensive Optimal Treatment [8] trial, a J-curve relationship was observed with respect to diastolic blood pressure and myocardial infarction in the sub-group with coronary disease treated with a dihydropyridine calcium channel blocking agent when the diastolic blood pressure was lowered to <70mm Hg **(Ib/A)**. It should be noted, however, that diabetics within this study clearly benefited when the diastolic blood pressure was <80mm Hg. In light of the uncertain relationship between diastolic blood pressure, antihypertensives, and coronary events, both the JNC 7 and the AHA have advised caution especially in reducing diastolic blood pressure to <60mm Hg, and particularly in patients >60 years of age.

While trials discussed so far suggested the existence of the J-curve, they enrolled only patients with established hypertension, and therefore did not address patients with IHD defined by the JNC 7 as being 'pre-hypertensive' or 'normal', despite data that risk for ischemic death is increased within these groups. The CAMELOT trial specifically addressed the effect of antihypertensive medications on cardiovascular events in patients with coronary disease and 'normal' blood pressure [9] **(Ib/A)**. In this double-blind, randomized, 24-month trial, nearly 2000 patients with angiographically documented coronary disease were randomized to 10mg of amlodipine, 20mg of enalapril or placebo. The mean systolic pressure was 129mm Hg; the mean diastolic pressure was 77mm Hg. During follow-up, the mean blood pressure increased 0.7/0.6mm Hg in the placebo group, with a significant drop (versus placebo) of approximately 5.0/2.5mm Hg in the treatment arms. The primary outcome of cardiovascular events was defined as cardiovascular death, non-fatal infarction, resuscitated cardiac arrest, coronary revascularization, hospitalization for angina or heart failure, stroke or transient ischemic attack, or a new diagnosis of peripheral arterial disease. Subjects treated with amlodipine had significantly fewer cardiovascular events than did those receiving placebo. While there was no significant outcome difference between the two treatment arms, enalapril did not demonstrate a significant difference from placebo. These findings suggested that in patients with documented coronary artery disease, lowering the systolic blood pressure well below the 140mm Hg goal of JNC 7 is associated with a reduction in cardiovascular risk, and without evidence of a J-curve.

Within CAMELOT, 274 patients completed an intravascular ultrasound (IVUS) substudy, with IVUS at study entry and upon completion of 24 months of treatment or placebo. Not surprisingly, the placebo arm demonstrated significant progression of coronary atherosclerosis of the study period. However, compared with baseline the amlodipine arm showed no progression by IVUS. Within this sub-study, 76 subjects met the JNC 7 definition of 'normal' (SBP <120mm Hg and DBP <80mm Hg), 157 were categorized as 'pre-hypertensive' (SBP 120-139mm Hg or DBP 80-89mm Hg), and 41 were defined as 'hypertensive' (SBP >140mm Hg, or DBP >90mm Hg) [10]. There were no significant differences in atheroma volume at inception to the study. While the hypertensive group showed significant increase in atheroma volume over the 24-month study period, there was no significant difference in the 'pre-hypertensive' group. Astoundingly, there was regression of atheroma volume in the 'normotensive' group to a degree greater than that seen in prior trials of high-dose 'statins'. Additionally, 'pre-hypertensive' patients to 'normal' also demonstrated a significantly lower rate of progression of atheroma volume as compared with 'pre-hypertensives' who did not change. These findings suggest that progression of atherosclerosis is related to blood pressure levels with ranges that would not carry an indication for treatment according to current guidelines, and that the target for treatment may be much lower than previously espoused. Additionally, these studies suggested that lowering the systolic blood pressure to 'normal' targets was not associated with adverse outcomes.

Chronic ischemic heart disease – specific antihypertensive agents

The ACC/AHA, in their guidelines for the management of patients with chronic stable angina, have recommended β-blockers as first-line therapy [11]. There is little argument regarding the benefit of β-blockade in patients who have sustained a myocardial infarction, and a meta-analysis of over 24,000 patients in the pre-thrombolytic era demonstrated that β-blockade conferred a 23% reduction in mortality [12] **(Ia/A)**. This effect may be due to a reduction in arrhythmic sudden cardiac death, and a reduction in re-infarction, rather than an effect on blood pressure. This type of robust data, however, is not available for patients who have not incurred infarction, and there are reasons to believe that β-blockade may not be optimal as monotherapy within this cohort. β-blockers have potential side effects that may make them less than optimal for patients with IHD but without prior infarction. In a meta-analysis of 22 clinical hypertension trials in which subjects did not have diabetes at inception, the risk of new onset of diabetes was greatest in those receiving β-blockade and thiazide diuretics [13] **(Ia/A)**. It should be noted, however, that not all β-blockers necessarily share this trait, and in the GEMINI trial (Glycemic Effects in Diabetes Mellitus Carvedilol-Metoprolol Comparison in Hypertensives) [14], treatment of hypertensive diabetics with carvedilol did not increase the hemoglobin A1c (as metoprolol did) **(Ib/A)**. The increased risk for development of diabetes may, in part, be due to reduced metabolic activity and weight gain, which have been reported in some studies [15]. Interestingly, patients treated with metoprolol in GEMINI demonstrated significant weight gain, while those treated with carvedilol did not. Additionally, left ventricular hypertrophy (LVH) is an important and independent predictor of cardiovascular mortality, and regression of LVH has been shown to be associated with itinerant reduction in risk [16]. While antihypertensive agents that affect the renin-angiotensin-aldosterone cascade reduce myocardial collagen content, β-blockers do not [17]. This was borne out in the Losartan Intervention for Endpoint reduction study (LIFE)[18] **(Ib/A)**, which compared losartan with atenolol, and again in a meta-analysis in which β-blockers incurred the least LVH regression as compared with other antihypertensive classes[19] **(Ia/A)**.

Several large-scale trials involving patients considered to be 'high risk' for cardiovascular events have compared different antihypertensive treatment regimens. The Antihypertensive and Lipid-Lowering Treatment to Prevent Heart Attack Trial (ALLHAT) [20] randomized over 33,000 patients with hypertension and at least one other IHD risk factor to receive chlorthalidone, amlodipine, or lisinopril, with a mean follow-up of 4.9 years. While a priori documentation of IHD was not requisite, approximately half of the subjects in each arm had some documentation of atherosclerotic cardiovascular disease. The primary outcome of combined fatal IHD and non-fatal infarction, and a secondary outcome of all-cause mortality, did not differ significantly between the three groups, leading the authors to conclude that thiazide diuretics should be considered as first-line therapy, in part due to the lower cost **(Ib/A)**. We should be careful, however, about generalizing this study to all patients with IHD.

The Anglo-Scandinavian Cardiac Outcomes Trial (ASCOT) [21] enrolled a high-risk cohort of patients aged 40-79 who had hypertension and at least three additional risk factors for cardiovascular disease. Patients with prior myocardial infarction or currently treated angina pectoris were excluded from this study, however. Subjects were randomized to receive either amlodipine (plus perindopril as needed), or atenolol (with the addition of a thiazide diuretic if needed). While there was no significant difference in the primary composite endpoint of cardiac death and non-fatal infarction, subjects randomized to amlodipine had significantly lower rates of stroke, development of diabetes, total cardiovascular events and procedures, and all-cause mortality, leading to premature termination of the study **(Ib/A)**. An interesting sub-study of ASCOT, the Conduit Artery Function Evaluation (CAFÉ) study [22], examined the relationship in the two treatment arms between treated peripheral blood pressure and central aortic pressure, as derived from radial tonometry and pulse wave analysis. Despite similar brachial pressures between the two groups, central aortic pressure was consistently and significantly lower in the amlodipine treatment arm as compared with the group receiving atenolol.

The INVEST [23] trial enrolled 22,576 patients aged 50 and older, all of whom were hypertensive and had documented IHD. Subjects were randomized to receive either sustained release verapamil or atenolol, with trandolapril / HCTZ added as needed for further blood pressure control. The primary outcome was a combined endpoint of death, non-fatal infarction or non-fatal stroke. After a mean follow-up of 2.7 years per patient, there was no statistically significant difference between the two groups with regards to either the primary outcome or the efficacy of blood pressure control. The authors concluded that a verapamil-trandolapril strategy was as effective as atenolol-HCTZ **(Ib/A)**. However, the verapamil-trandoplapril group had a lower frequency of angina, and fewer new diagnoses of diabetes mellitus. We should note that most patients in this trial required combination therapy to meet blood pressure goal, which limits comparison of the efficacy of single agents.

Lastly, a recent meta-analysis [24] addressed cardiac events as a function of heart rate in nine randomized controlled trials evaluating β-blockers for treatment of hypertension in patients without prior infarction **(Ia/A)**. While the incidence of IHD within the analysis is not clear, the information from the study must give us pause with regards to the common assumption that β-blockers derive a cardioprotective effect related to heart rate. Within this meta-analysis, a lower heart rate was associated with a significantly greater risk for all-cause mortality, cardiovascular mortality, myocardial infarction, stroke, and heart failure.

Acute coronary syndromes / myocardial infarction

Following acute myocardial infarction, there is little controversy regarding the role of β-blockade, although their benefit is likely independent of blood pressure (Table 1). In a meta-analysis of trials enrolling over 24,000 patients in the pre-thrombolytic era the use of β-blockade post-infarction yielded a 23% reduction in long-term mortalilty [12], most likely related to prevention of re-infarction, and an anti-arrhythmic effect **(Ia/A)**. In large part because of this data, there have been a number of trials devoted to evaluating the impact of early β-blockade during ST segment elevation infarction (STEMI). In the second Thrombolysis in Myocardial Infarction [25] (TIMI) study, patients without significant rales, heart block or asthma were randomized to receive either immediate β-blockade intravenously, followed by oral

Table 1. Summary of major trials of β-blockers / calcium channel blockers in acute infarction.

Trial	MI-type	Study medication	Acute mortality benefit	Delayed mortality benefit	Type of study
TIMI - II	STEMI	Metoprolol	No	Yes	P/R/DB/PC
ISIS - I	STEMI	Atenolol	No	Yes	P/R/DB/PC
COMMIT	STEMI	Metoprolol	No	Yes	P/R/DB/PC
INTERCEPT	STEMI	Diltiazem	No	No	P/R/DB/PC
DAVIT - II	STEMI / NSTEMI	Verapamil	No	Yes	P/R/DB/PC
Diltiazem Reinfarction Study Group	NSTEMI	Diltiazem	No	No, but reduction in non-fatal events over 2 weeks. Signal of harm in patients with clinical CHF	P/R/DB/PC
HINT	NSTEMI	Regular release nifedipine vs. metoprolol	No	No. Signal of harm in patients receiving nifedipine	P/R/DB

P = prospective; R = randomized; DB = double-blind; PC = placebo-control

therapy, or delayed oral therapy only, beginning on day 6 post-infarction. While there was no mortality difference, those receiving immediate β-blockade demonstrated a significantly lower incidence of re-infarction and recurrent chest pain **(Ib/A)**. Similar findings were demonstrated in the first International Study of Infarct Survival (ISIS) [26] **(Ib/A)**. The COMMIT trial, performed in China, subsequently randomized patients with STEMI to immediate intravenous β-blockade, followed by oral therapy, versus placebo [27]. At discharge, neither the primary composite outcome of death, in-hospital re-infarction, or cardiac arrest, nor the all-cause mortality was reduced by metoprolol **(Ib/A)**. Similar to ISIS-1 and TIMI-IIB, the incidence of re-infarction was significantly reduced with the administration of β-blockade. The use of β-blockade in the setting of STEMI for the treatment of hypertension carries an AHA/ACC Class I indication ("there is evidence and/or general agreement that a given procedure or treatment is beneficial, useful, and effective"). In large part, these studies have been generalized to the therapy of non-ST segment myocardial infarction (NSTEMI), although there are no large randomized trials to specifically address this issue.

Calcium channel blockers have generally been disappointing in the treatment of STEMI. There have been no large-scale trials of dihydropyridine calcium channel blockers in STEMI. The non-dihydropyridine calcium channel blocker, diltiazem, has been studied in patients without clinical heart failure treated for STEMI with thrombolysis. In this trial, 874 patients were randomized to receive either sustained release diltiazem 300mg, or placebo, beginning within 4 days of infarction and continued for up to 6 months [28]. Diltiazem did not reduce the cumulative occurrence of cardiac death, non-fatal re-infarction, or refractory ischemia, but did reduce a composite endpoint of non-fatal cardiac events, especially the need for myocardial revascularization **(Ib/A)**. Calcium channel blocking agents have been studied more rigorously in the setting of NSTEMI. The rate-limiting calcium channel blocker, diltiazem, was compared with placebo in the treatment of 576 patients who presented with NSTEMI [29]. Over a 2-week follow-up period, there was no difference in mortality, but diltiazem significantly reduced the risks of recurrent infarction and severe recurrent angina. Of note, sub-group analysis suggested that patients with clinical evidence of heart failure fared worse with the addition of calcium channel blockade **(Ib/A)**. In the Danish Verapamil Infarction Trial (DAVIT) [30] II, patients with myocardial infarction, but without congestive heart failure, were randomized to verapamil versus placebo and followed for a mean of 18 months. There was a significant reduction in mortality for patients receiving verapamil as compared with placebo in this trial **(Ib/A)**. The HINT [31] trial compared the use of regular release nifedipine with metoprolol in patients hospitalized for acute infarction, and demonstrated a potential increase in mortality in patients treated with this dihydropyridine calcium channel blocking agent **(Ib/A)**. The ACC/AHA have recommended β-blockers as first-line therapy for the treatment of hypertension in the setting of NSTEMI, with the use of non-dihydropyridine calcium channel blockers reserved for patients with contraindications to β-blockade who do not have left ventricular systolic dysfunction.

Hypertension, ischemic disease, and left ventricular dysfunction

Patients with left ventricular systolic dysfunction and symptoms of heart failure have been studied extensively, and there is little controversy regarding the survival benefit afforded to these patients by vasodilator therapy. Specifically, V-Heft-I [32] (the first Veteran's

Administration co-operative heart failure trial) demonstrated a significant reduction in mortality in New York Heart Association Class II-III heart failure patients with LVEF <0.40 with the use of a combination of hydralazine and nitrates **(Ib/A)**. V-Heft-II [33] demonstrated significantly better survival with enalapril as compared to this treatment regimen **(Ib/A)**. Similar findings were demonstrated with the use of ACE inhibition in the Studies of Left Ventricular Dysfunction (SOLVD) [34], and patients with Class IV NYHA CHF were found to have significant benefit with ACE inhibition in the CONSENSUS [35] trial **(both Ib/A)**. As powerful as these trials have been, we should recognize that they were focused solely on heart failure, included non-ischemic subjects, and that hypertension was not requisite for entry.

Several studies involving ACE inhibition have specifically enrolled subjects post-myocardial infarction, although hypertension was not necessary for entry. In the Acute Infarction Ramipril Efficacy study (AIRE) [36], subjects were randomized to receive either ramipril or placebo and were followed for an average of 15 months. All-cause mortality was reduced by 17% in the treatment arm **(Ib/A)**. In the TRACE [37] study (Trandolapril Cardiac Evaluation), patients with acute myocardial infarction and LVEF <0.35 were randomized to receive either trandolapril or placebo. Long-term treatment with trandolapril significantly reduced the risk of overall mortality, mortality from cardiovascular causes, sudden death, and the development of severe heart failure in patients with recent acute myocardial infarction and heart failure **(Ib/A)**.

Angiotensin receptor blockers have been rigorously studied in patients with heart failure and left ventricular dysfunction, and studies such as CHARM [38] (Candesartan in Heart Failure: Assessment of Reduction of Mortality and Morbidity), have demonstrated that for patients who can not tolerate an ACE-I, that the use of an ARB is associated with a significant reduction in cardiovascular death **(Ib/A)**. However, as with ACE inhibitors, there has not been a major randomized trial of patients with hypertension and ischemic left ventricular dysfunction.

In patients with left ventricular dysfunction, non-dihydropyridine calcium channel blockers should be avoided, as there has been no convincing demonstration of benefit, and there is potential for harm given the negative inotropic effects of these agents **(IV/C)**. The dihydropyridine calcium channel blocker, amlodipine, has been studied in patients with heart failure (including advanced heart failure) and appears to be safe [39] **(Ib/A)**.

There have been multiple, large-scale, randomized trials of β-blockers in the heart failure population, although these trials did not specifically enroll only patients with hypertension and ischemic LV dysfunction. Nevertheless, we should note the 34% reduction in mortality with metoprolol versus placebo in MERIT-HF[40], the 38% reduction in death with carvedilol versus placebo in the COPERNICUS [41] trial, and the 32% reduction in all-cause mortality with bisoprolol versus placebo in CIBIS-II [42]. Based upon this data, the use of a β-blocker should be strongly considered as part of a treatment regimen for hypertension in patients with ischemic LV dysfunction **(Ib/A)**.

Conclusions

Hypertension is a major risk factor for the development of ischemic heart disease, and treatment within our country currently misses a large population at risk. While the standard goals established by JNC 7 are reasonable starting points, current data suggest that the risks for development of ischemic heart disease might be reduced even further by much more aggressive goals, as the risks appear to increase above systolic blood pressure levels that have long been considered 'normal'. While there has been concern regarding adverse effects on coronary perfusion pressure, this has not been demonstrated in all studies, is debatable, and may be linked to the degree of coronary occlusion.

While β-blockers are a common choice as initial therapy in patients with ischemic heart disease, there is little data to support their superiority as monotherapy in patients with preserved left ventricular systolic function who have not suffered a myocardial infarction. Since many of these patients will require more than one drug to reach goal, especially if more stringent goals are applied, it seems prudent to include a β-blocker as part of a multi-therapeutic approach. There is, however, firm evidence to support the use of a β-blocker in patients with myocardial infarction.

Large-scale randomized trials have not specifically addressed hypertension in patients with ischemic left ventricular dysfunction. However, robust mortality data from multiple large-scale randomized trials form a compelling reason to use either an ACE inhibitor or an angiotensin receptor blocking agent as part of the medical regimen. Similar data strongly support the use of a β-blocking agent within this cohort. The strength of data for use of a β-blocking agent in the treatment of ischemic heart disease is most supportive in the setting of the complicated patient with prior infarction, reduced systolic function, arrhythmias, or uncontrolled hypertension. Superiority of these agents is much more difficult to demonstrate in uncomplicated cases (Figure 2).

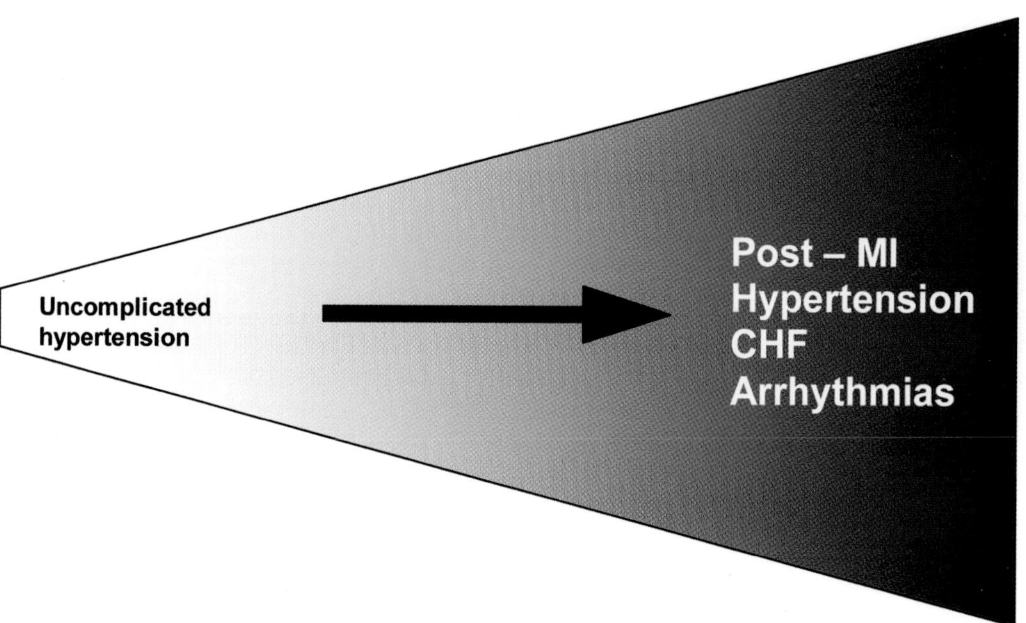

Figure 2. Evidence-based support for the use of β-blocking agents in ischemic heart disease. *Adapted from Bangalore S, et al* [43].

Key points	Evidence level
◆ Risk for fatal ischemic heart disease is related in a step-wise fashion to systolic blood pressure.	Ia/A
◆ Lowering diastolic blood pressure to <60mm Hg may be associated with worse outcomes in the elderly and those with ischemic heart disease.	Ib/A
◆ 'Pre-hypertensive' patients with ischemic heart disease may still benefit from reduction in systolic pressure.	Ib/A
◆ β-blocking agents reduce the risks of death and re-infarction in patients who have previously incurred an ST elevation myocardial infarction.	Ia/A
◆ Patients with hypertension and ischemic left ventricular dysfunction benefit from treatment with β-blocking agents and angiotensin converting enzyme inhibitors.	Ib/A

References

1. Neal B, MacMahon S, Chapman N. Blood Pressure Lowering Treatment Trialists' Collaboration. Effects of ACE inhibitors, calcium antagonists, and other blood-pressure lowering drugs: results of prospectively designed overviews of randomized trials. *Lancet* 2000; 356: 1955-64.
2. http://www.nhlbi.nih.gov/guidelines/hypertension/jnc7full.htm.
3. Guidelines on the management of stable angina pectoris: executive summary. The Task Force on the Management of Stable Angina Pectoris of the European Society of Cardiology. *Eur Heart J* 2006; 27: 1341-81.
4. Rosendorff C, Black H, Cannon C, *et al.* Treatment of hypertension in the prevention and management of ischemic heart disease. *Circulation* 2007; 115: 2761-88.
5. Lewington S, Clarke R, Qizilbash, N, Peto R, Collins R. Prospective studies collaboration. Age-specific relevance of usual blood pressure to vascular mortality: a meta-analysis of individual data for one million adults in 61 prospective studies. *Lancet* 2002; 360: 1903-13.
6. Pepine CJ, Handberg EM, Cooper-DeHoff RM, *et al.* A calcium antagonist vs a noncalcium antagonist hypertension treatment strategy for patients with coronary artery disease. The International Verapamil-Trandolapril Study (INVEST): a randomized controlled trial. *JAMA* 2003; 290: 2805-16.
7. Somes GW, Pahor M, Shorr, RI, Cushman WC, Applegate WB. The role of diastolic blood pressure when treating isolated systolic hypertension. *Arch Intern Med* 1999; 159: 2004-9.
8. Hansson L, Zanchetti A, Carruthers SG, *et al.* Effects of intensive blood-pressure lowering and low-dose aspirin in patients with hypertension. *Lancet* 1998; 351: 1755-62.
9. Nissen SE, Tuzcu EM, Libby P, *et al.* Effect of antihypertensive agents on cardiovascular events in patients with coronary disease and normal blood pressure. The CAMELOT study: a randomized controlled trial. *JAMA* 2004; 292: 2217-26.
10. Sipahi I, Tuzcu EM, Schoenhagen P, *et al.* Effects of normal, pre-hypertensive and hypertensive blood pressure levels on progression of atherosclerosis. *J Am Coll Cardiol* 2006; 48: 833-8.
11. Gibbons RJ, Chatterjee K, Daley J, *et al.* ACC/AHA/ACP-ASIM guidelines for the management of patients with chronic stable angina: a report of the American College of Cardiology / American Heart Association Task Force on Practice Guidelines (Committee on Management of Patients with Chronic Stable Angina). *J Am Coll Cardiol* 1999; 33: 2092-97.
12. Chae CU, Hennekens CH. Beta blockers. In: *Clinical Trials in Cardiovascular Disease: A companion to Braunwald's Heart Disease.* Hennekens CH, Ed. Philadelphia: WB Saunders, 1999: 76-94.

13. Elliot WJ, Meyer PM. Incident diabetes in clinical trials of antihypertensive drugs: a network meta-analysis. *Lancet* 2007; 369: 201-7.
14. Bakris GL, Fonseca V, Katholi RE, *et al.* Metabolic effects of carvedilol vs metoprolol in patients with type 2 diabetes mellitus and hypertension: a randomized controlled trial. *JAMA* 2004; 292: 2227-36.
15. Pischon T, Sharma AM. Use of beta-blockers in obesity hypertension: potential role of weight gain. *Obes Rev* 2001; 2: 275-80.
16. Okin PM, Devereaux RB, Jern S, *et al.* Regression of electrocardiographic left ventricular hypertrophy during antihypertensive treatment and the prediction of major cardiovascular events. *JAMA* 2004; 292: 2343-9.
17. Ciulla MM, Paliotti R, Esposito A, *et al.* Different effects of antihypertensive therapies based on losartan or atenolol on ultrasound and biochemical markers of myocardial fibrosis: results of a randomized trial. *Circulation* 2004; 110: 552-7.
18. Dahlof B, Devereux RB, Kjeldsen SE, *et al.* Cardiovascular morbidity and mortality in the Losartan Intervention For Endpoint reduction in hypertension study (LIFE): a randomised trial against atenolol. *Lancet* 2002; 359: 995-1003.
19. Dahlof B, Pennert K, Hansson L. Regression of left ventricular hypertrophy - a meta-analysis. *Clin Exp Hypertens A* 1992; 14: 173-80.
20. ALLHAT Officers and Coordinators for the ALLHAT Collaborative Research Group. The Antihypertensive and Lipid-Lowering Treatment to Prevent Heart Attack Trial. Major outcomes in high-risk hypertensive patients randomized to angiotensin-converting enzyme inhibitor or calcium channel blocker vs diuretic: The Antihypertensive and Lipid-Lowering Treatment to Prevent Heart Attack Trial (ALLHAT). *JAMA* 2002; 288: 2981-97.
21. Dahlof B, Sever PS, Poulter NR, *et al.* Prevention of cardiovascular events with an antihypertensive regimen of amlodipine adding perindopril as required versus atenolol adding bendroflumethiazide as required, in the Anglo-Scandinavian Cardiac Outcomes Trial-Blood Pressure Lowering Arm (ASCOT-BPLA): a multicentre randomised controlled trial. *Lancet* 2005; 366: 895-906.
22. Williams B, Lacy PS, Thorn SM, *et al.* Differential impact of blood pressure-lowering drugs on central aortic pressure and clinical outcomes. Principal results of the Conduit Artery Function Evaluation (CAFÉ) study. *Circulation* 2006; 113: 1213-25.
23. Pepine CJ, Handberg EM, Cooper-DeHoff RM, *et al.* A calcium antagonist vs a non-calcium antagonist hypertension treatment strategy for patients with coronary artery disease. The International Verapamil-Trandolapril Study (INVEST): a randomized controlled trial. *JAMA* 2003; 290: 2805-16.
24. Bangalore S, Sawhney S, Messerli FH. Relation of beta-blocker-induced heart rate lowering and cardioprotection in hypertension. *J Am Coll Cardiol* 2008; 52: 1482-9.
25. Roberts R, Rogers WJ, Mueller HS, *et al.* Immediate versus deferred β-blockade following thrombolytic therapy in patients with acute myocardial infarction. Results of the Thrombolysis in Myocardial Infarction (TIMI) II-B study. *Circulation* 1991; 83: 422-37.
26. First International Study of Infarct Survival Collaborative Group. Randomised trial of intravenous atenolol among 16,027 cases of suspected acute myocardial infarction: ISIS-1. *Lancet* 1986; 2: 57-66.
27. Chen ZM, Pan HC, Chen YP, *et al.* COMMIT Collaborative Group. Early intravenous then oral metoprolol in 45,852 patients with acute myocardial infarction: randomised placebo-controlled trial. *Lancet* 2005; 366: 1622-32.
28. Boden WE, van Gilst WH, Scheldewaert RG, *et al.* Diltiazem in acute myocardial infarction treated with thrombolytic agents: a randomised placebo-controlled trial: Incomplete Infarction Trial of European Research Collaborators Evaluating Prognosis post-Thrombolysis (INTERCEPT). *Lancet* 2000; 355: 1751-6.
29. Gibson RS, Boden WE, Theroux P, *et al.* Diltiazem and reinfarction in patients with non-Q wave myocardial infarction: results of a double-blind, randomized multicenter trial. *N Engl J Med* 1986; 315: 423-9.
30. The Danish Study Group on Verapamil in Myocardial Infarction. The effect of verapamil on mortality and major events after myocardial infarction. The Danish Verapamil Infarction Trial (DAVIT) II. *Am J Cardiol* 1990; 66: 779-85.
31. Early Treatment of Unstable Angina in the coronary care unit: a randomised, double blind, placebo controlled comparison of recurrent ischaemia in patients treated with nifedipine or metoprolol or both: report of the Holland Interuniversity Nifedipine/Metoprolol Trial (HINT) Research Group. *Br Heart J* 1986; 56: 400-13.
32. Cohn JN, Archibald DG, Ziesche S, *et al.* Effect of vasodilator therapy on mortality in chronic congestive heart failure. Results of a Veteran's Administration Cooperative Study. *N Engl J Med* 1986; 314(24): 1547-52.

33. Cohn JN, Johnson G, Ziesche S, *et al.* A comparison of enalapril with hydralazine - isosorbide dinitrate in the treatment of chronic congestive heart failure. *N Engl J Med* 1991; 325: 303-10.
34. The SOLVD Investigators. Effect of enalapril on survival in patients with reduced left ventricular ejection fractions and heart failure. *N Engl J Med* 1991; 325: 293-302.
35. The CONSENSUS Trial Study Group. Effects of enalapril on mortality in severe congestive heart failure. Results of the Cooperative North Scandinavian Enalapril Survival Study. *N Engl J Med* 1987; 316: 429-35.
36. Effect of ramipril on mortality and morbidity of survivors of acute myocardial infarction with clinical evidence of heart failure. The Acute Infarction Ramipril Efficacy (AIRE) Study Investigators. *Lancet* 1993; 342(8875): 821-8.
37. Kober L, Torp-Pederson C, Carlsen JE, *et al.* A clinical trial of the angiotensin-converting enzyme inhibitor trandolapril in patients with left ventricular dysfunction after myocardial infarction. Trandolapril Cardiac Evaluation (TRACE) Study Group. *N Engl J Med* 1995; 333: 1670-6.
38. Granger CB, McMurray JJ, Yusuf S, *et al.* Effects of candesartan in patients with chronic heart failure and reduced left ventricular function intolerant to angiotensin-converting-enzyme inhibitors: the CHARM-alternative trial. *Lancet* 2003; 362: 777-81.
39. O'Connor CM, Carson PE, Miller AB, *et al.* Effect of amlodipine on mode of death among patients with advanced heart failure in the PRAISE trial: Prospective Randomized Amlodipine Survivial Trial Evaluation. *Am J Cardiol* 1998; 82: 881-7.
40. MERIT-HF Study Group. Effect of metoprolol CR/XL in chronic heart failure: Metoprolol CR/XL Randomized Intervention Trial in Congestive Heart Failure (MERIT-HF). *Lancet* 1999; 353: 2001-7.
41. Packer M, Fowler MB, Roecker EB, *et al.* Carvedilol Prospective Randomized Cumulative Survival (COPERNICUS) Study Group. Effect of carvedilol on the morbidity of patients with severe chronic heart failure: results of the Carvedilol Prospective Randomized Cumulative Survival (COPERNICUS) Trial. *Circulation* 20002; 106: 2194-9.
42. CIBIS-II Investigators and Committees. The Cardiac Insufficiency Bisoprolol Study II (CIBIS-II): a randomised trial. *Lancet* 1999; 353: 9-13.
43. Bangalore S, Messerli FH, Kostis JB, Pepine CJ. Cardiovascular protection using beta-blockers. A critical review of the evidence. *J Am Coll Cardiol* 2007; 50: 563-72.

Chapter 11

Management of patients with left ventricular hypertrophy

Wallace R. Johnson, Jr, MD
Assistant Professor of Medicine
University of Maryland School of Medicine
Maryland, USA

Introduction

It has long been appreciated that hypertension has important structural and functional effects on the heart. In 1867, the great French physician, Auguste Laennec, described a relationship between cardiac hypertrophy and characteristics of the arterial circulation in noting [1]: "When affecting the left ventricle, I have seen its parietes more than an inch thick...the septum between the two ventricles becomes also notably thickened in the disease of the left ventricle...Symptoms are – a strong full pulse, strong and obvious pulsation of the heart...". Subsequently, the noted English clinician, Thomas Janeway, described congestive heart failure (CHF) as the manifestation of hypertensive cardiovascular disease [2]. Later, the relationship between hypertension and hypertrophy of the left ventricle was established in observations linking cardiac findings to the then new technique of indirect blood pressure (BP) measurement with sphygmomanometry.

Although left ventricular hypertrophy (LVH) was quickly associated with CHF, the relation of hypertension to cardiovascular morbidity and death is, in fact, complex. There is a complicated interplay between hypertension, atherosclerotic disease, diabetes, and abnormal lipid metabolism. Nonetheless, clinical and epidemiologic studies have convincingly demonstrated the independent predictive value of echocardiographically measured LVH for cardiovascular morbidity and mortality [3-5] and surrogate arrhythmic endpoints [6-8]. Measurement of LVH can be accomplished by a number of methods with the strengths and weaknesses of each noted in the following table (Table 1).

Table 1. LVH and clinical outcomes in hypertensive patients.

	ECG	M-mode echo-cardiography	2D echo-cardiography	Cardiac MRI
Sensitivity	Low	Moderate	High	High
Specificity	High	High	High	High
Cost	Low	Moderate	Moderate	High
Interpatient reproducibility	Moderate	Moderate	Moderate	High

Cardiac changes in hypertension: pathologic findings

Pathologic findings in hypertension have included increased left ventricular (LV) wall thickness, increased cardiac weight, perivascular and myocardial fibrosis, and increased myocyte diameter [9, 10]. Diabetes mellitus, which combines with hypertension in producing greater risk for CHF [11] and myocardial infarction (MI) [12] than would occur with either disease alone, also exacerbates the pathological effects of hypertension to a greater extent than would occur with either disease alone. Comparing autopsy findings in patients with hypertension, diabetes, and those with both diseases, it was found [10] that heart weight and fibrosis was greatest in diabetic hypertensive hearts. Moreover, findings of CHF were associated with the degree of myocardial fibrosis.

Prevalence of left ventricular hypertrophy in hypertension

The reported prevalence of LVH in hypertension [13-18] varies greatly, from about 10% to 60%, in part reflecting differences in study population (e.g. obesity, severity of hypertension) and criteria for LVH. In one of the earliest echocardiographic studies of LVH in hypertension, 51% of hypertensive participants (average systolic BP 150±20mm Hg in treated participants) in the Framingham cohort had LVH as defined by values of LV mass exceeding the 95% prediction interval derived from normotensive participants. Subsequently, investigators at Cornell [14], using cut-off values for LV mass of 110g/m^2 (body surface area [BSA]) in men and 134g/m^2 in women, found that 12% of borderline hypertensives and 20% of mild hypertensives had LVH. In the Treatment of Mild Hypertension Study [15] in which the mean systolic BP was 140±12mm Hg, the prevalence of LVH (Cornell criteria) was 13% in men and 20% in women. However, using criteria that adjust for height rather than BSA, and hence are more sensitive in the presence of obesity, the prevalence of LVH rose to 24% in men and 45% in women. Black participants did not have greater LV mass or prevalence of LVH than white participants.

In the Hypertension Genetic Epidemiology Network (HyperGen) study [17], which evaluated hypertensive members of sibships (two siblings with hypertension), many of whom were on treatment (with average BP 131/75mm Hg in overweight, 140/76mm Hg in obese subjects), the prevalence of LVH (Cornell criteria) was 14% in obese versus 19% in non-obese subjects. However, when body size was adjusted for by height [2, 7], the prevalence of LVH in non-obese versus obese subjects reversed to 20% and 32%, respectively. In a Veterans Affairs study [16] of 692 men with hypertension of somewhat greater severity than some other studies discussed here (average BP 150/100mm Hg), 63% met Framingham criteria and 46% met Cornell criteria for LVH. One study [18], which evaluated the relationship between hypertension control and LVH prevalence (Cornell criteria) in over 2000 participants, found a prevalence of 14% in untreated patients (average BP 148±16mm Hg), 19% in controlled hypertension (average systolic BP 128±8mm Hg) and 29% in uncontrolled patients (average systolic BP 158±19mm Hg). The take home message is that not all hypertensive patients get LVH, and conversely, all cases of LVH are not associated with elevated blood pressure **(Ia/A)**.

Left ventricular hypertrophy and risk

The importance of LVH in the morbidity of hypertensive disease has been underscored by the number of electrocardiographic and echocardiographic studies that have convincingly demonstrated its importance as a significant predictor of morbidity and mortality [3, 19-22] **(Ia/A)**. Not only does LVH, as a dichotomous variable, predict adverse outcome, but the magnitude of LV mass, as a continuous variable, is also associated with cardiovascular risk, even with values for LV mass within the normal range. In the Framingham Heart Study, it was shown [23] that, for each 50g/m^2 increase in LV mass (corrected for height), there was a relative risk for mortality of 1.73, even in subjects free of clinically apparent cardiovascular disease. It was also demonstrated that this risk was independent of blood pressure, age, antihypertensive treatment, and other cardiovascular risk factors **(Ia/A)**.

The close relationship between body size and LV mass in infancy and childhood decreases with age, possibly resulting from an increasing impact of hemodynamic factors on LV mass [24]. The amount of LV mass that exceeds what can be accounted for by body size and by hemodynamic load, has been termed inappropriate LV mass. Excess LV mass has shown prognostic value for cardiovascular events over and above that of traditional LV mass and predicts risk even in the absence of LVH defined in usual ways [25] **(Ib/A)**.

Additionally, the pattern of LVH and the magnitude of increase in LV mass are of importance in predicting the risk of LVH for cardiovascular morbidity (Figure 1). It has been reported [20] that individuals with a higher relative wall thickness at any value of LV mass,

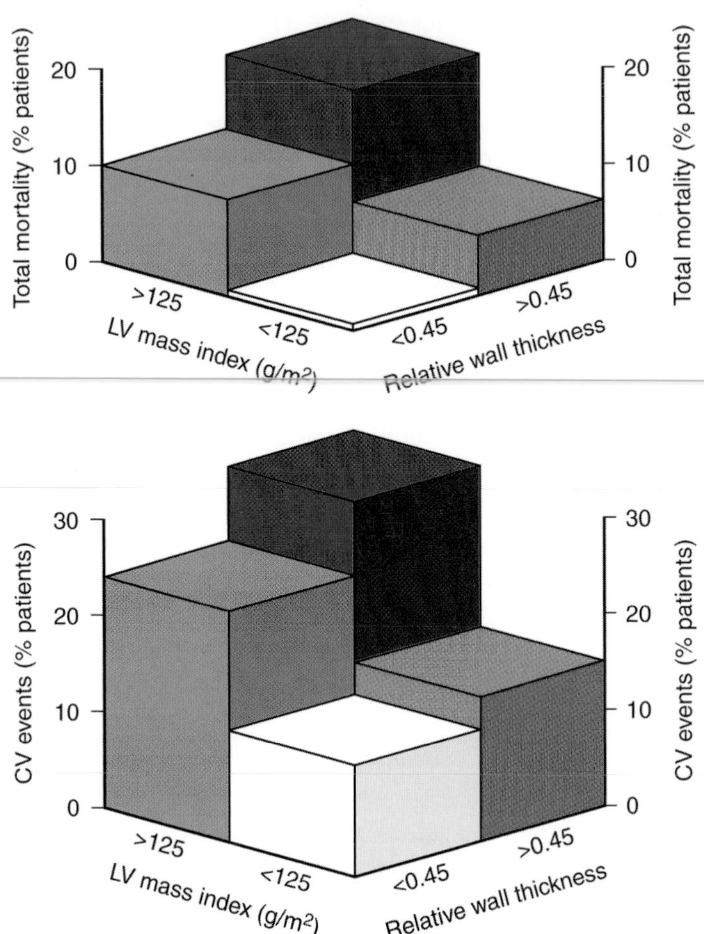

Figure 1. Relation of left ventricular (LV) architecture, left ventricular hypertrophy, and outcome. Increased mortality (top) and morbidity (bottom) are associated with increased relative wall thickness (>45) even in the absence of increased left ventricular mass (<125g/m^2), that is concentric remodeling. CV = cardiovascular. *Reproduced with permission from Koren MJ, et al* [20].

including values below the partition value for LVH (i.e. concentric remodeling) [20, 26], have greater risk of cardiovascular events. However, a more recent study [27] has suggested that the prognostic importance of concentric remodeling may not be independent of LV mass **(IIb/B)**.

Importantly, there is an association of LVH with complex ventricular arrhythmia, a possible precursor of sudden death in hypertensive patients, even in patients without coronary artery disease on angiography [8] **(Ib/A)**. In patients with reversible myocardial perfusion defects on thallium scintigraphy, both LVH and inducible ischemia are independently associated with ventricular arrhythmia [28] **(Ib/A)**. Research has also suggested that regression of LVH may be associated with reduction of arrhythmia [29] and improvement in electrophysiologic characteristics, such as QT dispersion [30], associated with arrhythmic risk **(Ib/A)**. Although there is comorbidity between hypertension, LVH, and coronary artery disease, LVH is nonetheless associated with an increase in mortality even in the absence of coronary disease on angiography [21] **(Ia/A)**.

Demographic and physiologic descriptors of left ventricular hypertrophy in hypertension

Although elevated blood pressure is considered an important factor promoting increase in LV mass and LVH, it has become clear that blood pressure only accounts for a portion of the observed variance in LV mass. Other clinical descriptors [15, 31-41] that have been implicated as contributing to LVH include obesity, age, race, dietary sodium intake, sleep apnea, insulin resistance, and other neurohormonal factors including adrenergic factors and the renin-angiotensin system (Table 2).

Table 2. Factors that affect left ventricular mass.

Demographic & physiologic variables	Hemodynamic workload	Non-hemodynamic factors
Age	Blood pressure	Renin-angiotensin system
Race	Vascular resistance or impedance	Parathyroid hormone
Gender	LV inotropy and geometry	Genetic susceptibility
Body size	Stress	Growth hormones
	Exercise	Salt intake
	Physiologic	Sleep apnea

Obesity and left ventricular hypertrophy

In the Framingham Heart Study [33, 34], which used echocardiography in a large population-based cohort, obesity measured by body mass index (BMI) or by skinfold thickness was associated with substantial increases in the prevalence of LVH in men. Although both hypertension and obesity were independently associated with LV mass and wall thickness, the associations were additive but not synergistic. Liebson and colleagues [15] noted that, in patients with mild hypertension and virtual absence of LVH on ECG, that body weight and body mass index were important predictors of LV wall thickness, LV mass, and hypertrophy on ECG.

In a study [16] of 692 male veterans with mild-moderate hypertension and a high prevalence (63% using Framingham criteria) of LVH, both LV wall thickness and LV cavity volume were greater in obese and overweight hypertensive men, than in those of normal weight **(Ib/A)**. Moreover, despite the importance of obesity in the cohort, even lean hypertensives with mild-moderate hypertension had a high prevalence of LVH in contrast to a previous study [36]. Also, relative wall thickness was equally increased in all adiposity groups.

However, in the Strong Heart Study, a population-based study of cardiovascular risk in American Indians, it was found [42] that LV mass was only marginally related to adipose mass, in contrast to having a stronger relationship with fat-free mass. Increases in LV mass in obesity might be a compensatory mechanism for increased workload. In a recent study of American Indian adolescents [43] from the Strong Heart Study, obese and overweight participants both had greater LV diameter, mass, and prevalence of LVH (34% and 12%, respectively) than those with normal weight (LVH=4%). However, there was a four-fold higher probability of obese adolescents having LV mass exceeding values compensatory for their cardiac workload, and this excess LV mass was associated with lower EF, myocardial contractility, and greater force developed by left atrium to complete LV filling. Obesity seems to have a complex but definite relationship to LVH **(Ib/A)**.

Race and left ventricular hypertrophy

The prevalence and severity of hypertension is greater in blacks than whites [44, 45], and ECG studies have suggested a greater prevalence of LVH (Figure 2) as well [46, 47]. An early echocardiographic study of a relatively small number of black and white hypertensives [48] found greater LV mass in blacks consequent to greater LV cavity size. However, possible racial differences in obesity, which is known to increase LV volume, were not controlled.

In the Jackson Heart Study [49], the prevalence of LVH (Framingham criteria) was as high as 83% in black women with diabetes, hypertension, and obesity and as low as 28% (still substantial) in black men without any of those risk factors. In contrast, the population-based prevalence of LVH in adults in the Framingham Heart Study [33], which had relatively few black participants but included hypertension and obesity, was 16% in men and 19% in women.

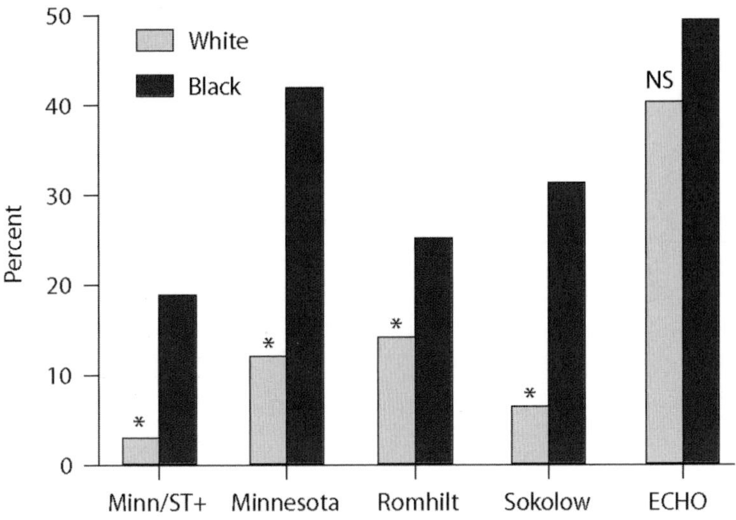

Figure 2. Influence of race on prevalence of left ventricular hypertrophy (LVH): echocardiographic (ECHO) versus various electrocardiographic criteria (Minnesota codes, Romhilt-Estes, Sokolow). Despite a statistically insignificant difference in LVH prevalence on echocardiogram, a markedly greater prevalence of LVH is present on electrocardiogram in black men with established hypertension with all criteria used (p=0.05 all comparisons). *Adapted from Gottdiener JS, et al* [16].

A recent population-based, cross-sectional study of 1439 African Americans in Jackson Mississippi [50] found that middle-aged African Americans with generalized and focal retinal arteriolar narrowing were more likely to have LVH. Retinal microvascular signs (other than diabetic retinopathy) were significantly associated with LVH, with an OR of 1.64 (95% CI 1.29-2.09) for generalized arteriolar narrowing; an OR of 1.82 (95% CI 1.33-2.50) for focal arteriolar narrowing; and an OR of 1.35 (95% CI 1.02-1.79) for AV nicking. Although this association was only partly explained by cardiovascular risk factors and hypertension, checking for retinal microvascular signs may prove to be a useful and cost effective way to select which patients may benefit from echocardiographic screening for suspected LVH **(III/B)**. Alternatively, hypertensive patients with pathological retinal microvascular signs could be selectively treated with antihypertensive therapy which has been proven to result in LVH regression or at least avoid drugs which tend to increase LVH such as direct vasodilators (III/B).

Other factors

Although theoretic and experimental observations in humans have indicated that inotropic properties of the left ventricle, LV geometry, and blood pressure are important in describing ideal LV mass [27, 31-41], non-hemodynamic factors remain an important consideration in the pathogenesis of LVH in human hypertension. Such considerations have included neurohumoral factors, genetic susceptibility, obstructive sleep apnea, neurobehavioral aspects, diet – particularly salt intake – and the interaction of hypertension with other pathologic processes, such as atherosclerosis and diabetes mellitus.

In support of the hypothesis that non-hemodynamic factors are an important consideration in the pathogenesis of left ventricular hypertrophy (LVH) related to human hypertension, both increased carotid intimal thickness and the presence of microalbuminuria have been associated with a higher prevalence of LVH (Table 3). A large number of investigators have established carotid intimal medial thickness and microalbuminuria as surrogate markers for cardiovascular outcomes. Further research will be needed to determine if carotid intimal medial thickness and microalbuminuria can be viewed as risk factors and/or strong indicators for which patients should be evaluated for the presence of LVH.

Renin-angiotensin system relation to left ventricular hypertrophy

Because angiotensin I and angiotensin II may stimulate myocardial protein synthesis [51, 52], and the renin-angiotensin system has been established as playing a role in some forms of hypertension, it is reasonable to suspect a direct link between the angiotensin-renin system and myocardial hypertrophy. Animal studies of regression of LVH in the spontaneously hypertensive rat have documented a parallel reduction of plasma renin activity and LV mass in animals treated with propranolol or alphamethyldopa, but an increase in both parameters in animals treated with minoxidil, producing similar blood pressure reduction [53]. Although these studies were not sufficient to demonstrate a direct link between angiotensin and LVH, angiotensin-converting enzyme (ACE) inhibiting drugs have consistently produced reductions of LV mass in clinical studies **(Ia/A)**. In addition, drugs that elevate plasma renin activity (hydralazine, diuretics) seem to less consistently induce regression of LVH than do drugs that inhibit renin activity [54] **(Ib/A)**. However, echocardiographic studies in patients with high renin versus low renin forms of hypertension have failed to show differences of LV mass [55].

Even though the relationship between renin-angiotensin activation and LV mass is uncertain, it appears that LV performance in hypertensive subjects is worse in high renin subgroups [56] **(IIb/B)**. Of note, a high renin profile has also been associated with a greater risk of MI in patients with hypertension [57]. While the mechanisms for these associations remain uncertain, it has been well documented that angiotensin has potent vasoconstrictive effects. Hence, these patients may have altered coronary reactivity with a propensity toward infarction and accelerated atherosclerosis perhaps related to smooth muscle hyperplasia [58, 59].

Left ventricular hypertrophy and salt intake

Although the role between salt intake, salt excretion, and blood pressure in hypertension has been well appreciated, the relationship between LV mass and sodium metabolism independent of blood pressure has been less well studied. Experimental studies have

Table 3. Studies in hypertensive populations demonstrating the association between LVH and other surrogate markers of cardiovascular outcome. *Adapted from Ruilope LM, Schmieder RE [104].*

First author	Inclusion criteria	n	Outcome
Agrawal [105] 1996	HPT, mean age 57 years, no DM	11,343 (17% with LVH)	44.2% of those with LVH had microproteinuria, compared with 28.7% of those without LVH
Roman [106] 1996	Untreated HPT 25-88 years	271	c-IMT was greater in those with concentric hypertrophy compared with those with normal geometry, concentric remodeling or eccentric hypertrophy
Saitoh [107] 1998	Untreated HPT	174	In those with echo LVH, 20% had proteinuria and 13% had grade III retinal vascular changes, compared to 8% and 0% of those with no LVH
Vaudo [108] 2000	Untreated HPT 18-54 years	96	Those with echo LVH (n=33) had a greater c-IMT and f-IMT compared with those with no LVH
Wachtell [109] 2002	Untreated HPT, LVH 55-80 years	8029	LVH on two consecutive ECGs (persistent LVH) was associated with a 1.6-fold increased prevalence of microalbuminuria and a 2.6-fold increased prevalence of macroalbuminuria compared with those without persistent ECG LVH
Leoncini [110] 2002	Untreated HPT no DM	346	Microalbuminuria was significantly correlated with LVMI
Tsioufis [111] 2002	Untreated essential HPT, 30-70 years no DM	249	LVMI was significantly and independently associated with log 24-hour urinary albumin excretion. The concentric LVH group had higher log 24-hour urinary albumin excretion levels than those with eccentric LVH, concentric LV remodeling or normal LV geometry
Dell'omo [112] 2003	Untreated HPT, male no DM	330	The prevalence of microalbuminuria was double in the LVH group vs. no LVH group. After adjustment for BP, the hazard ratio for microalbuminuria was 2.8 for concentric LVH vs. normal geometry

BP = blood pressure; c-IMT = carotid intima-media thickness; DM = diabetes mellitus; ECG = electrocardiogram; f-IMT = femoral intima-media thickness; HPT = hypertension; LIFE = Losartan Intervention for Endpoint Reduction study; LV = left ventricular; LVH = left ventricular hypertrophy; LVMI = left ventricular mass index

indicated a role for sodium intake in LVH. Despite failure to reverse hypertension, sodium restriction in rats with induced renal hypertension may produce reductions in heart weight [60]. In a clinical study, sodium excretion predicted not only increased LV mass consequent to an increase in LV volume – as might be expected with sodium-related volume overload – but was also a strong predictor of increased posterior wall thickness and relative wall thickness. In fact, it was the strongest predictor of all other non-hemodynamic determinants, including body mass index, hematocrit, and serum epinephrine [61] **(IIb/B)**. However, further work is needed to determine the independence of sodium intake from systolic blood pressure in the induction of LVH in hypertension patients.

Effects of antihypertensive therapy on the heart

Left ventricular mass

Although antihypertensive therapy has been shown to reduce LV mass and the prevalence of LV hypertrophy [62, 63], some studies [53, 64-66] indicate that not all drugs are equally effective in reducing LV mass, even with comparable reduction of blood pressure **(Ia/A)**. In particular, it has been suggested that diuretics and vasodilators may be ineffective in decreasing LV mass because of their failure to inhibit neurohumoral mechanisms responsible for LVH [53] **(Ib/A)**. However, much of the literature [62] on LV mass regression has been based on uncontrolled, short-term, and non-randomized studies with only one or two therapeutic arms and relatively small numbers of patients. Moreover, the influence of covariates other than drug selection known to affect LV mass [5, 16], such as obesity, the magnitude of weight loss, the extent of systolic blood pressure reduction, race, plasma renin, sodium excretion, and physical activity, have often not been evaluated.

Although thiazide diuretics are effective and inexpensive drugs for the therapy of mild-moderate hypertension, some studies [67-72] have suggested that diuretics are either completely ineffective for reduction of LV mass or produce only small decreases in LV mass, disproportionate to their effects on blood pressure **(Ib/A)**. Moreover, studies in animals and in humans [54, 68, 73-75] have provided a physiological basis for ineffective regression of LVH with diuretics, in contrast to that produced by other drugs. Although β-blockers, ACE inhibitors, calcium blockers, and centrally acting α-blockers reduce blood pressure and interfere with postulated neurohormonal mechanisms of hypertrophy, diuretics and peripheral vasodilators either produce no inhibition of these mechanisms or actually result in their reflex activation [76]. Therefore, despite reduction of blood pressure, diuretics and peripheral vasodilators might be expected to be associated with no decrease, or even increases in LV mass **(IIa/B)**.

Despite these considerations, a meta-analysis [77] suggested that diuretics can in fact produce decreases in LV mass [78-82] **(Ib/A)**. Although many studies of LV mass reduction have been criticized for methodologic limitations [67], including short duration, lack of controls, small sample sizes, and uncertain blinding, the Treatment of Mild Hypertension Study (TOMHS), avoided these methodologic shortcomings. TOMHS was a double-blind, placebo-controlled trial of 844 patients with mild hypertension and low prevalence of LVH, randomized to nutritional-hygienic intervention in combination with one of five classes of active antihypertensive drugs or placebo. Echocardiographic evaluation over 4 years showed decreased LV mass for all treatment groups including placebo and chlorthalidone. However, LV mass decreased more than placebo only in the chlorthalidone treatment group (p=0.03) based on longitudinal analyses adjusted for baseline LV mass [83] **(Ib/A)**.

The Veterans Affairs Trial of Monotherapy in Mild-Moderate Hypertension was a placebo-controlled, titration trial of monotherapy, employing six active drugs and placebo, to test the comparative efficacy of different classes of drugs for the lowering of diastolic blood pressure [84]. One objective of this study was to use echocardiography to assess the response of LV mass and its structural components over the 2-year period of antihypertensive monotherapy. Because the mechanisms responsible for LV hypertrophy, and presumably its regression, are multifactorial [15], the echocardiographic data were analyzed with adjustment for potentially contributory factors in addition to drug selection, such as body weight, the magnitude of blood pressure reduction, race, and age, using appropriate statistical methods [85]. Patients with mild to moderate hypertension (diastolic BP 95 to 109mm Hg) were randomly allocated to treatment with atenolol, captopril, clonidine, diltiazem, hydrochlorothiazide, prazosin, or placebo in a double-blinded trial in which medications were titrated to achieve a goal diastolic blood pressure of 90mm Hg. At 2 years, only hydrochlorothiazide was associated with reduction of LV mass **(Ib/A)**. The effect of hydrochlorothiazide persisted even after adjustment for covariates and was the result of decreased wall thickness. LV mass increased with atenolol. Presently, the efficacy of different monotherapy choices for reduction of LV mass is of less interest given the common use of multiple drug regimens to treat hypertension (see Table 6 below).

A recent study comparing the effects of the angiotensin receptor blocker (ARB), valsartan, with the calcium channel blocker, amlodipine [86], found that valsartan has BP-independent effects on LVH, reactive oxygen species (ROS) formation by monocytes, and CRP in patients with LVH. Participants in the cross-sectional and prospective study were randomly assigned to either 80mg valsartan or 5mg amlodipine and treated for 8 months. Both treatment groups experienced a similar reduction in blood pressure. After 8 months, valsartan reduced LVMI, but amlodipine had less effect (16% vs. 1.2%, n=50, p <0.01)**(Ib/A)**. Valsartan reduced formation of ROS by monocytes to a greater extent than amlodipine (28% vs. 2%, n=50, p<0.01). In addition, valsartan reduced CRP levels but amlodipine did not. This small 104 patient trial suggests more research is needed to assess the pleotrophic blood pressure independent effects of ARBs on hypertensive patients with LVH.

A brief review of some key studies looking at LVH and the potential effect of various anti-hypertensives is noted in Table 4.

Non-pharmacologic treatment

Non-pharmacologic treatment of hypertension has also been associated with reduction of LV mass. In one study [87], a greater trend in LV mass reduction was seen with weight loss than with drug therapy of hypertension, despite better reduction of blood pressure with drugs. Also, results of a study involving 38 morbidly obese adolescents [88] demonstrated that large weight loss after bariatric surgery improves predictors of cardiovascular morbidity, such as LV mass index, concentric LVH, diastolic function and cardiac workload **(IIa/B)**.

Table 4. Major comparative antihypertensive trials in hypertensives with LVH. *Adapted from Ruilope LM, Schmieder RE [104].*

Trial/first author	Study population	Comparators	Outcome
LIVE [113] Gosse 2000	505 hypertensives with echo LVH, ≥20 years	Indapamide SR 1.5mg; enalapril 20mg. If necessary, prazosin 5mg or doxazosin 2mg was added	After 48 weeks, indapamide SR significantly reduced LVMI but enalapril did not
PRESERVE [114] Devereux 2001	303 hypertensives with echo LVH, ≥50 years	Enalapril 10mg; nifedipine 30mg If necessary, doses were increased to 20mg/60mg respectively, then HCTZ 25mg was added, then atenolol 25mg was added	After 48 weeks, enalapril-based therapy and nifedipine-based therapy resulted in similar reductions in BP and LVMI
4E [115] Pitt 2003	153 hypertensives with echo or ECG LVH	Eplerenone 200mg; enalapril 40mg Eplerenone 200mg + enalapril 40mg	After 9 months, change in LVM (assessed by MRI) was -14.5 ±3.36g for eplerenone group, -19.7±3.2g for enalapril and -27.2±3.39g for eplerenone + enalapril group
LIFE [116] Okin 2003	9193 hypertensives with ECG LVH, 55-80 years	Losartan 50mg; atenolol 50mg. If necessary, HCTZ 12.5mg was added, then losartan/atenolol doses were doubled, then a CCB was added	After 6 months (adjusting for baseline LVH, baseline and in-treatment BP, and for diuretic therapy), losartan-based therapy was associated with greater regression of both Cornell product and Sokolow-Lyon voltage, than atenolol-based therapy. Greater regression of LVH persisted at each subsequent annual evaluation in the losartan-treated group
PICXEL [117] Dahlöf 2005	556 hypertensives with echo LVH ≥18 years	Perindopril 2mg /indapamide 0.625mg combination; enalapril 10mg. Doses were doubled if BP was inadequately controlled	After 1 year the LVMI decreased significantly more in the perindopril/indapamide group than the enalapril group (between group difference 9.3g/m^2)

BP = blood pressure; CCB = calcium channel blocker; ECG = electrocardiogram; HCTZ = hydrochlorothiazide; LIFE = Losartan Intervention for Endpoint Reduction study; LIVE = regression of left ventricular hypertrophy in hypertensive patients treated with indapamide SR 1.5mg vs. enalapril 20mg (the LIVE study); LVH = left ventricular hypertrophy; LVMI = left ventricular mass index; MRI = magnetic resonance imaging; PICXEL = Perindopril Indapamide combination in Controlled study Versus Enalapril; PRESERVE = Prospective Randomized Enalapril Study Evaluating Regression of Ventricular Enlargement; SR = sustained release

Salt restriction has also been associated with reduction of LV mass on echocardiography [89, 90] **(Ib/A)**. In contrast, although exercise has been successful in reducing blood pressure in patients with hypertension, it has been associated with increased LV mass on echocardiography [91], secondary to increased LV cavity size with no change in wall thickness **(Ib/A)**. This pattern of increase in LV mass, accompanied by preservation of diastolic LV function was considered consistent with physiologic hypertrophy.

In general, modifiable cardiovascular risk factors should all be addressed as a potential method of promoting LV regression. Interventions such as exercise, weight loss, CPAP therapy for sleep apnea, salt restriction, smoking cessation, lipid management and glucose management in appropriate patients would be expected to have a favorable impact on LVH but not all of these interventions have been evaluated by clinical trials. At present, it is suggested these interventions be implemented unless there are definite clinical contraindications **(IV/C)**.

Effects of antihypertensive therapy on left ventricular functions

Systolic function

Clinical studies that have evaluated ejection phase indices of LV function with echocardiography [62, 85, 92-94] have not demonstrated adverse effects of LV mass reduction on systolic function during or after antihypertensive therapy **(Ia/A)**. Studies employing ejection phase indices, such as velocity of circumferential fiber shortening, fractional shortening, and EF might not have been capable of detecting myocardial impairment because these indices are highly load dependent. The tendency for LV function to increase during the initial stages of therapy may, in fact, reflect the effects of reduced afterload [92]. A study of midwall fractional shortening relationships with end-systolic stress in patients with substantial reductions of LV mass during treatment also failed to disclose adverse effects [95].

Diastolic function

Conceivably, reduction of LV mass might be associated with adverse effects on diastolic LV function. This could occur if reduction of LV mass occurred without reduction in connective tissue mass. Then, with reduction of total LV mass, a relative increase in the collagen to LV weight ratio could result in decreased diastolic distensibility of the left ventricle. However, studies using Doppler echocardiography have failed to disclose worsened diastolic function with LVH regression [62, 96-98] **(Ia/A)**. Indeed, some studies have shown improvement in diastolic indices of LV filling on Doppler [96, 97].

Regression of left ventricular fibrosis

Fibrosis may account for a substantial portion of the effects of LVH on diastolic function. Therefore, it is important to know if reduction of LV mass includes regression in collagen and muscle. All hypertensive agents may not be equally effective in regression of the increased myocardial fibrosis, which accounts for part of the LV hypertrophic response to hypertension. In a human study [99] using endomyocardial biopsy to compare the effects of lisinopril with hydrochlorothiazide, ACE inhibition with lisinopril was associated with regression of fibrosis and improvement in diastolic function, whereas hydrochlorothiazide was not **(Ib/A)**. Notably, regression of LV mass occurred with diuretics but not with ACE inhibitors, possibly related to previous optimal blood pressure control in all patients, in combination with the added reduction of preload in association with diuretics.

Effect of left ventricular mass reduction on cardiovascular risk

Although reduction of LV mass with treatment of hypertension does not produce adverse effects on surrogate measures of outcome, such as LV function, there are no prospective controlled trials that test the hypothesis that reduction of LV mass is beneficial independently of reduction of blood pressure and the selected therapy. However, in an analysis of a cohort of hypertensive patients receiving drug therapy, Verdecchia and colleagues [100] showed that regression of LVH was associated with reduction in clinical events independently of the magnitude of blood pressure decrease. Moreover, in the Framingham study [101], reduction of ECG features of LVH were also independently associated with reduced risk for cardiovascular disease **(IIb/B)**. In a prospective study of hypertension patients with ECG LVH [102], achievement of lower LV mass after treatment was associated with a reduced rate of a composite endpoint (cardiovascular death, MI, stroke) independent of drug assignment or magnitude of blood pressure lowering **(IIb/B)**. It remains uncertain whether treatment targeted to reduction of LV mass, rather than to maximum reduction of blood pressure, would improve mortality and morbidity of hypertension (Table 5).

Clinical use of echocardiography in patients with hypertension

The value of echocardiography as a research tool in hypertension is uncontested. Although it has been suggested that treatment choices in individual patients should be guided by echocardiographic findings [103], the value of echocardiography in the clinical management of hypertension is unproved.

Potential impact on clinical management

The benefits of echocardiography depend on its value in affecting treatment decisions and in early identification and intervention in patients at risk who would not otherwise be treated (Table 2). Moreover, demonstration of value requires that the impact of echocardiography on clinical decisions is accompanied by improvement in patient outcome. Importantly, any consideration of the usefulness of echocardiography is contingent on its reliability for assessment of target measures, such as LV mass. However, little information is available on the impact of echocardiographic data on physician behavior or on patient outcomes in hypertension (see Table 2).

Table 5. Studies showing regression of LVH improves cardiovascular outcome. ***Adapted from Ruilope LM, Schmieder RE*** [104].

First author/ year	Inclusion criteria	n	Outcome
Verdecchia [118] 2003	HPT, mean age 45-51 years	1064	LVH regression was associated with a 59% reduction in the risk of cardiovascular events compared with persistence or new development of LVH. Those with normal LVM before and during treatment showed a 36% reduced risk of cardiovascular events compared with those with regresion of LVH
Okin [119] 2004	HPT, ECG LVH 55-80 years	9193	After 4 years of follow-up, adjusted hazard ratios for a 1 s.d. (1050mm x ms) decrease in the Cornell product were 0.86 for composite endpoint, 0.78 for CV deaths, 0.90 for MI, and 0.90 for stroke. Corresponding values for a 1 s.d. (10.5mm) decrease in the Sokolow-Lyon voltage were 0.83, 0.90, 0.81, and 0.89
Devereux [120] 2004	HPT, ECG LVH 55-80 years	941	After 1 year of treatment (and independent of baseline LVMI, study treatment and BP lowering), hazard ratios per 1 s.d. decrease in LVMI (25.3g/m^2) were 0.74 for composte endpoint (CV death, MI or stroke), 0.57 for CV mortality, 0.88 for MI, 0.78 for stroke, and 0.7 for all-cause mortality
Verdecchia [121] 2006	HPT, mean age 48 years	880	The risk of cerebrovascular events was 2.8-times higher in those with a lack of regression or new development of LVH, compared with those with LVH regression or persistently normal LVM. This effect was independent of age and 24-hour SBP

BP = blood pressure; ECG = electrocardiogram; HPT = hypertension; LIFE = Losartan Intervention for Endpoint Reduction study; LVH = left ventricular hypertrophy; LVM = left ventricular mass; LVMI = left ventricular mass index; MI = myocardial infarction; PIUMA = Progetto Ipertensione Umbria Monitoraggion Ambulatoriale; SBP = systolic blood pressure

Before formulating strategies for using echocardiography in the management of hypertension, it is helpful to specifically consider which echocardiographic assessments are likely to be of value and then consider clinical situations in which the findings of those assessments might influence clinical decision making. For example, pertinent echocardiographic assessments might include quantitation of LV mass, determining the presence or absence of LVH, assessment of LV architecture (e.g. relative wall thickness, concentric remodeling), and measurement of LV systolic and diastolic function. Because of the comorbidity of hypertension and coronary artery disease, assessment of regional wall motion abnormality also is an appropriate goal of echocardiography in the evaluation of patients with hypertension. Another targeted echocardiographic assessment in elderly patients with hypertension is age-related degenerative valvular disease, principally aortic stenosis, which may have clinical interactions with hypertensive LVH. Also, inappropriately small LV cavity size and markedly thickened LV walls (hypertensive HCM) may contribute to orthostatic hypotension in older patients, particularly with usage of diuretics or vasodilators. Hence, echocardiography may be of particular importance in the management of hypertension in the elderly.

Another way to look at the potential application of echocardiography in clinical hypertension is to consider how the findings might affect management of certain clinical subsets or hemodynamic profiles. Table 6 summarizes this potential strategy. The results of assessment of LV mass and architecture, according to this schema, could have clinical impact on management choices in established hypertension, 'white coat hypertension', and borderline hypertension. For example, marginally elevated blood pressure, or intermittently elevated blood pressure in the physician's office in the presence of concentric remodeling or clear-cut LVH, might result in drug therapy with agents believed to be effective for reduction of LV mass. In contrast, the absence of cardiac abnormality might suggest the feasibility of close follow-up, perhaps coupled with nutritional-hygienic management (e.g. weight loss, exercise, salt restriction).

The effects of treatment on LVM in essential hypertension

A recent meta-analysis of double-blind trials that measured the effects of antihypertensive therapy on left ventricular mass [118] demonstrated that antihypertensive medications have different effects, but it remains to be determined if reduction of LVM actually results in better clinical outcomes. After adjusting for treatment duration and change in diastolic blood pressure, there was a significant difference ($p=0.004$) among medication classes. LVM index decreased by 13% with angiotensin II receptor antagonists; by 11% with calcium antagonists; by 10% with ACE inhibitors; by 8% with diuretics; and by 6% with β-blockers. When compared directly, angiotensin II receptor antagonists, calcium antagonists, and ACE inhibitors were more effective in reducing LVM than were β-blockers (all $p < 0.05$).

Table 6. Hypothetical impact of echocardiography on clinical management (III/B).

Clinical subset	Echocardiographic target	Finding	Possible impact
Established hypertension	LV mass or LVH	No LVH	Diuretics and vasodilators can be used
		Unequivocal	Neurohormonal blockade (ACE inhibitors/ARB); Calcium blockers?
		Persistent LVH with therapy	Change drugs
Borderline hypertension: 'white-coat' hypertension	LV mass or LVH	No LVH	Follow closely
		Equivocal or mild LVH	Nutritional Rx
		Unequivocal LVH	Drug Rx
Hemodynamic profile	Cardiac output and total peripheral resistance	High output-low resistance	β-blockers, diuretics, calcium blockers
		High resistance-low output	ACE inhibitors, vasodilators
High risk for coronary artery disease	RWMA	RWMA present	Prior infarct – ? stress test
		RWMA and poor LV function	?Angiography; drug selection – 'anti-ischemic' antihypertensive drugs
Hypertension in the elderly	Valvular disease, LV architecture	Mitral annular calcification	Avoid vasodilators, diuretics, ?calcium blockers
	LV outflow tract dynamic gradient	Aortic stenosis, relative wall thickness, small LV cavity, LV outflow tract obstruction	Avoid diuretics; avoid vasodilators; ?β-blockers

ACE = angiotensin-converting enzyme; LV = left ventricular; LVH = left ventricular hypertrophy; Rx = therapy; RWMA = regional wall motion abnormality

Conclusions

The management of left ventricular hypertrophy (LVH) is related mainly to management of the modifiable factors which affect left ventricular mass **(IIb/A)**. The modifiable factors, namely blood pressure, body size, stress (exercise-related and physiologic), renin-angiotensin activity, parathyroid hormone activity, salt intake, and sleep apnea should be the primary focus of any efforts to manage LVH in the opinion of myself and others already cited in this publication **(III/C)**. A suggested practical clinical approach to LVH identification and subsequent management probably should include the following:

- a baseline history and physical exam as well as electrocardiogram (ECG); if LVH is found by these methods then implement modifiable risk factor management;
- if the retinal vascular changes like AV-nicking and/or urinary microalbuminuria are found, the probability that LVH is present increases, and one could treat the patient as a 'LVH-equivalent' **(III/B)**;
- patients without LVH easily identified by ECG could undergo a 2-D echocardiogram; again if LVH is identified then appropriate risk factor management would occur **(IIb/B)**;
- if non-pharmacologic measures fail to achieve therapeutic targets strongly consider the use of renin-angiotensin modulators, namely ACE inhibitors and angiotensin receptor blockers as first-line therapy with the addition of other agents based on guideline-based recommendations of achieving risk factor control **(IV/C)**.

In summary, LVH increases cardiovascular morbidity and mortality and screening by EKG and 2-D echo will allow one to use medications along with lifestyle changes in order to promote LV regression **(Ia/A)**.

Key points	Evidence level
◆ Reduction of LVH is associated with reduction of risk.	Ib/A
◆ LV mass or geometry is affected by factors other than blood pressure, including body weight, obesity, age, and race.	Ib/A
◆ The relation between LV mass and hypertension is bidirectional, that is, both are predicted by the other.	Ib/A
◆ Cardiac effects of hypertension involve all chambers of the heart and the aorta.	Ia/A
◆ Virtually all regimens, which are effective for treating hypertension, have in some study, been shown to be associated with reduction of LV mass.	Ia/A
◆ Reduction of LV mass does not produce impairment of diastolic or systolic LV function.	Ib/A
◆ Echocardiography shows many of the effects of hypertension on the heart, including LVH, LA enlargement, aortic dilation, and some of the effects of comorbidities (e.g. atherosclerosis), such as segmental LV wall motion abnormality.	Ia/A
◆ Despite the foregoing, the use of echocardiography in clinical practice to monitor effects of antihypertensive treatment on LV mass, LVH, and direct therapy accordingly is not supported by current data.	Ib/A
◆ Renin-angiotensin system (RAAS) antagonists have been proven as preferred agents in the management of LVH associated with hypertension.	Ib/A

References

1. Laennec R. *Of Hypertrophia, or Simple Enlargement of the Heart, A Treatise on the Diseases of the Chest.* Philadelphia: James Webster, 1823.
2. Janeway TC. A clinical study of hypertensive cardiovascular disease. *Arch Intern Med* 1913; 12: 755.
3. Casale PN, Devereux RB, Milner M. Value of echocardiographic measurement of left ventricular mass in predicting cardiovascular morbid events in hypertensive men. *Ann Intern Med* 1986; 105: 173-8.
4. Drizel T, Dannenberg AL, Engel A. Blood pressure levels in persons 18-74 years of age in 1978-80 and trends in blood pressure from 1960 to 1980 in the United States. NCHS Series II #234. Washington, DC: US Government Printing Office, 1986.
5. Rowland M, Roberta J. Blood pressure levels and hypertension in persons ages 6-74 years: United States, 1976-1980. National Center for Health Statistics, 1993.
6. McLenachan JM, Dargie HJ. Ventricular arrhythmias in hypertensive left ventricular hypertrophy: relationship to coronary artery disease, left ventricular dysfunction, and myocardial fibrosis. *Am J Hypertens* 1990; 3: 735-40.
7. Levy D, Anderson KM, Savage DD. Risk of ventricular arrhythmias in left ventricular hypertrophy: the Framingham Heart Study. *Am J Cardiol* 1987; 60: 560-5.
8. Ghali JK, Kadakia S, Cooper RS, Liao YL. Impact of left ventricular hypertrophy on ventricular arrhythmias in the absence of coronary artery disease. *J Am Coll Cardiol* 1991; 17: 1277-82.
9. Burt VL, Whelton P, Roccella EJ, *et al.* Prevalence of hypertension in the US adult population. Results from the Third National Health and Nutrition Examination Survey, 1988-1991. *Hypertension* 1995; 25: 305-13.
10. van Hoeven KH, Factor SM. A comparison of the pathological spectrum of hypertensive, diabetic, and hypertensive-diabetic heart disease. *Circulation* 1990; 82: 850-5.
11. Stearns S, Schlesinger MJ, Rudy A. Incidence and clinical significance of coronary artery disease in diabetes mellitus. *Arch Int Med* 1947; 80: 463-74.
12. Assman G, Schulte H. The prospective cardiovascular munster (PROCAM) study: prevalence of hyperlipidemia in persons with hypertension and/or diabetes mellitus and the relationship to coronary artery disease. *Am Heart J* 1980; 116: 1713-24.
13. Savage DD, Drayer JI, Henry WL, *et al.* Echocardiographic assessment of cardiac anatomy and function in hypertensive subjects. *Circulation* 1979; 59: 623-32.
14. Hammond IW, Devereux RB, Aldermann MA. The prevalence and correlates of echocardiographic left ventricular hypertrophy among employed patients with uncomplicated hypertension. *J Am Coll Cardiol* 1986; 7: 639-50.
15. Liebson PR, Grandits G, Prineas R, *et al.* Echocardiographic correlates of left ventricular structure among 844 mildly hypertensive men and women in the Treatment Of Mild Hypertension Study (TOMHS). *Circulation* 1993; 87: 476-86.
16. Gottdiener JS, Reda DJ, Materson BJ, *et al.* Importance of obesity, race and age to the cardiac structural and functional effects of hypertension. *J Am Coll Cardiol* 1994; 24: 1492-8.
17. Palmieri V, De Simone G, Arnett DK, *et al.* Relation of various degrees of body mass index in patients with systemic hypertension to left ventricular mass, cardiac output, and peripheral resistance (The Hypertension Genetic Epidemiology Network Study). *Am J Cardiol* 2001; 88: 1163-8.
18. Mancia G, Carugo S, Grassi G, *et al.* Prevalence of left ventricular hypertrophy in hypertensive patients without and with blood pressure control: Data from the PAMELA population. Pressioni Arteriose Monitorate E Loro Associazioni. *Hypertension* 2002; 39: 744-9.
19. Messerli FH, Ventura HO, Elizardi DJ. Hypertension and sudden death: increased ventricular ectopic activity in left ventricular hypertrophy. *Am J Med* 1984; 77: 18.
20. Koren MJ, Devereux RB, Casale PN. Relation of left ventricular mass and geometry to morbidity and mortality in uncomplicated essential hypertension. *Ann Intern Med* 1991; 114: 345-52.
21. Ghali JK, Liao Y, Simmons B, *et al.* The prognostic role of left ventricular hypertrophy in patients with or without coronary artery disease. *Ann Intern Med* 1992; 117: 831-6.
22. Devereux RB, Roman MJ, O'Grady MJ, *et al.* Differences in echocardiographic findings and systemic hemodynamics among non-diabetic American Indians in different regions. The Strong Heart Study [In Process Citation]. *Ann Epidemiol* 2000; 10: 324-32.
23. Levy D, Garrison RJ, Savage DD, *et al.* Prognostic implications of echocardiographically determined left ventricular mass in the Framingham Heart Study. *N Engl J Med* 1990; 322: 1561-6.

24. De Simone G, Devereux RB, Kimball TR, *et al.* Interaction between body size and cardiac workload: influence on left ventricular mass during body growth and adulthood. *Hypertension* 1998; 31: 1077-82.
25. De Simone G, Verdecchia P, Pede S, *et al.* Prognosis of inappropriate left ventricular mass in hypertension: the MAVI Study. *Hypertension* 2002; 40: 470-6.
26. Verdecchia P, Schillaci G, Borgioni C, *et al.* Adverse prognosis significance of concentric remodeling of the left ventricle in hypertensive patients with normal left ventricular mass. *J Am Coll Cardiol* 1995; 25: 871-8.
27. Krumholz HM, Larson M, Levy D. Prognosis of left ventricular geometric patterns in the Framingham Heart Study. *J Am Coll Cardiol* 1995; 25: 879-84.
28. Szlachcic J, Tubau JF, O'Kelly B. What is the role of silent coronary artery disease and left ventricular hypertrophy in the genesis of ventricular arrhythmias in men with essential hypertension? *J Am Coll Cardiol* 1992; 19: 803-8.
29. Papademetriou V, Narayan P, Kokkinos P. Effects of diltiazem, metoprolol, enalapril and hydrochlorothiazide on frequency of ventricular premature complexes. *Am J Cardiol* 1994; 73: 242-6.
30. Karpanou EA, Vyssoulis GP, Psichogios A, *et al.* Regression of left ventricular hypertrophy results in improvement of QT dispersion in patients with hypertension. *Am Heart J* 1998; 136: 765-8.
31. Egan B, Fitzpatrick MA, Juni J, *et al.* Importance of overweight in studies of left ventricular hypertrophy and diastolic function in mild systemic hypertension. *Am J Cardiol* 1989; 64: 752-5.
32. Hammond IW, Devereux RB, Alderman MH, Laragh JH. Relation of blood pressure and body build to left ventricular mass in normotensive and hypertensive employed adults. *J Am Coll Cardiol* 1988; 12: 996-1004.
33. Levy D, Anderson KM, Savage DD, *et al.* Echocardiographically detected left ventricular hypertrophy: prevalence and risk factors. The Framingham Heart Study. *Ann Intern Med* 1988; 108: 7-13.
34. Dannenberg AL, Levy D, Garrison RJ. Impact of age on echocardiographic left ventricular mass in a healthy population (the Framingham Study). *Am J Cardiol* 1989; 64: 1066-8.
35. Messerli FH, Nunez BD, Ventura HO, Snyder DW. Overweight and sudden death: increased ventricular ectopy in cardiopathy of obesity. *Arch Intern Med* 1987; 147: 1725-8.
36. Messerli FH, Sungaard-Riise K, Reisin ED, *et al.* Dimorphic cardiac adaptation to obesity and arterial hypertension. *Ann Intern Med* 1983; 99: 757-61.
37. Hammond IW, Alderman MH, Devereux RB, *et al.* Contrast in cardiac anatomy and function between black and white patients with hypertension. *J Natl Med Assoc* 1984; 76: 247-55.
38. Chaturvedi N, Athanassopoulos G, McKeigue PM, *et al.* Echo-cardiographic measures of left ventricular structure and their relation with rest and ambulatory blood pressure in blacks and whites in the United Kingdom. *J Am Coll Cardiol* 1994; 24: 1499-505.
39. Koren MJ, Mensah GA, Blake J, *et al.* Comparison of left ventricular mass and geometry in black and white patients with essential hypertension. *Am J Hypertens* 1993; 6: 815-23.
40. Sasson Z, Rasooly Y, Bhesania T, Rasooly I. Insulin resistance is an important determinant of left ventricular mass in the obese. *Circulation* 1993; 88: 1431-6.
41. Dahlof B. Factors involved in the pathogenesis of hypertensive cardiovascular hypertrophy. A review. *Drugs* 1988; 35 (Suppl 5): 6-26.
42. Bella JN, Devereux RB, Roman MJ, *et al.* Relations of left ventricular mass to fat-free and adipose body mass: the Strong Heart Study. The Strong Heart Study Investigators. *Circulation* 1998; 98: 2538-44.
43. Chinali M, De Simone G, Roman MJ, *et al.* Impact of obesity on cardiac geometry and function in a population of adolescents: the Strong Heart Study. *J Am Coll Cardiol* 2006; 47: 2267-73.
44. Hypertension Detection and Follow-Up Program Cooperative Group (HDFP). Race, education and prevalence of hypertension. *Am J Epidemiol* 1977; 106: 351-61.
45. Freis ED. Age, race, sex and other indices of risk in hypertension. *Am J Med* 1073; 55: 275-80.
46. Kannel WB, Dannenberg AL. Prevalence and natural history of electrocardiographic left ventricular hypertrophy. In: *The Heart and Hypertension.* Messerli FH, Ed. New York: York Medical Books, 1987: 53-62.
47. Lee DK, Marantz PR, Devereux RB, *et al.* Left ventricular hypertrophy in black and white hypertensives. Standard electrocardiographic criteria overestimate racial differences in prevalence. *J Am Med Assoc* 1992; 267: 3294-9.
48. Dunn FG, Oigman W, Sungaard-Riise K. Racial differences in cardiac adaptation to essential hypertension determined by echocardiographic indexes. *J Am Coll Cardiol* 1983; 5: 1348-51.
49. Arnett DK, Skelton TN, Liebson PR, *et al.* Comparison of m-mode echocardiographic left ventricular mass measured using digital and strip chart readings: The Atherosclerosis Risk in Communities (ARIC) study. *Cardiovasc Ultrasound* 2003; 1: 8.

50. Tikelis G, Arnett DK, Skelton TN, Taylor HW, *et al.* Retinal arteriolar narrowing and left ventricular hypertrophy in African-Americans, the Atherosclerosis Risk in Communities (ARIC) study. *Am J Hypertens* 2008; 21(3): 352-9.
51. Robertson AL Jr, Khairallah PA. Angiotensin II: rapid localization in nuclei of smooth and cardiac muscle. *Science* 1971; 172: 1138-9.
52. Roth RH, Hughes J. Acceleration of protein biosynthesis by angiotensin's correlation with angiotensin's effect on catecholamine biosynthesis. *Biochem Pharmacol* 1972; 21: 3182-7.
53. Tarazi RC, Sen S, Fouad FM, Wicker P. Regression of myocardial hypertrophy: conditions and sequelae of reversal in hypertensive heart disease. In: *Perspectives in Cardiovascular Research*, 7th ed. Alpert NR, Ed. New York: Raven Press, 1983: 637.
54. Devereux RB, Pennert K, Cody RJ. Relation of renin-angiotensin system activity to left ventricular hypertrophy and function in experimental and human hypertension. *J Clin Hypertens* 1987; 13: 87-103.
55. Devereux RB, Savage DD, Drayer JIM. Left ventricular hypertrophy and function in high-, normal-, and low-renin forms of essential hypertension. *Hypertension* 1982; 4: 524-31.
56. Vensel LA, Devereux RB, Pickering TG. Cardiac structure and function in renovascular hypertension produced by unilateral and bilateral renal artery stenosis. *Am J Cardiol* 1986; 58: 575-82.
57. Alderman MH, Madhavan S, Ooi WL. Association of the reninsodium profile with the risk of myocardial infarction in patients with hypertension. *N Engl J Med* 1991; 324: 1098-104.
58. Meyer P. Similarities in cellular proliferative mechanisms in hypertension and neoplasia. In: *Hypertension: Pathophysiology, Diagnosis and Management.* Laragh JH, Brenner BM, Eds. New York: Raven Press, 1990: 541-5.
59. Marban E, Koretsune Y. Cell calcium, oncogenes, and hypertrophy. *Hypertension* 1990; 15: 652-8.
60. Lindpainter K, Sen S. Role of sodium in hypertensive cardiac hypertrophy. *Circ Res* 1985; 57: 610.
61. Schmeider RE, Messerli FH, Garavaglia GE. Dietary salt intake: a determinant of cardiac involvement in essential hypertension. *Circulation* 1988; 78: 951-6.
62. Liebson PR. Clinical studies of drug reversal of hypertensive left ventricular hypertrophy. *Am J Hypertens* 1990; 3: 512-7.
63. Trimarco B, Wikstrand J. Regression of cardiovascular structural changes by antihypertensive treatment. Functional consequences and time course of reversal as judged from clinical studies. *Hypertension* 1984; 6(suppl 3): III-150.
64. Schulman SP, Weiss JL, Becker LC, *et al.* The effects of antihypertensive therapy on left ventricular mass in elderly patients. *N Engl J Med* 1990; 322: 1350-6.
65. Sen S. Regression of cardiac hypertrophy. Experimental animal model. *Am J Med* 1983; 75(suppl 3A): 87.
66. Fouad-Tarazi F, Liebson PR. Echocardiographic studies of regression of left ventricular hypertrophy in hypertension. *Hypertension* 1987; 4(Suppl 2): 65-8.
67. Massie BM. Effect of diuretic therapy on hypertensive left ventricular hypertrophy. *Eur Heart J* 1992; 13 (Suppl G): 53-60.
68. Pfeffer MA, Pfeffer JM. Reversing cardiac hypertrophy in hypertension. *N Engl J Med* 1987; 322: 1388-90.
69. Devereux RB, Savage DD, Sachs I, Laragh JH. Effect of blood pressure control on left ventricular hypertrophy and function in hypertension. *Circulation* 1980; 62(suppl 3): 36.
70. Wollam GL, Hall WD, Porter VD, *et al.* Time course of regression of left ventricular hypertrophy in treated hypertensive patients. *Am J Med* 1983; 26: 100-10.
71. Drayer JIM, Gardin JM, Weber MA, Aronow WS. Changes in ventricular septal thickness during diuretic therapy. *Clin Pharmac Therap* 1982; 32: 283-8.
72. Giles TD, Sander GE, Roffidal LC, *et al.* Comparison of nitrendipine and hydrochlorothiazide for systemic hypertension. *Am J Cardiol* 1987; 60: 103-6.
73. Pfeffer MA, Pfeffer JM. Pharmacologic regression of cardiac hypertrophy in experimental hypertension. *J Cardiovasc Pharmacol* 1984; 6(suppl 6): S865.
74. Pegram BL, Ishise S, Frohlich ED. Effects of methyldopa, clonidine and hydralazine on cardiac mass and haemodynamics in Wistar Kyoto and spontaneously hypertensive rats. *Cardiovasc Res* 1982; 16: 40.
75. Plotnick GD, Fisher ML, Wohl B. Improvement in depressed cardiac function in hypertensive patients during pindolol treatment. *Am J Cardiol* 1984; 76: 25.
76. Burnier M, Brunner HR. Neurohormonal consequences of diuretics in different cardiovascular syndromes. *Eur Heart J* 13 1992; (Suppl G): 28-33.

77. Dahlof B, Pennert K, Hansson L. Reversal of left ventricular hypertrophy in hypertensive patients: a meta-analysis of 109 treatment studies. *Am J Hypertens*1992; 5: 95-110.
78. Reichek N, Franklin BB, Chandler T, *et al.* Reversal of left ventricular hypertrophy by antihypertensive therapy. *Eur Heart J* 1982; 3: 165-9.
79. Cherchi A, Sau F, Seguro C. Regression of left ventricular hypertrophy after treatment of hypertension by chlorthalidone for one year and other diuretics for two years. *J Hypertens* 1983; 1(suppl 2): 278-80.
80. Ferrara LA, De Simone G, Mancini M, *et al.* Changes in left ventricular mass during a double-blind study with chlorthalidone and slow-release nifedipine. *Eur J Clin Pharmacol* 1984; 27: 525-8.
81. Mace PJE, Littler WA, Glover DR, *et al.* Regression of left ventricular hypertrophy in hypertension: comparative effects of three different drugs. *J Cardiovasc Pharmacol* 1985; 7: S52-5.
82. Sami M, Haichin R. Regression of left ventricular hypertrophy in hypertension with indapamide. *Am Heart J* 1991; 122: 1215-8.
83. Neaton JD, Grimm RJ Jr, Prineas RJ, *et al.* Treatment of Mild Hypertension Study. Final results. Treatment of Mild Hypertension Study Research Group. *J Am Med Assoc* 1993; 270: 713-24.
84. Materson BJ, Reda DJ, Cushman WC, *et al.* Single-drug therapy for hypertension in men. A comparison of six antihypertensive agents with placebo. The Department of Veterans Affairs Cooperative Study Group on Antihypertensive Agents. *N Engl J Med* 1993; 328: 914-21.
85. Gottdiener JS, Reda DJ, Massie BM, *et al.* Effect of single-drug therapy on reduction of left ventricular mass in mild to moderate hypertension: Comparison of six antihypertensive agents. The Department of Veterans Affairs Cooperative Study Group on Antihypertensive Agents. *Circulation* 1997; 95: 2007-14.
86. Yasunari K, Maeds K, Watanbe T, Nakamura M, *et al.* Comparative effects of valsartan versus amlodipine on left ventricular mass and reactive oxygen species formation by monocytes in hypertensive patients with left ventricular hypertrophy. *J Am Coll Cardiol* 2004; 43(11): 2116-23.
87. Fagerberg B, Berglund A, Andersson OK, *et al.* Cardiovascular effects of weight reduction versus antihypertensive drug treatment: a comparative, randomized, 1-year study of obese men with mild hypertension. *J Hypertens* 1991; 9: 431-9.
88. Ippisch HM, Inge TH, Daniels SR, *et al.* Reversibility of cardiac abnormalities in morbidly obese adolescents. *J Am Coll Cardiol* 2008; 51(14): 1-9. Available at: www.medscape.com/viewarticle/571363.
89. Ferrara LA, De Simone G, Pasanisi F, Mancini M. Left ventricular mass reduction during salt depletion in arterial hypertension. *Hypertension* 1984; 6: 755-9.
90. Jula AM, Karanko HM. Effects on left ventricular hypertrophy of long-term nonpharmacological treatment with sodium restriction in mild-to-moderate essential hypertension. *Circulation* 1994; 89: 1023-31.
91. Kelemen MH, Effron MB, Valenti SA, Stewart KJ. Exercise training combined with antihypertensive drug therapy: effects on lipids, blood pressure, and left ventricular mass. *J Am Med Assoc* 1990; 263: 2766-71.
92. Khatri IM, Gottdiener JS, Notargiacomo AV, Freis E. The effect of therapy on left ventricular function in hypertension. *Clin Sci* 1980; 59: 435s-9.
93. Phillips RA, Ardeljan M, Shimabukuro S. Normalization of left ventricular mass and associated changes in neurohormones and atrial natriuretic peptide after 1 year of sustained nifedipine therapy for severe hypertension. *J Am Coll Cardiol* 1991; 17: 1595-602.
94. Oren S, Messerli FH, Grossman E, *et al.* Immediate and short-term cardiovascular effects of fosinopril, a new angiotensin-converting enzyme inhibitor, in patients with essential hypertension. *J Am Coll Cardiol* 1991; 17: 1183-7.
95. Aurigemma GP, Gottdiener JS, Gaasch WH, *et al.* Ventricular and myocardial function following regression of hypertensive left ventricular hypertrophy. *J Am Coll Cardiol* 1995; (Special Issue) February: 251A.
96. Trimarco B, DeLuca N, Rosiello G. Improvement of diastolic function after reversal of left ventricular hypertrophy induced by long-term antihypertensive treatment with tertatolol. *Am J Cardiol* 1989; 64: 745-51.
97. Muiesan ML, Agabiti-Rosei E, Romanelli G. Improved left ventricular systolic and diastolic function after regression of cardiac hypertrophy, treatment withdrawal, and redevelopment of hypertension. *J Cardiovasc Pharmacol* 1991; 17(suppl 2): S179-81.
98. Gottdiener JS. Measuring diastolic function. *J Am Coll Cardiol* 1991; 18: 83-4.
99. Brilla CG, Funck RC, Rupp H. Lisinopril-mediated regression of myocardial fibrosis in patients with hypertensive heart disease [see comments]. *Circulation* 2000; 102: 1388-93.
100. Verdecchia P, Schillaci G, Borgioni C, *et al.* Prognostic significance of serial changes in left ventricular mass in essential hypertension. *Circulation* 1998; 97: 48-54.

101. Levy D, Salomon M, D'Agostino RB, *et al.* Prognostic implications of baseline electrocardiographic features and their serial changes in subjects with left ventricular hypertrophy. *Circulation* 1994; 90: 1786-93.
102. Devereux RB, Wachtell K, Gerdts E, *et al.* Prognostic significance of left ventricular mass change during treatment of hypertension. *J Am Med Assoc* 2004; 292: 2350-6.
103. De Simone G, Ganau A, Verdecchia P, Devereux RB. Echocardiography in arterial hypertension: when, why and how? *J Hypertens* 1994; 12: 1129-1136.
104. Ruilope LM, Schmieder RE. Left ventricular hypertrophy and clinical outcomes in hypertensive patients. *Am J Hypertension* 2008; 21(5): 500-8.
105. Agrawal B, Berger A, Wolf K, Luft FC. Microalbuminuria screening by reagent strip predicts cardiovascular risk in hypertension. *J Hypertens* 1996; 14: 223-8.
106. Roman MJ, Pickering TJ, Schwartz JE, Pini R, Devereux RB. Relation of arterial structure and function to left ventricular geometric patterns in hypertensive adults. *J Am Coll Cardiol* 1996; 28: 751-6.
107. Saitoh M, Matsu K, Nomoto S, Kondoh T, Yanagawa T, Katoh Y, Hasegawa K. Relationship between left ventricular hypertrophy and renal and retinal damage in untreated patients with essential hypertension. *Intern Med* 1998; 37: 576-80.
108. Vaudo G, Schillaci G, Evangelista F, Pasqualini L, Verdeccia P, Mannarino E. Arterial wall thickening and its association with left ventricular hypertrophy in newly diagnosed essential hypertension. *Am J Hypertens* 2000; 13: 324-31.
109. Wachtell K, Olsen MH, Dahlöf B, Devereux RB, Kjeldsen SE, Nieminen MS, Okin PM, Papademetriou V, Mogensen CE, Borch-Johnsen K, Ibsen H. Microalbuminuria in hypertensive patients with electrocardiographic left ventricular hypertrophy: The LIFE study. *J Hypertens* 2002; 20: 405-12.
110. Leoncini G, Sacchi G, Ravera M, Viazzi F, Ratto E, Vettoretti S, Parodi D, Bezante GP, Del Sette M, Deferrari G, Pontremolli R. Microalbuminuria is an integrated marker of subclinical organ damage in primary hypertension. *J Hum Hypertens* 2002; 16: 399-404.
111. Tsioufis C, Stefanadis C, Toutouza M, Kallikazaros I, Tousoulis D, Pitsavos C, Papademetriou V, Toutouzas P. Microalbuminuria is associated with unfavourable geometric adaptations in essential hypertensive subjects. *J Hum Hypertens* 2002; 16: 249-54.
112. Dell'omo G, Giorgi D, Di Bello V, Mariani M, Pedrinelli R. Blood pressure independent association of microalbuminuria and left ventricular hypertrophy in hypertensive men. *J Intern Med* 2003; 254: 76-84.
113. Gosse P, Sheridan DJ, Zannad F, Dubourg O, Guéret P, Karpov Y, de Leeuw PW, Palma-Gamiz JL, Pessina A, Motz W, Degaute JP, Chastant C. Regression of left ventricular hypertrophy in hypertensive patients treated with indapamide SR 1.5mg versus enalapril 20mg: the LIVE study. *J Hypertens* 2000; 18: 1465-75.
114. Devereux RB, Palmieri V, Sharpe N, De Quattro N, Bella JN, de Simone G, Walker JF, Hahn RT, Dahlöf B. Effects of once-daily angiotensin-converting enzyme inhibition and calcium channel blockade-based antihypertensive treatment regimens on left ventricular hypertrophy and diastolic filling in hypertension: the Prospective Randomized Enalapril Study Evaluating Regression of Ventricular Enlargement (PRESERVE) trial. *Circulation* 2001; 104: 1248-54.
115. Pitt B, Reichek N, Willenbrook R, Zannad F, Phillips RA, Roniker B, Kleiman J, Krause S, Burns D, Williams GH. Effects of eplerenone, enalapril and eplerenone/enalapril in patients with essential hypertension and left ventricular hypertrophy. The 4E-left ventricular hypertrophy study. *Circulation* 2003; 108: 1831-8.
116. Okin PM, Devereux RB, Jern S, Kjeldsen SE, Julius S, Nieminen MS, Snapinn S, Harris KE, Aurup P, Edelman JM, Dahlof B; Losartan Intervention For Endpoint reduction in hypertension study investigations. Regression of electrocardiographic left ventricular hypertrophy by losartan versus atenolol. The Losartan Intervention For Endpoint reduction in hypertension (LIFE) study. *Circulation* 2003; 108: 684-90.
117. Dahlöf B, Gosse P, Gueret P, Dubourg O, de Simone G, Schmieder R, Karpov Y, García-Puig J, Matos L, De Leeuw PW, Degaute JP, Magometschnigg D; The PICXEL Investigators. Perindopril/indapamide combination more effective than enalapril in reducing blood pressure and left ventricular mass: the PICXEL study. *J Hypertens* 2005; 23: 2063-70.
118. Verdecchia P, Angeli F, Borgioni C, Gattobigio R, de Simone G, Devereux RB, Porcellati C. Changes in cardiovascular risk by reduction of left ventricular mass in hypertension: a meta-analysis. *Am J Hypertens* 2003; 16: 895-9.
119. Okin PM, Devereux RB, Jern S, Kjeldsen SE, Julius S, Nieminen MS, Snapinn S, Harris KE, Aurup P, Edelman JM, Dahlof B; LIFE Study Investigators. Regression of electrocardiographic left ventricular hypertrophy during antihypertensive treatment and the prediction of major cardiovascular events. *JAMA* 2004; 292: 2343-9.

120. Devereux RB, Wachtell K, Gerdts E, Boman K, Nieminen MS, Papademitriou V, Rokkedal J, Harris K, Aurup P, Dahlöf B. Prognostic significance of left ventricular mass change during treatment of hypertension. *JAMA* 2004; 292: 2350-6.
121. Verdecchia P, Angeli F, Gattobigio R, Sardone M, Pede S, Reboldi GP. Regression of left ventricular hypertrophy and prevention of stroke in hypertensive subjects. *Am J Hypertens* 2006; 19: 493-9.

Chapter 12

Management of hypertension in left ventricular systolic dysfunction

Faisal Siddiqi MD, Fellow, Cardiology
Kristin Thanavaro MD, Resident, Internal Medicine
Mandeep R. Mehra MD, Professor of Medicine and Head of Cardiology
University of Maryland School of Medicine
Division of Cardiology, Baltimore, Maryland, USA

Introduction

Heart failure is a progressive disorder characterized by fluid retention and symptoms of dyspnea and exercise intolerance. Heart failure patients are divided between those with reduced left ventricular function and those with preserved function.

Hypertension contributes to the pathogenesis of both systolic and diastolic heart failure and more than two thirds of patients with heart failure have a past or previous history of hypertension. Analysis from the Framingham Heart Study indicated that hypertension accounted for 39% of heart failure cases among men and 59% among women [1]. This concern is heightened by the fact that despite advances in antihypertensive drug therapy, the prevalence of hypertension continues to increase worldwide [2]. Treatment of hypertension can reduce the incidence of heart failure by 50% [3]. Guidelines for the diagnosis and management of hypertension have been established in the most recent JNC 7 report. Preference is given to thiazide diuretics, dihydropyridine calcium channel blockers and ACE inhibitors [4]. Beta-blockers are discouraged for first-line treatment due to a lack of overall mortality benefit and associated increase in stroke risks [5].

However, guidelines established for the management of left ventricular systolic dysfunction emphasizes the role of ACE inhibitors (ACE-Is), angiotensin receptor blockers (ARBs), and β-blockers. In select groups, aldosterone antagonists and combinations of nitrates and hydralazine are also recommended.

The focus of this chapter will be the management of hypertension in the setting of left ventricular systolic dysfunction.

Pathophysiology

Our understanding of the pathophysiology of heart failure has gradually evolved over the past few decades predicated on the results of numerous large, randomized clinical trials. Initial focus was on the hemodynamic and cardiocirculatory models that addressed the basic needs of symptom management and hemodynamic improvement. The contemporary hypothesis is that heart failure is a progressive disorder of left ventricular remodeling that develops as a consequence of the up-regulation of endogenous neurohormones and sympathetic activation following an initial insult (i.e. myocardial infarction, myocarditis, etc.) [6]. This concept, known as the neurohormonal model, has provided therapeutic targets for symptom relief, halting disease progression and increasing survival [7].

Myocardial hypertrophy occurs in hypertension as a compensatory mechanism to increasing pressure and left ventricular wall stress. Over time, this beneficial remodeling is exhausted and chamber dilation leads to eventual depression in myocardial performance and heart failure. Transition from left ventricular hypertrophy to hypertensive heart failure occurs through related mechanisms of neurohormonal activation that imposes hemodynamic stress on the left ventricle through sodium retention, peripheral vasoconstriction and direct toxic effects on myocardial cells [8]. The primary hormones implicated in this process are renin, angiotensin, aldosterone, and catecholamines, all of which are elevated in heart failure patients. By this same process, hypertension can also accelerate the process of ventricular remodeling among patients with other forms of cardiomyopathies. The end result of cardiac remodeling is the development of symptoms and/or death from progressive heart failure.

Management of hypertension and left ventricular systolic dysfunction

Current therapy focuses on ACE-Is, ARBs, β-blockers, aldosterone antagonists, and combinations of hydralazine/nitrates designed to interrupt the renin-angiotensin-aldosterone system (RAAS) and sympathetic systems. Numerous trials have demonstrated the efficacy of these agents and formed the basis of treatment guidelines published by the American College of Cardiology/American Heart Association (ACC/AHA), Heart Failure Society of America (HFSA), and European Society of Cardiology (ESC) [9]. Interestingly, drug classes preferred in the management of essential hypertension without heart failure have not conferred the same benefits in patients with systolic dysfunction. Therefore, thiazide diuretics and calcium channel blockers are discouraged before appropriate implementation of evidenced-based therapies.

Heart failure is staged according to the ACC/AHA classification scheme or the familiar New York Heart Association (NYHA) functional class system (see Figure 1). A basic understanding of the staging of heart failure is a crucial aspect of managing patients with heart failure with systolic dysfunction. In general, all patients with Stage B (NYHA Class I) or greater should be treated with ACE-Is and β-blockers unless contraindicated. Additional recommendations are based on continued signs and symptoms of disease. It should be noted that patients characteristically demonstrate fluctuation in their symptoms and NYHA Class

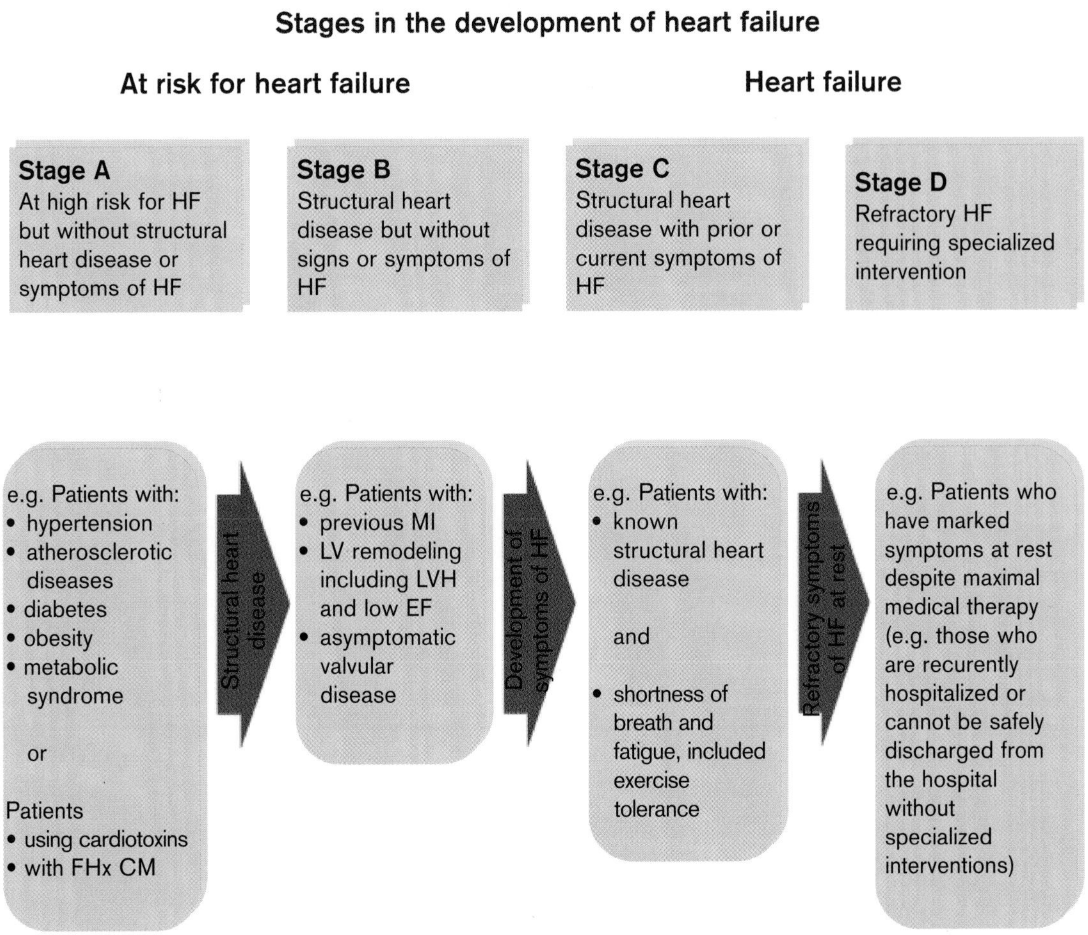

Stages in the development of heart failure

At risk for heart failure | **Heart failure**

Stage A
At high risk for HF but without structural heart disease or symptoms of HF

Stage B
Structural heart disease but without signs or symptoms of HF

Stage C
Structural heart disease with prior or current symptoms of HF

Stage D
Refractory HF requiring specialized intervention

e.g. Patients with:
- hypertension
- atherosclerotic diseases
- diabetes
- obesity
- metabolic syndrome

or

Patients
- using cardiotoxins
- with FHx CM

Structural heart disease

e.g. Patients with:
- previous MI
- LV remodeling including LVH and low EF
- asymptomatic valvular disease

Development of symptoms of HF

e.g. Patients with:
- known structural heart disease

and

- shortness of breath and fatigue, included exercise tolerance

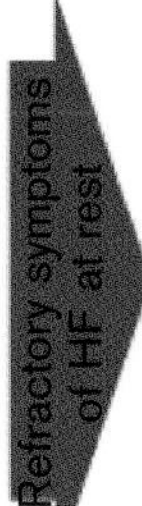

e.g. Patients who have marked symptoms at rest despite maximal medical therapy (e.g. those who are recurently hospitalized or cannot be safely discharged from the hospital without specialized interventions)

Figure 1. ACC/AHA Heart Failure Classification Scheme. *Reproduced with permission from Circulation 2009; 119: e391-e479. © 2009, American Heart Association, Inc.*

over time; however, sustained improvement is dependent on treatment and therefore should be continued indefinitely, except in rare circumstances [10].

Unfortunately, despite readily available guidelines, there has been under-utilization of drugs that have been shown to improve quality of life and improve mortality in left ventricular systolic dysfunction (Figure 2) [11]. Accounting for patient-related factors (i.e. renal insufficiency, advanced lung disease) that influence hospital discharge medications, these numbers remain unsatisfactory. Recently published data indicate a higher compliance with recommended therapy in outpatient cardiology practices. However, this adherence to recommended therapy differs greatly between age groups [12]. Current guidelines do not distinguish recommendations based on age or gender differences.

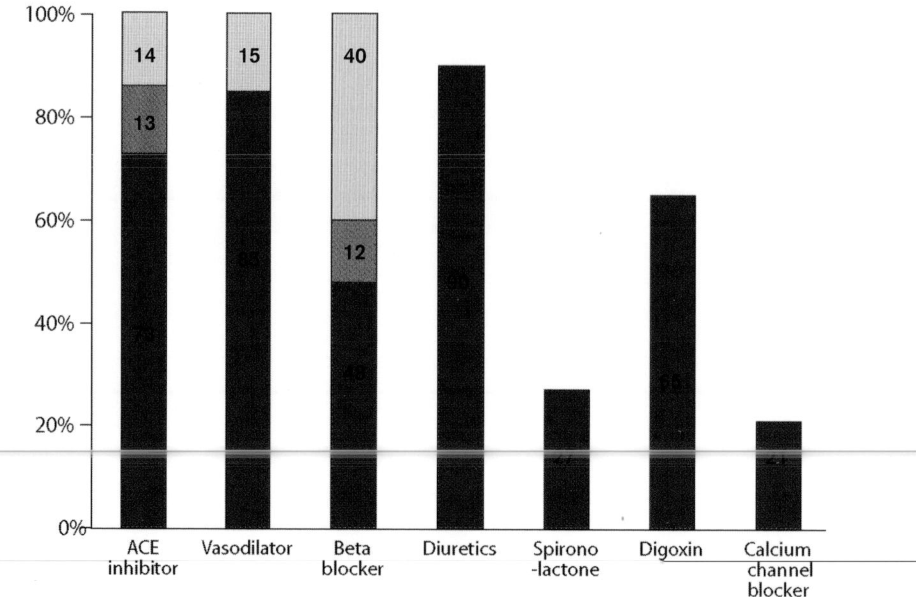

Figure 2. Medication use among 494 managed Medicare and Medicaid patients with HF due to moderate-to-severe left ventricular dysfunction. Numbers in bars = percentages; purple-shaded bars = percentage prescribed; pink-shaded bars = percentage of ACE inhibitor vasodilators and β-blockers with a documented contraindication; yellow-shaded bars = quality gap.

Therapeutic strategies

As mentioned, guidelines exist regarding the management of hypertension and heart failure separately [10, 13-15]. However, there are no separate guidelines for the specific management of coexisting hypertension in heart failure. Therefore, recommendations are based on consensus opinions extrapolated from large trials of anti-heart failure medications that also reduce blood pressure. In treating left ventricular systolic dysfunction, relief of symptoms and survival benefits are often independent of blood pressure effects. As such, ACE-Is, β-blockers, and aldosterone antagonists are preferred in this patient population over other antihypertensive medications, despite their potential weaker effects on blood pressure.

Even less clear is the target for blood pressure in patients with heart failure. According to the JNC 7, hypertensive patients without co-existing heart failure should be treated to a blood pressure less than 140/90mm Hg with more aggressive targets for patients with diabetes and chronic kidney disease. Many heart failure specialists go beyond normotension and titrate medications to reach the lowest possible blood pressure possible without causing symptoms or signs of hypoperfusion [16]. Retrospective studies and registries have questioned this method in light of evidence suggesting an inverse relationship between systolic blood pressure and survival in patients with acute and chronic heart failure [16-19]. However, this inverse correlation is likely because more severe cardiac dysfunction causes a decline in systemic blood pressures, making low blood pressure a marker for more advanced heart failure [20]. Clinicians should attempt to use doses that have been shown to reduce the risks of cardiovascular events in clinical trials (Table 1)[10] **(IV/C)**.

Table 1. ACC/AHA guidelines for initial and target doses of evidence-based drug therapies in systolic heart failure [10]. *Reproduced with permission from Circulation 2009; 119: e391-e479. © 2009, American Heart Association, Inc.*

Inhibitors of the renin-angiotensin-aldosterone system and beta-blockers commonly used for the treatment of patients with heart failure and low ejection fraction

Drug	Initial daily dose(s)	Maximum dose(s)
ACE inhibitors		
Captopril	6.25mg 3 times	50mg 3 times
Enalapril	2.5mg twice	10 to 20mg twice
Fosinopril	5 to 10mg once	40mg once
Lisonopril	2.5 to 5mg once	20 to 40mg once
Perindopril	2mg once	8 to 16mg once
Quinapril	5mg twice	20mg twice
Ramipril	1.25 to 2.5mg once	10mg once
Trandolapril	1mg once	4mg once
Angiotensin receptor blockers		
Candesartan	4 to 8mg once	32mg once
Losartan	25 to 50mg once	50 to 100mg once
Valsartan	20 to 40mg twice	160mg twice
Aldosterone antagonists		
Spironolactone	12.5 to 25mg once	25mg once or twice
Eplerenone	25mg once	50mg once
Beta-blockers		
Bisoprolol	1.25mg once	10mg once
Carvedilol	3.125mg twice	25mg twice 50mg twice for patients >85kg
Metoprolol succinate extended release (metoprolol CR/XL)	12.5 to 25mg once	200mg once

ACE = angiotensin-converting enzyme; mg = milligrams; kg = kilograms

ACE inhibitors (ACE-Is)

ACE-Is are the best studied class of agents in left ventricular systolic dysfunction and form the cornerstone of therapy. Large prospective therapies have validated the efficacy of ACE-Is in reducing total mortality and heart failure admissions [21-24]. ACE-Is achieve their beneficial effects on mortality by antagonizing the effects of angiotensin II on vasoconstriction, inhibiting vascular smooth muscle cell proliferation, and improving endothelial function. Additionally, ACE-Is possess growth inhibitory properties and collagen modulating effects that reduce left ventricular remodeling [7]. Collectively, ACE-Is have been evaluated in randomized, placebo-controlled trials encompassing greater than 20,000 patients with left ventricular systolic dysfunction (EF <40%). In addition to reductions in all-cause mortality and heart failure admissions, ACE-Is also alleviated symptoms, improved NYHA class, and enhanced overall sense of well-being [21-25]. More significantly, their benefits were seen across all causes and stages of HF. As such, ACE-Is are recommended for all patients, asymptomatic and symptomatic, with reduced left ventricular function [10] **(Ia/A)**.

Unlike some other anti-heart failure medications, ACE-Is are considered to have a class effect with no differences in efficacy among available ACE-Is. However, it is recommended to consider agents that have been well-studied (captopril, enalapril, lisinopril, ramipril, trandolapril) because these studies have defined target doses [10]. Target doses for ACE-Is have historically been based on those used in large clinical trials. In practice, however, clinicians commonly prescribe doses well below these goals. In the ATLAS trial, high-dose lisinopril (32.5-35mg of daily) was compared to low-dose lisinopril (2.5-5mg daily) among 3164 patients with advanced heart failure [21]. High-dose ACE-Is had a 15% lower risk of the combined endpoint – death or hospitalization (p=0.002) [26]. Therefore, clinicians should attempt to titrate ACE-I doses to those used in clinical trials despite normotensive blood pressure measurements (Table 1).

In prescribing ACE-Is, careful attention should be paid to serum creatinine levels (>2.5mg/dL), potassium levels and a history suggestive of angioedema. Treatment should be initiated at low doses then titrated to evidence-based doses if tolerated. Renal function and potassium levels should be checked 1 to 2 weeks following initiation or dosing changes. A significant increase in serum creatinine (>0.3mg/dL) occurs in 15-30% of patients and will often improve gradually or with reduced doses of diuretic therapy. Every effort should be made to continue ACE-I treatment even if it requires tolerating mild to moderate azotemia. Angioedema occurs in less than 1% of patients taking ACE-Is but justifies discontinuation of ACE-I therapy. The development of a cough is the most common reason for discontinuation of ACE-I therapy and is often done inappropriately. The cough is dry, develops within 1 month of initiation of treatment, and clears 1 to 2 weeks after discontinuation. However, it is important to exclude all other causes of cough before discontinuing ACE-Is. A re-challenge with an alternative ACE-I is recommended and alternative therapy (such as angiotensin receptor blockers) should be considered only if symptoms recur.

Angiotensin receptor blockers (ARBs)

Although ACE-Is reduce morbidity and mortality in patients with LV systolic dysfunction, blockade of RAAS remains incomplete with continued production of hormones from alternative pathways. ARBs were developed in the hopes that angiotensin receptor blockade would provide superior interruption of the neurohormonal axis in heart failure [27]. ELITE II was a double-blind, randomized controlled trial comparing the effects of losartan with captopril on all-cause mortality in patients with reduced LV function and advanced heart failure. There was no significant difference in the effect of losartan compared with captopril on the primary endpoint (HR 1.13; p=0.16) [28]. A meta-analysis comparing ACE-Is and ARBs also found no significant difference on all-cause mortality or HF hospitalizations [29]. Although ARBs did not have the survival benefits seen with ACE-Is, the data suggested ARBs could be safely used as alternative therapy in ACE-I-intolerant patients. As such, ARBs are strongly recommended for treatment of left ventricular dysfunction among patients with intolerance to ACE-Is [10] **(Ia/A)**.

A separate issue is the effect of combining ACE-Is with ARBs on mortality and morbidity in patients with left ventricular dysfunction. A meta-analysis including Val-HeFT and CHARM-Added showed that the combination of ARB and ACE-I compared with ACE-Is alone had no additional benefit on all-cause mortality (OR 0.97, 95% CI 0.87-1.08). However, the combination was associated with a significant 23% reduction in hospitalizations due to heart failure [29]. Individually, the CHARM-Added randomized trial did find significant reductions in cardiovascular mortality with the addition of ARBs to background ACE-I therapy [30]. The ACC/AHA guidelines state that the addition of an ARB to a regimen that already includes an ACE-I and a β-blocker is a Class IIb recommendation among patients with persistent symptoms. The routine combined use of ACE-Is, aldosterone antagonists, and ARBs is strongly discouraged [10] **(IV/C)**.

Initiation of ARBs involves similar risks of renal dysfunction and hyperkalemia as seen with ACE-Is and therefore titration is done with careful monitoring. However, ARBs can be safely administered to patients with history of intolerance to ACE-Is including those with angioedema.

β-blockers

β-blockers are a mainstay of treatment in systolic heart failure by further targeting the neurohormonal pathways that cause ventricular dysfunction and remodeling. Like ACE-Is, the evidence showing survival benefit with β-blockers is so strong that all patients with heart failure, regardless of their blood pressure, should be taking a β-blocker unless contraindicated [10] **(Ia/A)**. This is because certain β-blockers, namely bisoprolol, metoprolol and carvedilol, have been shown to improve survival and decrease cardiovascular events across all stages of systolic heart failure [31-34]. These positive effects are augmented when used with other heart failure medications such as ACE-Is [1-4]. The negative chronotropic and inotropic properties of β-blockers also reduce systemic blood pressure. These properties along with the survival benefits make β-blockers ideal for treating hypertension in patients with systolic heart failure.

There are three general classes of β-blockers currently available. The first generation is non-selective – examples include propranolol and timolol. The second generation agents are β-1 selective and include metoprolol, atenolol and bisoprolol. Both the first and the second generation β-blockers have no vasodilation properties. Third generation β-blockers, such as carvedilol and labetalol, are β-non-selective with adjunctive α-receptor blockade.

Second generation β-blockers are commonly used in the treatment in systolic heart failure. However, unlike ACE-Is and ARBs, which are believed to have a class effect, β-blockers have important differences in efficacy. Selective agents such as metoprolol XL and bisoprolol have been shown to decrease mortality in patients with heart failure [31, 32]. In the CIBIS-II study, patients taking bisoprolol were less likely to die (11.8% vs. 17.3%), have cardiovascular events (12% vs. 9%) or be admitted to the hospital (39% vs. 33%) as compared to those patients taking placebo [31]. Metoprolol has also been extensively studied in heart failure. Earlier studies did not show a mortality benefit with short-acting metoprolol tartrate and therefore its use is not recommended for patients with systolic heart failure. However, the MERIT-HF trial showed that the extended-release version of metoprolol succinate, when added to standard heart failure medications, decreased all-cause mortality (7.2% vs. 11%), death from cardiovascular causes, and sudden cardiac death (SCD) [32].

It must be noted that although these non-selective β-blockers have been shown to decrease mortality in heart failure, their lack of vasodilatation properties leads to only a modest effect on systemic blood pressure. Therefore, patients with severe hypertension may benefit from additional therapy with other anti-heart failure medications or substitution with carvedilol because of its additional α-blockade effect. Two landmark studies have shown that carvedilol reduces mortality and SCD, when used in the treatment of systolic heart failure [33, 34]. A once-daily preparation of carvedilol has also become available and demonstrates similar efficacy [35].

A novel third generation β-blocker, nebivolol, has recently been approved by the FDA for the treatment of hypertension. This agent has been used successfully in Europe for many years. Its mechanism of action is unique because of its β-1 specificity and nitric oxide-mediated vasodilatation. Studies have shown that nebivolol reduces blood pressure as well as bisoprolol without the usual hemodynamic side effects of other β-blockers [36]. More studies are still needed to examine the role of nebivolol in heart failure, though European trials suggested that it was effective in treating heart failure in the elderly [37].

Initiation of a β-blocker should be done at the lowest dose and if tolerated, doubled every 2 weeks. Some patients, especially those with severe heart failure, may become symptomatic from the negative inotrope. Effects may include increased lower extremity edema, fatigue, weakness, and in some cases cardiogenic shock. Generally, most of these symptoms can be alleviated with a transient decrease in β-blocker dosage and/or an increase in diuretics.

Patients in frank shock should immediately discontinue β-blockers. As noted before, target dosages are those used in clinical trials (Table 1).

Hydralazine and nitrates

The combination of hydralazine and nitrates in addition to standard therapy has proven to be very effective among African American patients. The A-HeFT trial specifically compared a fixed-dose combination of nitrate and hydralazine with placebo in African American patients with Class III or IV heart failure. The combination significantly improved survival by 43% [38], providing strong support for its use among African American patients. The distinct benefit among black individuals is thought to be related to endothelial dysfunction and a decreased ability to produce endogenous nitric oxide, which makes them particularly responsive to nitrates. Hydralazine acts as both a vasodilator and as an antioxidant that prevents nitrate tolerance [39]. The combination's reduction of blood pressure also likely played a role in survival benefit and makes it particularly attractive in hypertensive patients. Less is known about the benefit of nitrates plus hydralazine in patients who do not identify themselves as black; however, another trial did demonstrate a 34% reduction in mortality ($p<0.038$) with the combination versus placebo among all groups [40]. The combination is recommended as part of standard therapy for all African American patients with left ventricular systolic dysfunction and NYHA Class III or IV heart failure [10, 14] **(Ib/A)**. It should also be considered for all other patients with persistent symptoms despite standard therapy [10] (II/B).

Aldosterone antagonists

Many clinicians assumed ACE-Is and ARBs would block both angiotensin II and aldosterone. However, suppression of aldosterone is not maintained long term, which has had several consequences. Aldosterone increases sodium retention, potassium and magnesium loss, and myocardial fibrosis and hypertrophy [7]. Blocking its effects significantly improved survival among patients with reduced systolic function and NYHA Class III or IV heart failure [41]. The 30% reduction in mortality included a reduction in death due to both progressive heart failure and sudden cardiac death. Based on these results, aldactone is recommended for all patients with reduced LV function and NYHA Class III or IV heart failure [10] **(Ib/A)**.

Among resistant hypertensive patients, the addition of aldosterone antagonists can decrease the mean systolic blood pressure by more than 25mmHg and diastolic pressure by 10mmHg [42]. In another trial, the selective aldosterone blocker, eplerenone, offered a significant mortality reduction among patients with an EF <40% following an MI. Additionally, there were significant reductions in blood pressure and greater improvements demonstrated among individuals with a history of hypertension [43]. These findings supported the notion that aldosterone antagonists can be an additional tool in the control of blood pressure among patients with advanced heart failure.

Initiation of aldosterone antagonists should be reserved for carefully selected patients with reduced left ventricular function (EF <40%) and advanced heart failure or a recent myocardial infarction. Renal function and serum potassium levels must also be considered. Aldosterone antagonists are not recommended for patients with serum creatinine levels >2.5mg/dL or potassium levels greater than 5.0mEq/L.

Diuretics

Thiazide diuretics have long been used in the treatment of essential hypertension, but generally are not used in the treatment of left ventricular systolic dysfunction due to a lack of mortality benefit. Furthermore, in volume overloaded states and decreased renal function, thiazide diuretics are not efficacious due to low bioavailability. Instead, loop diuretics are the preferred agents to rapidly reverse fluid congestion and associated symptoms. Relief of fluid retention by diuretics also positively affects the response of other drugs given for the treatment of heart failure; these medications should be maintained until fluid retention is eliminated [10] **(IV/C)**.

Loop diuretics demonstrate a dose-response curve that is linear and determined by the fluid status and renal function. Furosemide is the most commonly used loop diuretic and dose adjustments are made based on relief of congestion. In some cases, patients may become unresponsive to even high doses of loop diuretic despite persistent fluid overload. In these instances, a distal blocking agent, such as chlorothiazide or metolazone, can be added to increase response in the outpatient setting.

Unfortunately, diuretic therapy has been associated with up-regulation of the neurohormonal axis involved with disease progression in heart failure. It is not clear if this is a direct response to diuretic therapy or a marker of advanced heart failure. However, it is recommended that once fluid congestion is relieved, every effort should be made to discontinue diuretic therapy. This should not discourage use of diuretics in individuals who are clearly volume overloaded. Besides increasing the efficacy of ACE-Is, aldosterone antagonists, and β-blockers, diuretics also relieve volume overload and thus decrease blood pressure. Volume expansion is the most frequent pathogenic cause of resistant hypertension [44] and appropriate diuretic use is the cornerstone of therapy.

Calcium channel blockers and other drugs

Non-dihydropyridine use is discouraged in patients with left ventricular dysfunction due to their negative inotropic effects and increased likelihood of causing CHF exacerbation [45].

Dihydropyridines (amlodipine and felodipine) have no effect on mortality outcomes in patients with heart failure [46] and therefore are only used in patients with persistent hypertension despite appropriate use of all evidence-based therapies.

α-blockers (doxazosin and prazosin) are not routinely used in the treatment of heart failure based on results from the ALLHAT trial indicating increased relative risks for the development of heart failure. Central acting agents (clonidine and minoxidil) are avoided based on evidence of harm in patients with heart failure [42]. The addition of aliskiren, a direct renin inhibitor, to standard heart failure therapy has demonstrated favorable neurohormonal effects without compromising safety and holds promise as another therapeutic agent [47].

Elderly

Chronic heart failure has become a major public health issue due in large part to the increasing elderly population. Unfortunately, there has been reluctance in the community to treat these individuals with proven heart failure medications. This reluctance is multifactorial and includes fear of decreased efficacy, concerns about increased side effects, and inappropriate use of complicated regimens [48]. However, sub-group analysis of many of the pivotal trials of ACE-Is, ARBs, β-blockers, and aldosterone antagonists among the elderly (>65 years of age) have demonstrated consistent efficacy of these medications [49]. From these results, it appears that elderly patients derive similar benefits from anti-heart failure medications as younger patients and should be actively treated by clinicians.

Conclusions

Hypertension is often a coexisting illness in patients with left ventricular systolic dysfunction and plays an important role in disease progression. Treatment involves important modifications in the standard hypertension therapy to address not only elevated blood pressures, but also to mitigate the neurohormonal activation responsible for ventricular remodeling. Doing so will improve morbidity and mortality in these patients. Furthermore, targeting the renin-angiotensin-aldosterone system is beneficial across the spectrum of disease severity and clinicians are encouraged to employ evidence-based therapies for all appropriate patients including the elderly.

Key points	Evidence level
◆ Angiotensin-converting enzyme inhibitors should be used in all patients with a reduced LVEF, unless contraindicated.	Ia/A
◆ Use of one of the three β-blockers (i.e. bisoprolol, carvedilol, and sustained release metoprolol succinate) is recommended for all patients with a reduced LVEF.	Ia/A
◆ Diuretics are indicated in patients with current or prior symptoms of HF and reduced LVEF who have evidence of fluid retention.	IV/C
◆ Angiotensin II receptor blockers are recommended in patients with current or prior symptoms of HF and reduced LVEF who are ACE-I-intolerant.	Ia/A
◆ Aldosterone antagonists are recommended in selected patients with moderately severe to severe symptoms of HF and reduced LVEF.	Ib/A
◆ The combination of hydralazine and nitrates is recommended to improve outcomes for patients self-described as African Americans, with moderate-severe symptoms already on optimal therapy with ACE-Is, β-blockers, and diuretics.	Ib/A
◆ The addition of a combination of hydralazine and a nitrate is reasonable for any patient with reduced LVEF who is already taking an ACE-I and β-blocker for symptomatic HF and who has persistent symptoms.	II/B
◆ The addition of an ARB may be considered in persistently symptomatic patients with reduced LVEF who are already being treated with ACE-Is and β-blockers.	II/B
◆ Routine combined use of an ACE-I, ARB, and aldosterone antagonist is not recommended for patients with current or prior symptoms of HF and reduced LVEF.	IV/C
◆ Calcium channel blocking drugs are not indicated as routine treatment of heart failure.	Ia/A
◆ Clinicians should attempt to titrate evidence-based therapies to doses that have been shown to reduce the risks of cardiovascular events in clinical trials (Table 1) [10].	IV/C

Adapted from the ACC/AHA 2009 Focused Update on the Guidelines for the "Diagnosis and Management of Heart Failure in Adults".

References

1. Lloyd-Jones DM, Larson MG, Leip EP, *et al.* Lifetime risk for developing congestive heart failure: the Framingham Heart Study. *Circulation* 2002; 106: 3068-72.

2. Chobanian AV. The hypertension paradox-more uncontrolled disease despite improved therapy. *N Engl J Med* 2009; 361: 878-87.
3. Baker DW. Prevention of heart failure. *J Card Fail* 2002; 8: 333-46.
4. Chobanian AV. Does it matter how hypertension is controlled? *N Engl J Med* 2008; 359(23): 2485-8.
5. Bangalore S, Sawhney S, Messerli FH. Relation of beta-blocker-induced heart rate lowering and cardioprotection in hypertension. *J Am Coll Cardiol* 2008; 52: 1482-9.
6. Francis GS, Tang WH. Pathophysiology of congestive heart failure. *Rev Cardiovasc Med* 2003; 4 Suppl 2: S14-20.
7. Mehra MR, Uber PA, Potluri S. Renin angiotensin aldosterone and adrenergic modulation in chronic heart failure: contemporary concepts. *Am J Med Sci* 2002; 324(5): 267-75.
8. Mitchell JA, Ventura HO, Mehra MR. Early recognition and treatment of hypertensive heart disease. *Curr Opin Cardiol* 2005; 20(4): 282-9.
9. Uddin N, Patterson JH. Current guidelines for treatment of heart failure: 2006 update. *Pharmacotherapy* 2007; 27(4 Pt 2): 12S-7.
10. Hunt SA, Abraham WT, Chin MH, Feldman AM, Francis GS, Ganiats TG, Jessup M, Konstam MA, Mancini DM, Michl K, Oates JA, Rahko PS, Silver MA, Stevenson LW, Yancy CW; American College of Cardiology Foundation; American Heart Association. 2009 Focused update incorporated into the ACC/AHA 2005 Guidelines for the Diagnosis and Management of Heart Failure in Adults - A Report of the American College of Cardiology Foundation/American Heart Association Task Force on Practice Guidelines Developed in Collaboration With the International Society for Heart and Lung Transplantation. *J Am Coll Cardiol* 2009; 53(15): e1-90.
11. Bertoni AG, Duren-Winfield V, Ambrosius WT, McArdle J, Sueta CA, Massing MW, Peacock S, Davis J, Croft JB, Goff DC Jr. Quality of heart failure care in managed Medicare and Medicaid patients in North Carolina. *Am J Cardiol* 2004; 93(6): 714-8.
12. Yancy CW, Fonarow GC, Albert NM, Curtis AB, Stough WG, Gheorghiade M, Heywood JT, McBride ML, Mehra MR, O'Connor CM, Reynolds D, Walsh MN. Influence of patient age and sex on delivery of guideline-recommended heart failure care in the outpatient cardiology practice setting: findings from IMPROVE HF. *Am Heart J* 2009; 157(4): 754-62.
13. Chobanian AV, Bakris GL, Black HR, Cushman WC, Green LA, Izzo JL Jr, Jones DW, Materson BJ, Oparil S, Wright JT Jr, Roccella EJ; National Heart, Lung, and Blood Institute Joint National Committee on Prevention, Detection, Evaluation, and Treatment of High Blood Pressure; National High Blood Pressure Education Program Coordinating Committee. The Seventh Report of the Joint National Committee on Prevention, Detection, Evaluation, and Treatment of High Blood Pressure: the JNC 7 report. *JAMA* 2003; 289(19): 2560-72.
14. Heart Failure Society of America. Managing patients with hypertension and heart failure. *J Card Fail* 2006; 12(1): e112-4.
15. European Society of Cardiology; Heart Failure Association of the ESC (HFA); European Society of Intensive Care Medicine (ESICM). ESC guidelines for the diagnosis and treatment of acute and chronic heart failure 2008: the Task Force for the diagnosis and treatment of acute and chronic heart failure 2008 of the European Society of Cardiology. Developed in collaboration with the Heart Failure Association of the ESC (HFA) and endorsed by the European Society of Intensive Care Medicine (ESICM). *Eur J Heart Fail* 2008; 10(10): 933-89.
16. Thohan V, Little WC. Is a higher blood pressure better in heart failure? *Heart* 2009; 95(1): 4-5.
17. Abraham WT, Fonarow GC, Albert NM, *et al.* Predictors of in-hospital mortality in patients hospitalized for heart failure: insights from the Organized Program to Initiate Lifesaving Treatment in Hospitalized Patients with Heart Failure (OPTIMIZE-HF). *J Am Coll Cardiol* 2008; 52: 347-56.
18. Raphael CE, Whinnett ZI, Davies JE, *et al.* Quantifying the paradoxical effect of higher systolic blood pressure on mortality in chronic heart failure. *Heart* 2009; 95: 56-62.
19. Yancy CW, Fonarow GC; ADHERE Scientific Advisory Committee. Quality of care and outcomes in acute decompensated heart failure: The ADHERE Registry. *Curr Heart Fail Rep* 2004; 1(3): 121-8.
20. Kalantar-Zadeh K, Block G, Horwich T, Fonarow GC. Reverse epidemiology of conventional cardiovascular risk factors in patients with chronic heart failure. *J Am Coll Cardiol* 2004;4 3(8): 1439-44.
21. The CONSENSUS Trial Study Group. Effects of enalapril on mortality in severe congestive heart failure: results of the Cooperative North Scandinavian Enalapril Survival Study (CONSENSUS). *N Engl J Med* 1987; 316 (23): 1429-35.

22. The SOLVD Investigators. Effect of enalapril on survival in patients with reduced left ventricular ejection fractions and congestive heart failure. *N Engl J Med* 1991; 325 (5): 293-302.
23. Cohn JN, Johnson G, Ziesche S, *et al.* A comparison of enalapril with hydralazine-isosorbide dinitrate in the treatment of congestive heart failure. *N Engl J Med* 1991; 325: 302-10.
24. Flather MD, Yusuf S, Kober L, *et al.* Long-term ACE inhibitor therapy in patients with heart failure or left-ventricular dysfunction: a systematic overview of data from individual patients. *Lancet* 2000; 355: 1575-81.
25. Demers C, Mody A, Teo KK, McKelvie RS. ACE inhibitors in heart failure: what more do we need to know? *Am J Cardiovasc Drugs* 2005; 5(6): 351-9.
26. Packer M, Poole-Wilson A, Armstrong PW, *et al.* Comparative effects of low and high doses of the angiotensin-converting enzyme inhibitor, lisinopril, on morbidity and mortality in chronic heart failure: the ATLAS Study Group. *Circulation* 1999; 100: 2312-8.
27. Mehra MR, Uber PA, Francis GS. Heart failure therapy at a crossroad: are there limits to the neurohormonal model? *J Am Coll Cardiol* 2003; 41(9): 1606-10.
28. Pitt B, Poole-Wilson PA, Segal R, *et al.* Effect of losartan compared with captopril on mortality in patients with symptomatic heart failure: randomized trial. Losartan Heart Failure Survival Study ELITE II: the ELITE II investigators. *Lancet* 2000; 355: 1582-7.
29. Lee VC, Rhew DC, Dylan M, *et al.* Meta-analysis: angiotensin-receptor blockers in chronic heart failure and high-risk acute myocardial infarction. *Ann Intern Med* 2004; 141: 693-704.
30. McMurray JJV, Östergren J, Swedberg K, *et al.* Effects of candesartan in patients with chronic heart failure and reduced left-ventricular systolic function taking angiotensin-converting-enzyme inhibitors: the CHARM-Added trial. *Lancet* 2003; 362: 767-11.
31. CIBIS-II Investigators and Committees. The Cardiac Insufficiency Bisoprolol Study II (CIBIS-II): a randomized trail. *Lancet* 1999; (353): 9-13.
32. MERIT-HF Study Group. Effect of metoprolol CR/XL in chronic heart failure: Metoprolol CR/XL Randomised Intervention Trial in Congestive Heart Failure (MERIT-HF). *Lancet* 1999; (353): 2001-7.
33. Packer M, Bristow MR, Cohn JN, Colucci WS, Fowler MB, Gilbert EM, Shusterman NH, For the U.S Carvedilol Heart Failure Group Study. The effect of carvedilol on morbidity and mortality in patients with chronic heart failure. *N Engl J Med* 1996; (334)21: 1349-55.
34. Macdonald PS, Kogh AM, Aboyoun CL, Lund M, Amor A, McCaffrey DJ. Tolerability and efficacy of carvedilol in patients with New York Heart Association Class IV heart failure. *JACC* 1999; (33)4: 924-31.
35. Greenberg BH, Mehra M, Teerlink JR, Ordronneau P, McCollum D, Gilbert EM. COMPARE: comparison of the effects of carvedilol CR and carvedilol IR on left ventricular ejection fraction in patients with heart failure. *Am J Cardiol* 2006; 98(7A): 53L-9.
36. Czuriga I, Riecansky I, Bodnar J, Fulop T, Kruzsicz V, Kristof E, Edes I, for the NEBIS Investigators; NEBIS Investigators Group. Comparison of the new cardioselective beta-blocker nebivolol with bisoprolol in hypertension: the Nebivolol, Bisoprolol Multicenter Study (NEBIS). *Cardiovasc Drugs Ther* 2003; 17(3): 257-63.
37. Weber MA. The role of the new beta-blockers in treating cardiovascular disease. *Am J Hypertens* 2005; 18: 169S-76.
38. Taylor AL, Ziesche S, Yancy C, Carson P, D'Agostino R, Ferdinand K, Taylor M, Adams K, Sabolinski M, Worcel M, Cohn J; for the African-American Heart Failure Trial Investigators. Combination of isosorbide dinitrate and hydralazine in blacks with heart failure. *N Engl J Med* 2004; 351: 2049-57.
39. Elkayam U, Bitar F. Effects of nitrates and hydralazine in heart failure: clinical evidence before the African American Heart Failure Trial. *Am J Cardiol* 2005; 96(7B): 37i-43.
40. Cohn JN, Archibald DG, Ziesche S, Franciosa JA, Harston WE, Tristani FE, Dunkman WB, Jacobs W, Francis GS, Flohr KH. Effect of vasodilator therapy on mortality in chronic congestive heart failure: results of a Veterans Administration Cooperative Study (V-HeFT). *N Engl J Med* 1986; 314: 1547-52.
41. Pitt B MD, Zannad F MD, Remme WJ MD, Cody R MD, Castaigne A MD, *et al.* The effect of spironolactone on morbidity and mortality in patients with severe heart failure. *N Engl J Med* 1999; 341(10): 709-17.
42. Manickavasagam S, Merla R, Koerner MM, Fujise K, Kunapuli S, Rosanio S, Barbagelata A. Management of hypertension in chronic heart failure. *Expert Review of Cardiovascular Therapy* 2009; 7(4): 423-33.
43. Pitt B, Remme W, Zannad F, *et al.* Eplerenone Post-Acute Myocardial Infarction Heart Failure Efficacy and Survival Study Investigators: eplerenone, a selective aldosterone blocker, in patients with left ventricular dysfunction after myocardial infarction. *N Engl J Med* 2003; 348: 1309-21.

44. Sarafidis PA, Bakris GL. Resistant hypertension: an overview of evaluation and treatment. *J Am Coll Cardiol* 2008; 52(22): 1749-57.
45. Mohan JC, Mohan V. Management of hypertension in heart failure: striking lack of evidence for a common problem. *Indian Heart J* 2008; 60(2): 139-43.
46. O'Connor CM, Carson PE, Miller AB, Pressler ML, Belkin RN, Neuberg GW, Frid DJ, Cropp AB, Anderson S, Wertheimer JH, DeMets DL. Effect of amlodipine on mode of death among patients with advanced heart failure in the PRAISE trial. Prospective Randomized Amlodipine Survival Evaluation. *Am J Cardiol* 1998; 82(7): 881-7.
47. Solomon SD, McMurray J, *et al.* Safety and tolerability profile of aliskiren added to optimized therapy in elderly and very elderly patients with heart failure. *Eur Heart J* 2009; 30: 165.
48. Komajda M, Follath F, Swedberg K, *et al.* The EuroHeart Failure Survey programme - a survey on the quality of care among patients with heart failure in Europe. Part 2: treatment. *Eur Heart J* 2003; 24: 464-74.
49. Dulin BR, Krum H. Drug therapy of chronic heart failure in the elderly: the current state of clinical-trial evidence. *Curr Opin Cardiol* 2006; 21(4): 393-9.

Chapter 13

Treatment of hypertension with cerebrovascular disease: what is the evidence?

William J. Elliott MD PhD, Professor of Preventive Medicine
Internal Medicine and Pharmacology
Pacific Northwest University of Health Sciences
Yakima, Washington, USA

Introduction

Current guidelines **(Ia/A)** unanimously agree that elevated blood pressure (BP) is a major risk factor for incident cerebrovascular disease (especially acute stroke) [1, 2]. From a population-based perspective **(Ia/A)**, lowering blood pressure is likely to be the most effective method of preventing cerebrovascular disease and acute stroke [3]. Nonetheless, great controversy currently exists (**IV/B** against vs. **Ib/B** for), at least in the United States (US), about whether blood pressure-lowering should ever be considered (much less attempted or recommended) for a patient with an acute 'stroke-in-evolution' [4, 5]. Even more contentious **(IV/B)** is the level to which blood pressure should be controlled once rehabilitation from the acute stroke has been completed [6, 7]. This chapter's objective is to review the available evidence and treatment options for abnormal blood pressures in patients with cerebrovascular disease.

Epidemiology and differential diagnosis of high and low blood pressures in patients with acute cerebrovascular disease

Elevated blood pressure (to ≥140/90mm Hg) occurs in about 75% of patients presenting with an acute stroke. A systolic blood pressure (SBP) ≥180mm Hg is observed in about 60%, with a somewhat greater prevalence among individuals with prior hypertension, hemorrhagic stroke, and greater stroke severity. In the US, about 87% of strokes are ischemic in origin, 10% are intracerebral hemorrhages, and about 3% are subarachnoid hemorrhages [8]. In most acute stroke patients with hypertension, the blood pressure nearly always falls without intervention, during the first day to weeks, reflecting the fact that the elevated blood pressures are often attributable to other causes, e.g. pain, distended bowel or bladder, psychological stress, physiological reaction to generalized or cerebral hypoxia, or increased intracerebral pressure (the 'Cushing reflex') [9]. A recent systematic review of 32 observational studies (that included more than 10,000 patients) **(IIb/B)** concluded that, among all stroke patients, high systolic or diastolic blood pressure (defined using various criteria in each study) was associated with a 1.5- to 5-fold increase in the risks of death, or the potentially more important composite of death or dependency [10, 11]. In another large database **(IIb/B)**, every 10mm Hg elevation in SBP over 180mm Hg increased the risk of neurological deterioration by 40%, and the risk of a poor outcome by 23% [12]. Although hypertension is vastly more common in acute stroke patients, hypotension predicts a poor prognosis: in the same database **(IIb/B)**, a BP <100/70mm Hg was associated with significantly poorer outcomes than a BP between 100/70 and 150/90mm Hg [13]. The differential diagnosis for hypotension in the face of an acute neurological event is important, because many of its underlying causes are reversible if treated. Thus, volume depletion (particularly in the setting of dysphagia), blood loss, decreased cardiac output due to myocardial ischemia, dysrhythmias (especially atrial fibrillation with a rapid ventricular response), and aortic dissection can all be improved, which generally leads to an improved neurological examination acutely and a better long-term prognosis. In general, a U-shaped curve is seen in the correlation of initial blood pressures and outcomes (all-cause mortality or the composite outcome of death or dependency) in ischemic stroke patients. For example, in the first International Stroke Trial **(IIa/B)**, the best outcomes occurred among ischemic stroke patients with modestly raised or high-normal blood pressure (optimum SBP around 150mm Hg). Higher blood pressures were independently associated with an increased risk of death from presumed cerebral edema, whereas lower blood pressures were associated with severe clinical stroke syndromes and an excess of deaths from coronary heart disease [12].

Acute treatment options for abnormal blood pressure in patients with cerebrovascular disease

Acutely lowering blood pressure is controversial

There are many theoretical reasons why lowering elevated blood pressures in an acute stroke might be beneficial, including: reducing brain edema, reducing the risk of hemorrhagic transformation of an ischemic event, preventing further damage to blood vessels, and reducing the risk of early recurrent stroke. Very few, if any, of these have been demonstrated in large-scale randomized clinical trials, perhaps because the traditional teaching in the US **(IV/C)** has been that antihypertensive treatment is warranted in the acute phase of stroke ONLY if the blood pressure is 'very high', or the patient has another reason to mandate blood pressure reduction (e.g. hypertensive encephalopathy, acute pulmonary edema, aortic dissection, etc.) [4]. Many older neurologists are very concerned about the risks of acute blood pressure lowering, including worsening of the neurological defects because of decreasing perfusion pressure to watershed areas of the ischemic penumbra [4].

These concerns about the adverse effects of lowering blood pressure in patients with cerebrovascular disease were largely supported by the results of several randomized trials **(Ib/A)** of nimodipine (vs. placebo) in acute stroke. As this drug offered proven beneficial effects in subarachnoid hemorrhage, it seemed reasonable to test its effects in other stroke subtypes. Unfortunately, no benefit of the drug was seen (across all randomized patients)**(Ib/A)**, and post hoc analyses showed poorer outcomes in nimodipine-treated patients with large infarcts and high pre-treatment blood pressures [13]. An analysis of 115 consecutive ischemic stroke patients **(III/B)** found that each 10mm Hg reduction in SBP during the first 24 hours was associated with an 89% increased risk of poor outcomes [14]. A subsequent post hoc report **(III/B)** concluded that early lowering of SBP by >20mm Hg with nimodipine increased the risk of worsened neurological status early, and infarcted brain volume and death later on [11]. Because of the current focus of many neurologists on the early use of thrombolytic agents (which are typically contraindicated if BP >185/110mm Hg), current US stroke guidelines **(IV/C)** recommend antihypertensive therapy ONLY to achieve a blood pressure that would allow intravenous thrombolytic therapy, or, otherwise, ONLY if the BP exceeds 180-230/105-120mm Hg [4]. The wide range of this threshold is evidence of the lack of agreement on what physicians should do about such blood pressures in the acute setting.

A number of uncontrolled or small trials have used ACE inhibitors, β-blockers, calcium antagonists, and nitrates in the acute stroke setting. Although few adverse effects have been reported, a recent systematic review **(Ia/A)** suggests there is little evidence of benefit, either [15]. A systematic review **(Ia/A)** of cerebral blood flow and flow velocity in patients with acute ischemic stroke showed no major diminution in these parameters [16], but current US guidelines **(IV/C)** still recommend withholding antihypertensive therapy from most patients for the first 24 hours after the stroke [4].

Perhaps the most famous of the randomized clinical trials **(Ia/A)** that began an antihypertensive agent AFTER the first 24 hours of an acute ischemic stroke compared candesartan, given at 4-16mg/d, titrated to 32mg/d (if BP >160/100mm Hg on day 2) vs. placebo for the first week, and thereafter added other antihypertensive medications, as needed, in both randomized treatment arms [17]. This multicenter trial planned to enroll 500 patients, but accrual was discontinued after 339, as there was already a significant benefit of the early candesartan regimen on combined cardiovascular events (the difference in recurrent stroke was not significant: 13 of 173 vs. 19 of 165). A smaller study **(IIb/B)** saw lowered blood pressures and somewhat improved short-term stroke outcomes when ischemic stroke patients with elevated blood pressures were given either amlodipine or captopril, again beginning 24 hours after stroke onset [18]. In contrast, bendrofluazide (the thiazide diuretic used most often in Great Britain) did not lower blood pressure very well in a small British trial [19] **(Ib/A)**.

These data, taken together, demonstrate the therapeutic equipoise needed to launch clinical trials in which one group of hypertensive acute stroke victims could ethically receive relatively long-acting antihypertensive drugs, and the other could receive whatever 'standard-of-care' regimen was in place at the time. The pilot phases of two such trials have recently been reported; neither showed an adverse effect of acute antihypertensive treatment, and therefore enrollment in the larger, definitive trial has been started in each case.

Recent trials suggesting potential benefit of acute lowering of blood pressure

The INTEnsive blood pressure Reduction in Acute Cerebral hemorrhage Trial (INTERACT)**(Ib/A)** was planned as a pilot study, with a primary endpoint of change in hematoma volume by computed tomography (a surrogate endpoint) at 24 hours after randomization to either an intensive blood pressure-lowering strategy (target SBP of 140mm Hg) or a 'conventional treatment' group (target SBP of 180mm Hg) [20]. There were no restrictions on the drug (or drugs) used; most investigators in this Australasian trial used furosemide or urapadil as first-line agents. The intensively treated group had a 10.8mm Hg lower SBP (from 1-24 hours after randomization), significantly smaller hematoma growth (13.7% vs. 36.3%, p=0.04) at 24 hours, although this became non-significant after pre-specified adjustment for baseline differences in initial hematoma volume and time between the onset of symptoms and the initial computed tomographic scan of the head. The authors extrapolated their observed difference in absolute hematoma size to about a 12% relative risk reduction for death or dependency. Only nine subjects suffered hypotension, and the 'severe' form was actually more common in the 'conventional' group. The authors therefore concluded that acute blood pressure reduction in intracranial hemorrhage is feasible, well-tolerated, and worthy of study in a much larger trial (INTERACT-2).

In the pilot phase of the Controlling Hypertension and Hypotension Immediately Post-Stroke (CHHIPS) trial **(Ib/A)**, 179 patients with acute ischemic or hemorrhagic strokes within the previous 36 hours, who had SBP >160mm Hg were randomized to placebo (n=63), labetalol (n=58) or lisinopril (n=58), the doses of which could be escalated for the first 2 weeks until the SBP was <150mm Hg [21]. For patients with dysphagia, antihypertensive drug therapy was given by the intravenous or sublingual route. There were significant decreases in blood pressure in the two actively treated groups during the first 24 hours (-21 vs. -11mm Hg), as well as at 2 weeks (-31mm Hg vs. -24mm Hg). The primary endpoint, death or dependency at 14 days after stroke, did not differ significantly (61% vs. 59%, p=0.82). However, neither early deterioration nor adverse events was worse in the actively treated group; in fact, 3 months after treatment, the risk of death was more than halved (9.7% vs. 20.3%, p=0.05). These optimistic results (involving small numbers of subjects) will be tested further in a similar trial that will enroll 2050 subjects.

Several large, outcome-based randomized trials of antihypertensive drugs for lowering blood pressure during acute stroke are ongoing **(Ib/A)**. The two largest of these include: the Continue or Stop post-Stroke Antihypertensives Collaborative Study (COSSACS; 2900 patients with stroke, randomized to stop or continue pre-existing antihypertensive drugs for 2 weeks after stroke) [22], and the Efficacy of Nitric Oxide in Stroke Trial (ENOS; 5000 patients with stroke, randomized to transdermal nitroglycerine patch or not for 7 days after stroke onset) [23].

Trials investigating acutely raising blood pressure in ischemic stroke-in-evolution

A very different approach has been advocated by other investigators, who believe that increasing blood pressure will improve brain oxygenation and outcomes in the acute stroke patient. A retrospective review **(III/B)** and a pilot study **(III/C)** from the Massachusetts General Hospital suggested that 1-6 days of phenylephrine infusion, titrated to raise SBP by 20% (but not to exceed 200mm Hg), resulted in improved neurological status at hospital discharge [24]. Similarly, a comparison **(III/B)** of 15 stroke patients with diffusion-perfusion mismatch on magnetic resonance imaging showed better NIH Stroke Scale scores, cognitive scores, and less hypoperfused brain tissue if they received drugs to mildly raise blood pressure at presentation [25]. The most recent systematic review **(Ib/B)** of this treatment option suggests that, although apparently safe and effective, the numbers of patients in the few small trials completed so far is insufficient to warrant a general recommendation for use [26], an opinion shared by the most recent American Stroke Association guidelines [4] **(IV/C)**.

Epidemiology and differential diagnosis for abnormal blood pressure weeks after a stroke

The amount and quality of clinical trial and epidemiological outcome data increase as the amount of time between the acute stroke increases, prompting a different set of much more optimistic guidelines **(Ia/A)** from the American Stroke Association [6]. As compared to primary prevention, fewer data exist between blood pressure and secondary stroke prevention **(Ia/A)**, but the direct relationship between blood pressure and stroke risk still holds [27]. There are no formal surveys of the prevalence of hypertension or hypotension among long-term stroke survivors, but it is likely that hypertension should be more common in this than in the general population. As a result, the differential diagnosis of an abnormal blood pressure in a stroke survivor is likely not different than what is considered in people without a stroke, except that other manifestations of atherosclerosis (including renovascular hypertension as a potential cause of hypertension) are more likely. The evaluation of a stroke survivor with abnormal blood pressure should likely follow the recommendations of JNC 7 **(IV/C)**[1], which has de-emphasized the role of extensive evaluations for secondary causes of hypertension unless there is a good clinical reason to do so (e.g. history of excessive dietary sodium consumption, presence of an abdominal bruit, unprovoked hypokalemia).

Treatment options for elevated blood pressure weeks after a stroke

Antihypertensive therapy to prevent recurrent cerebrovascular disease events

Although a large amount of clinical trial evidence suggests that antihypertensive drugs prevent stroke recurrence **(Ia/A)** [28], and a number of recent trials have suggested that the benefit is independent of the initial blood pressure, there may well be differences in the effectiveness of different classes of antihypertensive drugs in secondary prevention of cerebrovascular disease. Teasing out specific data about secondary stroke prevention from reports of many clinical trials is difficult, because subgroup analyses (reporting the numbers of patients who experienced second strokes) have infrequently been reported for trials that enrolled some, but not all, individuals who had suffered a first stroke. Fortunately, the Individual Data Analysis of Antihypertensive Intervention Trials (INDANA) investigators have gathered these data from trials completed prior to 1996 **(Ia/A)** [29]; sadly, many recent, large and important trials, such as the Antihypertensive and Lipid-Lowering to prevent Heart Attack Trial, have not yet reported data about secondary prevention. The data that have been reported [30-44] are summarized in Table 1. Unfortunately, a traditional Mantel-Haenszel meta-

Table 1. Trials of chronic antihypertensive drugs in secondary stroke prevention.

Trial	'Control' treatment	# of recurrent strokes /# at risk	Test agent	# of recurrent strokes /# at risk
Carter [30]	Placebo	21/49	Diuretic	10/50
HSCSG [31]	Placebo	42/219	Diuretic	37/233
EWPHE [29]	Placebo	9/28	Diuretic	5/35
Coope & Warrender [29]	No treatment	1/6	β-Blocker	2/11
HDFP [29]	'Usual care'	16/138	Diuretic	15/136
SHEP [29]	Placebo	7/40	Diuretic	8/59
STOP-1 [29]	Placebo	4/35	β-Blocker (or diuretic)	1/31
Dutch TIA [32]	Placebo	62/741	β-Blocker	52/732
PATS [33]	No treatment?	217/2824	Diuretic	159/2841
TEST [34]	Placebo	75/384	β-Blocker	81/372
HOPE [35]	Placebo	51/513	ACE-I	43/500
PROGRESS [36]	Placebo (±placebo)	420/3054	ACE-I (±diuretic)	307/3051
MOSES [37]	CCB	89/695	ARB	80/710
SCOPE [38]	Placebo	15/97	ARB	6/97
PRoFESS [39]	Placebo	934/10,186	ARB	880/10,146

HSCSG = Hypertension-Stroke Cooperative Study Group; EWPHE = European Working Party on Hypertension in the Elderly; HDFP = Hypertension Detection and Follow-Up Program; SHEP = Systolic Hypertension in the Elderly Program; STOP-1 = Swedish Trial in Old Patients #1; TIA = Transient Ischemic Attack; PATS = Post-stroke Antihypertensive Treatment Study; TEST = [atenolol] Evaluation in Stroke Trial; HOPE = Heart Outcomes Prevention Evaluation; ACE-I = angiotensin-converting enzyme inhibitor; PROGRESS = Perindopril pROtection aGainst REcurrent Stroke Study; MOSES = MOrbidity and mortality after Stroke-Eprosartan vs. nitrendipine in Secondary prevention; ARB = angiotensin II receptor blocker; CCB = calcium channel blocker; SCOPE = Study on COgnition and Prognosis in the Elderly; PRoFESS = Prevention Regimen [o] For Effectively avoiding Second Strokes

analysis (using a fixed-effects model) of the trials involving 'any active drug' vs. 'placebo/no treatment' displays significant inhomogeneity (p<0.02). Some of the inhomogeneity can be linked to the disagreement between the very positive overall results of PROGRESS [36] **(Ib/A)**, which showed a highly significant 26% reduction in recurrent stroke with perindopril±indapamide vs. placebo±placebo), and the non-significant 6% reduction seen in the comparison of an ARB vs. placebo in the larger PRoFESS [39] **(Ib/A)**. The results of a random-effects model (of DerSimonian and Laird [40]) are shown in Figure 1, the overall result

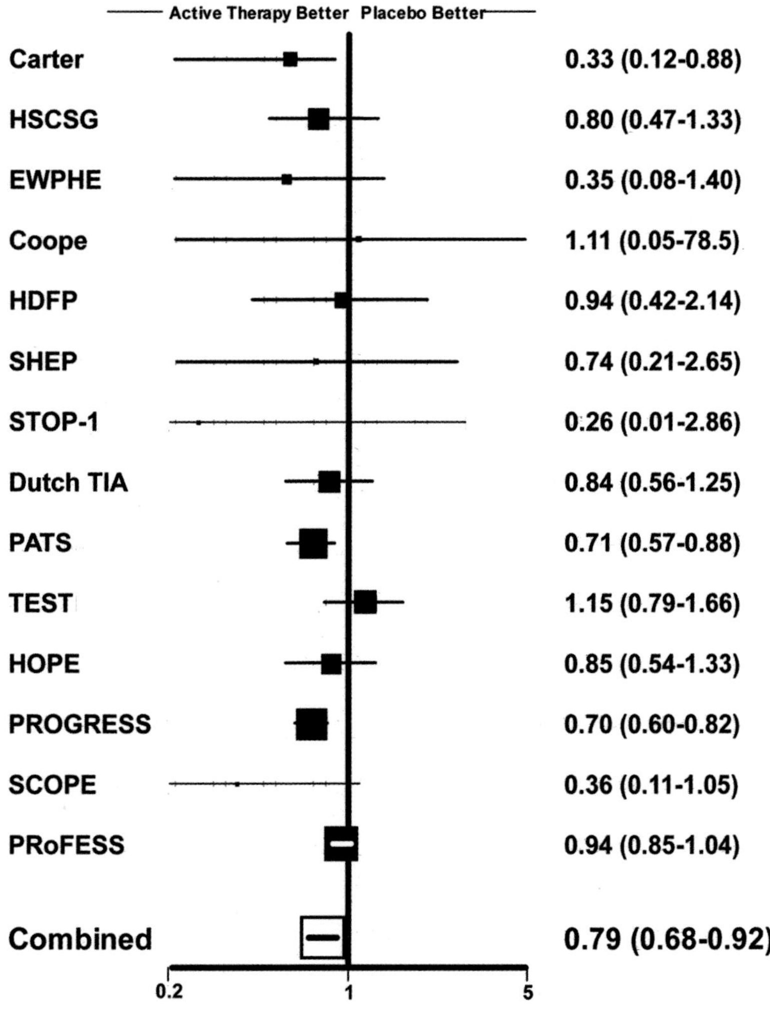

Figure 1. Results of a meta-analysis (using a random-effects model) of active antihypertensive agents vs. placebo/no treatment in the prevention of fatal or recurrent non-fatal stroke in patients with cerebrovascular disease. The overall pooled odds ratio for active treatment was 0.79, with a 95% confidence interval of 0.68-0.92, p<0.002. As customary, the area of each 'box' (corresponding to the effect size) is inversely proportional to the variance of each trial; the horizontal lines correspond to the 95% confidence limits for the odds ratio for each trial.

of which is a significant reduction in recurrent stroke by 21% (95% confidence interval: 0.58-0.92, p<0.002). The limitations and inhomogeneity of this dataset are further illustrated in Figure 2, which shows the results of pair-wise meta-analytic (direct) comparisons of the various initial antihypertensive drug classes used in these trials, including MOSES [37] **(Ib/A)**. Overall, a diuretic or an ACE inhibitor showed significant benefit (compared to placebo) in

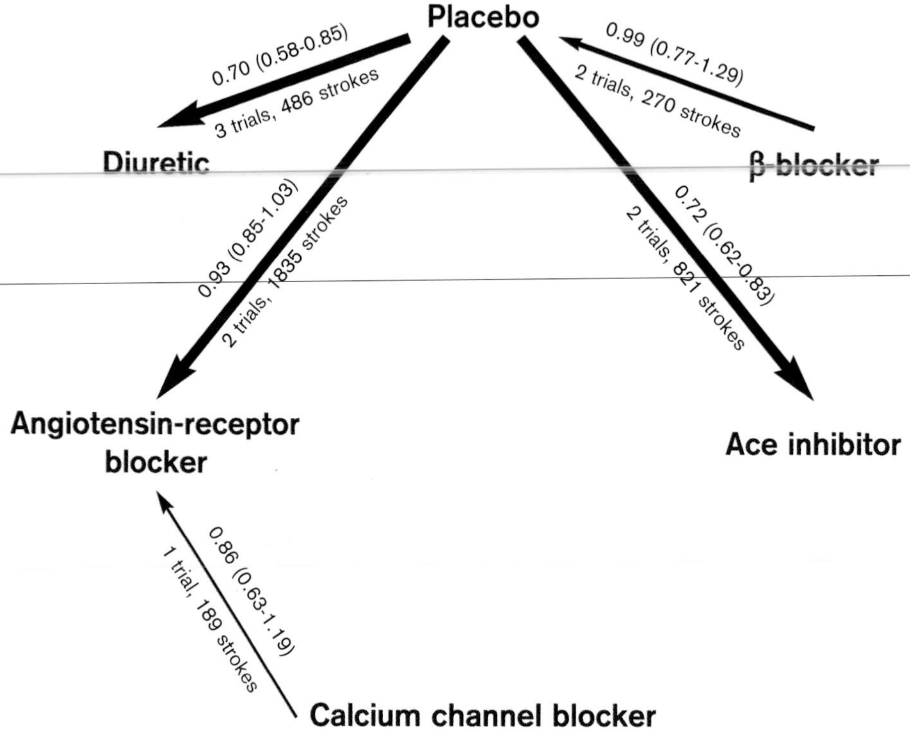

Figure 2. 'Network' summarizing comparative trials involving placebo and/or different antihypertensive drug classes in clinical trials for prevention of stroke in patients with cerebrovascular disease. The arrowhead points to the drug class with the lower risk of recurrent stroke; the breadth of the line is proportional to the number of recurrent strokes in the pair-wise meta-analytic comparison of the two entries. The summary odds ratio and 95% confidence limits are shown above the line between each entry; the number of trials and recurrent strokes in each meta-analysis are shown below the line. Note that the 'network meta-analysis' of these data results in a large 'incoherence', presumably because of the limited number of studies comparing two active drug classes.

preventing a second stroke, whereas neither a β-blocker nor an ARB was significantly better than placebo. Only one comparison involved a calcium channel blocker, and it was inferior in preventing the first recurrent stroke than the ARB, which was in turn not significantly better than placebo. Although there has not been a comparison of an ACE inhibitor vs. a diuretic in secondary stroke prevention, their indirect comparison (each vs. placebo) suggests they would not be much different (relative risk for the diuretic vs. ACE inhibitor: 0.97, with 95% confidence limits of 0.73-1.21) [41]. Similarly, an indirect comparison of a diuretic vs. ARB suggests superiority of the former (relative risk: 0.75, 95% CI: 0.54-0.96). The similarity of the effects of a β-blocker and placebo is seen, even without including the data of the Beta-blocker Evaluation in Stroke Trial (BEST), which reported only a larger number of deaths among subjects randomized to a β-blocker (vs. placebo), and no information about recurrent strokes [42]. The paucity of trials comparing calcium channel blockers with any other treatment (active or placebo) greatly widens confidence intervals for both direct and indirect comparisons involving this class of drugs, and makes the results of 'network meta-analysis' of the secondary stroke data incoherent (ω=1.65) [43]. These conclusions, based on many more data than were available in 2006, echo the conclusions of the guidelines from the American Stroke Association: "The optimal [antihypertensive] drug regimen remains uncertain" [6].

Antihypertensive therapy to prevent first cardiovascular disease events

What is less controversial is that chronic antihypertensive drug therapy, overall, prevents recurrent stroke (Figure 1), and perhaps more importantly, major adverse cardiovascular events in patients with a history of cerebrovascular disease [1, 2, 6, 7, 44]. In several recent trials, including PROGRESS [36], HOPE [35], and SCOPE [38], these benefits were independent of the initial blood pressure, and (at least in PROGRESS) directly related to the difference in SBP between the randomized groups [44].

What should the optimal blood pressure be for patients with cerebrovascular disease?

Evidence from blood pressure lowering in the setting of acute stroke-in-evolution

As discussed above, the concept of attempting to control blood pressure during the acute phase of a 'stroke-in-evolution' is a relatively new one, and quite controversial [4, 5]. There have, to date, been no trials that have compared outcomes in groups of acute stroke patients randomized to achieve various levels of blood pressure (as, for example was the intent in the Hypertension Optimal Treatment study). Current US guidelines **(IV/C)**, based primarily on experience and post hoc analyses of data from clinical trials **(IIa/B)** and epidemiological studies **(IIa/B)**, suggest that physicians allow the blood pressure in acute stroke patients to remain undisturbed unless the SBP exceeds 180mm Hg [4].

Evidence from blood pressure lowering in patients weeks removed from an acute stroke

There are also no prospective randomized trials to determine the optimal blood pressure for patients who are weeks removed from their acute stroke. Retrospective analyses of PROGRESS **(Ib/B)** suggest that the lowest risk of stroke recurrence was seen in those in the lowest quartile of achieved blood pressure (~112/72mm Hg), and rose progressively with higher follow-up blood pressures [44]. Rashid *et al* have performed meta-regression

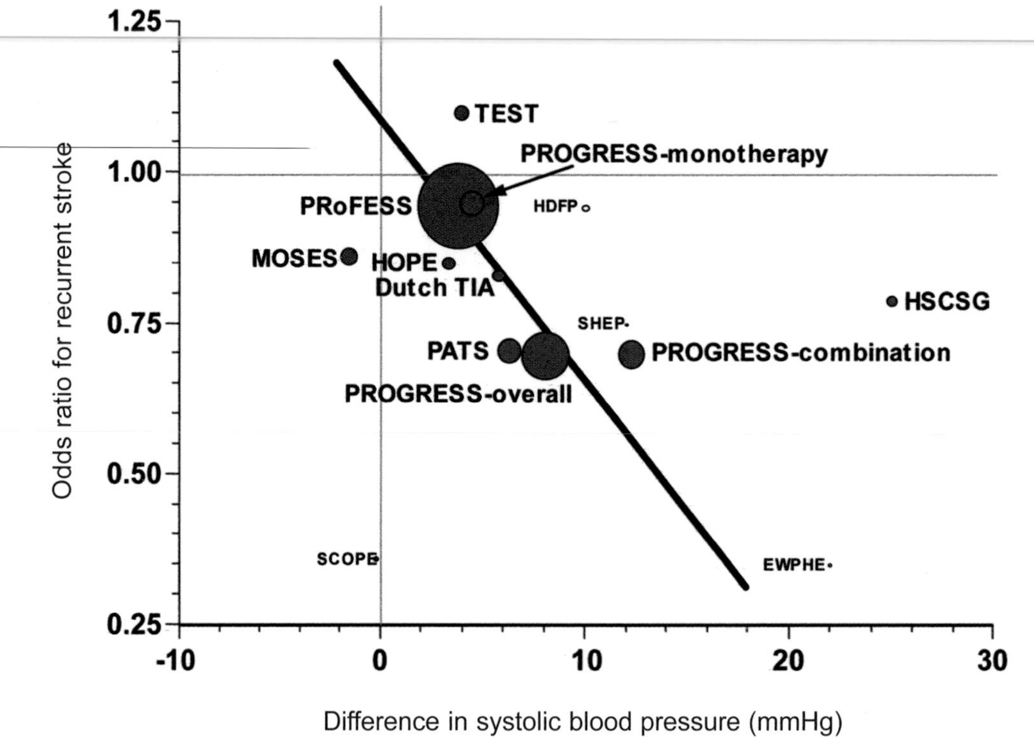

Figure 3. Plot of the significant relationship between the difference in systolic blood pressure between randomized arms during follow-up and the relative risk reduction for recurrent stroke in the clinical trials in Table 1. These data are consistent with the hypothesis that the benefit in recurrent stroke is proportional to the difference in achieved systolic BP between treatment arms. As is customary, the circle corresponding to each trial is drawn in proportion to the number of recurrent strokes observed. Trials that observed less than 10 recurrent strokes have circles that are too small to see at the resolution of the Figure. Acronyms of trials are expanded in the footnote to Table 1. *Updated from data of Rashid et al* [45].

analyses (see Figure 3 for an update), and concluded that there is a direct relationship between the relative risk reduction in recurrent stroke and the difference in achieved SBP between treatment arms [45]. These data are consistent with the general observation **(Ib/A)** and subsequent recommendation **(IV/C)** that higher-risk patients do better with a lower target blood pressure [1, 2], although the evidence to support such a recommendation specifically in patients with a history of cerebrovascular disease are similar in quality to those in patients with established heart disease, but clearly weaker than those in diabetics or chronic kidney disease.

Should blood pressure ever be raised in the patient with an evolving stroke?

Current US guidelines **(IV/C)** recognize the high risk associated with hypotension in acute stroke patients [4], and acknowledge the importance of considering its differential diagnosis, particularly since many of the possibilities are remediable. Thus, a patient with an evolving stroke who is volume depleted, suffering from an aortic dissection or cardiac ischemia, should have these conditions treated, which is likely to (secondarily) raise the blood pressure. The idea of using short-acting vasoconstrictors (e.g. phenylephrine) in acute stroke patients appears to be meritorious in some, but more information is needed on how this can be done safely, and easily and quickly reversed if neurological deterioration or other adverse experiences occur [4, 24-26].

Is a specific antihypertensive drug class better than others for the secondary prevention of stroke?

As discussed above, the current clinical trials database is not extensive enough to allow clear or useful conclusions to be drawn from fixed-effects or network meta-analyses. It appears that β-blockers are not very effective to prevent recurrent stroke. Overall, compared to placebo, β-blocker therapy was associated with a numerically, albeit non-significantly, higher risk of death in three studies: BEST [42], Dutch TIA [32], and TEST [34], odds ratio: 1.06, 95% confidence interval: 0.83-1.35, p=0.64. Some would argue that the very large and statistically powerful PRoFESS trial **(Ib/A)** clearly demonstrated that an ARB is not significantly better than placebo in preventing recurrent stroke, but others would suggest that adding an ARB to an ACE inhibitor (already being taken at randomization by 37% of the subjects) may have limited its effectiveness. Based primarily on the PROGRESS results [36] **(Ib/A)**, the most recent US guidelines **(IV/C)** conclude that "the available data support the use of diuretics and the combination of a diuretic and an ACE inhibitor **(I/A)**. The choice of specific drugs and targets should be individualized" [4].

Which patients are at risk for post-stroke dementia?

Many epidemiological studies **(IIa/B)** have attempted to identify risk factors for post-stroke dementia [46, 47]. The major ones include: younger age, pre-existing cognitive decline (without dementia), lower pre-stroke functional status, severity of the initial neurological deficit, and presence of silent infarcts or cerebral atrophy on CT or MRI done immediately after stroke [46].

The role of blood pressure lowering and antihypertensive drugs in the prevention of dementia, with or without a preceding stroke, is controversial **(Ib/A & III/B)** [48, 49]. The most recent meta-analysis of data from four trials involving 23,505 subjects **(Ia/A)** showed a non-significant 20% (95% confidence interval: -2 to 37%, p=0.07) relative risk reduction in dementia or cognitive decline in those randomized to active antihypertensive therapy [49]. The PROGRESS investigators **(Ib/B)** reported a non-significant (p=0.20) 12% reduction in dementia, but a significant decrease in cognitive decline (19%, p=0.01), as well as the composite outcomes of recurrent stroke or dementia and recurrent stroke or cognitive decline [50], which may have been influenced by pre-existing diseases [51]. These and other data do give hope to many that 'tight' control of blood pressure may prevent not only recurrent stroke and major adverse cardiovascular events, but also dementia and cognitive decline.

Conclusions

The evidence base for treatment of hypertension post-stroke is limited, but will soon be growing due to a number of important clinical trials that will soon be completed. In the USA, current guidelines for acute stroke suggest lowering blood pressure ONLY if systolic blood pressure exceeds 180mm Hg, but small studies suggest that careful lowering of blood pressure may be beneficial. In the days-to-weeks after stroke, clinical trial data exist for both points of view, and are difficult to reconcile. Many studies agree that lowering blood pressure more than a month after a stroke can prevent recurrent stroke; the combination of a diuretic + angiotensin-converting enzyme inhibitor can be recommended. Whether lowering blood pressure after stroke prevents dementia and/or cognitive decline is uncertain.

Key points	Evidence level
◆ Treatment of hypertension in the acute post-stroke period is controversial, but large randomized trials are underway.	IV/C
◆ Current recommendations are to consider lowering blood pressure only if the systolic exceeds 180mm Hg.	IIb/B
◆ However, several recent randomized trials have hinted that careful reduction in blood pressure with long-acting antihypertensive agents, often after a brief (e.g. 1 week) period of observation, may be beneficial.	Ia/A
◆ Small trials suggest that raising blood pressure in the acute stroke setting may be beneficial for some.	IIb/B
◆ Treatment of hypertension beginning in the days-weeks following an acute stroke is supported by data from a variety of randomized clinical trials.	Ia/A
◆ The largest and most recent of these trials did not show a significant benefit.	Ib/A
◆ Overall, however, blood pressure-lowering drugs appear to prevent recurrent stroke.	Ia/A
◆ Some data suggest (but do not prove [52]) that the greater the achieved blood pressure difference between the two randomized groups, the better the prevention.	IIb/B
◆ Current US guidelines recommend a diuretic or a diuretic and an ACE inhibitor for the chronic treatment of hypertensive patients with a history of cerebrovascular disease.	Ib/B
◆ Whether such interventions decrease the incidence of dementia and/or cognitive decline is still uncertain.	

References

1. Chobanian AV, Bakris GL, Black HR, *et al.* Seventh Report of the Joint National Committee on Prevention, Detection, Evaluation and Treatment of High Blood Pressure. National High Blood Pressure Education Program Coordinating Committee. *Hypertension* 2003; 42: 1206-52.
2. Mancia G, De Backer G, Dominiczak A, *et al.* 2007 Guidelines for the Management of Arterial Hypertension: The Task Force for the Management of Arterial Hypertension of the European Society of Hypertension (ESH) and the European Society of Cardiology (ESC). *J Hypertens* 2007; 25: 1105-87.
3. Goldstein LB, Adams R, Alberts MJ, *et al.* Primary Prevention of Ischemic Stroke: A Guideline from the American Heart Association/American Stroke Association Stroke Council: Cosponsored by the Atherosclerotic Peripheral Vascular Disease Interdisciplinary Working Group; Cardiovascular Nursing Council; Clinical Cardiology Council; Nutrition, Physical Activity, and Metabolism Council; and the Quality of Care and Outcomes Research Interdisciplinary Working Group. The American Academy of Neurology affirms the value of this guideline. *Stroke* 2006; 37: 1583-633.
4. Adams HP, del Zoppa G, Alberts MJ, *et al.* Guidelines for the early management of adults with ischemic stroke: A guideline from the American Heart Association/American Stroke Association Stroke Council, Clinical

Cardiology Council, Cardiovascular Radiology and Intervention Council, and the Atherosclerotic Peripheral Vascular Disease and Quality of Care Outcomes in Research Interdisciplinary Working Groups. *Stroke* 2007; 38: 1655-711.

5. Bath P, Chalmers J, Powers W, *et al*, for the International Society of Hypertension Writing Group. International Society of Hypertension (ISH): statement on the management of blood pressure in acute stroke. *J Hypertens* 2003; 21: 665-72.
6. Sacco RL, Adams R, Albers G, *et al*. Guidelines for prevention of stroke in patients with ischemic stroke or transient ischemic attack: a statement for healthcare professionals from the American Heart Association/American Stroke Association Council on Stroke; Co-sponsored by the Council on Cardiovascular Radiology and Intervention; The American Academy of Neurology affirms the value of this guideline. *Stroke* 2006; 37: 577-617; reprinted in *Circulation* 2006; 113: e409-49.
7. Gorelick PB, Broder MS, Crowell RM, *et al*. Determining the appropriateness of selected surgical and medical management options in recurrent stroke prevention: a guideline for primary care physicians from the National Stroke Association Work Group on Recurrent Stroke Prevention. *J Stroke Cerebrovasc Dis* 2004; 13: 196-207.
8. Lloyd-Jones D, Adams R, Carnethon M, *et al*. Heart Disease and Stroke Statistics, 2009 Update. A Report from the American Heart Association Statistics Committee and Stroke Statistics Subcommittee. *Circulation* 2009; 119: e1-e161. Available on the Internet at: http://circ.ahajournals.org/cgi/reprint/CIRCULATIONAHA.108.191261, accessed 16 July 2009.
9. Qureshi AI. Acute hypertensive response in patients with stroke: pathophysiology and management. *Circulation* 2008; 118: 176-87.
10. Willmot M, Leonardi-Bee J, Bath PM. High blood pressure in acute stroke and subsequent outcome: a systematic review. *Hypertension* 2004; 43: 18-24.
11. Castillo J, Leira R, Garcia MM, Serena J, Blanco M, Davalos A. Blood pressure decrease during the acute phase of ischemic stroke is associated with brain injury and poor stroke outcome. *Stroke* 2004; 35: 520-6.
12. Leonardi-Bee J, Bath PM, Phillips SJ, Sandercock PA. Blood pressure and clinical outcomes in the International Stroke Trial. IST Collaborative Group. *Stroke* 2002; 33: 1315-26.
13. Fogelholm R, Palomaki H, Erila T, Rissanen A, Kaste M. Blood pressure, nimodipine, and outcome of ischemic stroke. *Acta Neurol Scand* 2004; 109: 200-4.
14. Oliviera-Filho J, Silva SC, Trabuco CC, Pedreira BB, Sousa EU, Bacellar A. Detrimental effect of blood pressure reduction in the first 24 hours of acute stroke onset. *Neurology* 2003; 61: 1047-51.
15. Geeganage C, Bath PMW. Interventions for deliberately altering blood pressure in acute stroke. Cochrane Database Systematic Reviews. 2008, Issue 4. Art #CD000039: DOI: 10.1002/14651858. CD000039.pub2. Available on the Internet at: http://mrw.interscience.wiley.com/cochrane/clsysrev/articles/CD000039/fraom.html, accessed 5 January 2009.
16. Sare GM, Gray LJ, Bath PMW. Effect of antihypertensive agents on cerebral blood flow and flow velocity in acute ischaemic stroke: systemic review of controlled studies. *J Hypertens* 2008; 26: 1058-64.
17. Schrader J, Luders S, Kulschewski A, *et al*, for the Acute Candesartan Cilexitil Therapy in Stroke Survivors Study Group. The ACCESS Study: Evaluation of Acute Candesartan Cilexitil Therapy in Stroke Survivors. *Stroke* 2003; 34: 1699-703.
18. Rodriguez-Garcia JL, Botia E, de La Sierra A, Villaneuva MA, Gonzales-Spinolta J. Significance of elevated blood pressure and its management on the short-term outcome of patients with acute ischemic stroke. *Am J Hypertens* 2005; 18: 379-84.
19. Eames PJ, Robinson TG, Panerai RB, Potter JF. Bendrofluazide fails to reduce elevated blood pressure levels in the immediate post-stroke period. *Cerebrovasc Dis* 2005; 19: 253-9.
20. Anderson CS, Huang Y, Wang JG, *et al*, for the INTERACT Investigators. INTEnsive blood pressure Reduction in Acute Cerebral hemorrhage Trial (INTERACT): a randomized pilot trial. *Lancet Neuro* 2008; 7: 391-9.
21. Potter JF, Robinson TG, Ford GA, *et al*. Controlling Hypertension and Hypotension Immediately Post-Stroke (CHHIPS): a randomised, placebo-controlled, double-blind pilot trial. *Lancet Neurol* 2009; 8: 48-56.
22. COSSACS Trial Group. COSSACS (Continue or Stop post-Stroke Antihypertensives Collaborative Study): rationale and design. *J Hypertens* 2005; 23: 455-8.
23. Bath PMW, on behalf of the ENOS Investigators. Efficacy of Nitric Oxide in Stroke: The ENOS Trial. Available on the Internet at: http://asa.scientificposters.com/epsView.cfm?pid=CTP15&yr=2008, accessed 5 June 2009.

24. Rordorf G, Koroshetz WJ, Ezziddine MA, Siegel AZ, Buonanno FS. A pilot study of drug-induced hypertension in acute stroke. *Neurology* 2001; 56: 1210-3.
25. Hillis AE, Ulatowski JA, Parker PB, *et al.* A pilot randomized trial of induced blood pressure elevation: Effects on function and focal perfusion in acute and subacute stroke. *Cerebrovasc Dis* 2003; 16: 236-46.
26. Mistri AK, Robinson TG, Potter JF. Pressor therapy in acute ischemic stroke: systematic review. *Stroke* 2006; 37: 1565-71.
27. Lawes CMM, Bennett DA, Feigin VL, Rogers A. Blood pressure and stroke: an overview of published studies. *Stroke* 2004; 35: 776-85.
28. Rashid P, Leonardi-Bee J, Bath P. Blood pressure reduction and secondary prevention of stroke and other vascular events: a systematic review. *Stroke* 2003; 34: 2741-8.
29. Gueyffier F, Boissel JP, Boutitie F, *et al.* Effect of antihypertensive treatment in patients having already suffered from stroke: gathering the evidence. The INDANA Project Collaborators. *Stroke* 1997; 28: 2557-62.
30. Carter AB. Hypotensive therapy in stroke survivors. *Lancet* 1970; i: 485-9.
31. Hypertension-Stroke Cooperative Study Group. Effect of antihypertensive treatment on stroke recurrence. *JAMA* 1974; 229: 409-18.
32. The Dutch TIA Trial Study Group. Trial of secondary prevention with atenolol after transient ischemic attack or nondisabling ischemic stroke. *Stroke* 1993; 24: 543-8.
33. PATS Collaborating Group. Post-stroke antihypertensive treatment study. A preliminary result. *Chin Med J* 1995; 108: 710-7.
34. Eriksson S, Olofsson BO, Wester PO, for the TEST Study Group. Atenolol in secondary prevention after stroke. *Cerebrovasc Dis* 1995; 5: 21-5.
35. Bosch J, Yusuf S, Pogue J, *et al.* Use of ramipril in preventing stroke: double blind randomised trial. *BMJ* 2002; 324: 699-702.
36. PROGRESS Collaborative Group. Randomized trial of a perindopril-based blood-pressure-lowering regimen among 6105 individuals with previous stroke or transient ischemic attack. *Lancet* 2001; 358: 1033-41.
37. Schrader J, Luders S, Kulschewski A, *et al.* Morbidity and Mortality after Stroke: Eprosartan Compared with Nitrendipine for Secondary Prevention: principal results of a prospective randomized controlled study (MOSES). *Stroke* 2005; 36: 1218-26.
38. Trenkwalder P, Elmfeldt D, Hofman A, *et al*, for the Study on Cognition and Prognosis in the Elderly (SCOPE) Investigators. The Study on Cognition and Prognosis in the Elderly: major cardiovascular events and stroke in subgroups of patients. *Blood Press* 2005; 14: 31-7.
39. Yusuf S, Diener H-C, Sacco RL, *et al*, for the PRoFESS Study Group. Telmisartan to prevent recurrent stroke and cardiovascular events. *N Engl J Med* 2008; 359: 1225-37.
40. DerSimonian R, Laird N. Meta-analysis in clinical trials. *Controlled Clin Trials* 1986; 7: 177-88.
41. Bucher H, Guyatt G, Griffith L, Eccles M. The results of direct and indirect treatment comparisons in meta-analysis of randomized controlled trials. *J Clin Epidemiol* 1997; 50: 683-91.
42. Barer DH, Cruickshank JM, Ebrahim SB, Mitchell JRA. Low-dose beta-blockade in acute stroke ('BEST' trial): an evaluation. *BMJ* 1988; 296: 737-41.
43. Lumley T. Network meta-analysis for indirect treatment comparisons. *Stat Med* 2002; 21: 2313-24.
44. Arima H, Chalmers J, Woodward M, *et al*, for the PROGRESS Collaborative Group. Lower target blood pressures are safe and effective for the prevention of recurrent stroke: the PROGRESS trial. *J Hypertens* 2006; 24: 1201-8.
45. Rashid P, Leonardi-Bee J, Bath P. Blood pressure reduction and secondary prevention of stroke and other vascular events: a systematic review. *Stroke* 2003; 34: 2741-8.
46. Hénon H, Pasquier F, Leys D. Poststroke dementia. *Cerebrovasc Dis* 2006; 22: 61-70.
47. Sachdev PS, Bordaty H, Valenzuela MJ, *et al.* Clinical determinants of dementia and mild cognitive impairment following ischaemic stroke: The Sydney Stroke Study. *Dement Geriatr Cogn Disord* 2006; 21: 275-83.
48. Pickering TG. Does treating hypertension prevent dementia? *J Clin Hypertens* (Greenwich) 2008; 10: 866-70.
49. Feigin V, Ratnasabapathy Y, Anderson C. Does blood pressure lowering treatment prevent dementia or cognitive decline in patients with cardiovascular and cerebrovascular disease? *J Neurol Sci* 2005; 229-30: 151-5.
50. Effects of blood pressure lowering with perindopril and indapamide therapy on dementia and cognitive decline in patients with cerebrovascular disease. The PROGRESS Collaborative Group. *Arch Intern Med* 2003; 163: 1069-75.

51. Arima H, Tzourio C, Butcher K, *et al.* Prior events predict cerebrovascular and coronary outcomes in the PROGRESS trial. *Stroke* 2006; 37: 1497-502.
52. Geeganage CM, Bath PMW. Relationship between therapeutic changes in blood pressure and outcomes in acute stroke. *Hypertension* 2009; 54: 775-81.

Chapter 14

What is the optimal blood pressure treatment for patients with chronic kidney disease and/or albuminuria?

Rigas Kalaitzidis MD, Senior Registrar in Nephrology
University Hospital of Ioannina
Ioannina, Greece

George Bakris MD, Professor of Medicine; Director, Hypertensive Diseases Center
Section of Endocrinology, Diabetes and Metabolism, University of Chicago Pritzker School of Medicine, Chicago, Illinois, USA

Introduction

Hypertension is a well known independent risk factor for cardiovascular disease (CVD) [1] and development of chronic kidney disease (CKD) [2]. This is best exemplified by data from the Multiple Risk Factor Intervention Trial (MRFIT) where the level of blood pressure predicted development of end-stage renal disease (ESRD) in more than 330,000 middle-aged men over a 16-year period [3]. In 2008, hypertensive nephrosclerosis is the second most common cause of ESRD after diabetic nephropathy [4].

According to the National Kidney Foundation (NKF)-Kidney Disease Outcomes Quality Initiative (KDOQI) Working Group guidelines, the goals of antihypertensive therapy in patients with CKD are to lower blood pressure, reduce the risk of CVD in patients with or without hypertension, and slow the progression of kidney disease in patients with or without hypertension [5].

There has been much written about the level to which blood pressure should be reduced as well as the effects of proteinuria reduction on CKD progression [6, 7]. In spite of this, the percent of people with CKD achieving guideline blood pressure levels remains below 50% [8]. Moreover, very few physicians assess whether the proper blood pressure medications are prescribed and titrated to reduce proteinuria, maximally, in patients with CKD. This coupled with other factors has led over the past two decades to a worldwide epidemic of CKD.

Eight million people in the United States had an estimated GFR (eGFR) <60ml/min/1.73m^2 [9]. The estimated prevalence of CKD is about 14.8% of the general population [10]; the largest increase was in Stage 3 nephropathy with a 7.7% increase [9]. Both the incidence and prevalence of kidney failure treated by dialysis and transplantation continue to increase. Since 1999, the incident rates of those starting dialysis have been relatively stable, ranging from 333.1 per million populations in 1999 to 347.1 in 2005, a number almost four times higher than that in 1980 [10]. By the year 2030, more than 2.2 million individuals will require treatment for ESRD [10]. Patients with CKD have significant morbidity, and an increased risk of cardiovascular disease [11], progression to ESRD and death [12].

It is important to assess not only blood pressure but presence of albuminuria among those with CKD, since even small amounts of albuminuria, i.e. microalbuminuria, is associated with a much higher cardiovascular risk in CKD patients [13]. Moreover, increases in albuminuria, over time, to levels >300mg/day indicate presence of nephropathy and should be addressed urgently [13] **(IIa/B)**. In primary care practice, microalbuminuria (>30<300mg/day) is a common finding. In a normal functioning kidney, the amount of albuminuria is <30mg/day. There are several ways to measure albuminuria. While the traditional way is a 24-hour urine collection, a more practical and equally accurate way is an albumin to creatinine ratio on a spot collection of morning urine in a fasting state [14]. Guidelines recommend screening for albuminuria in hypertensive patients [15] especially in diabetes and CKD.

Blood pressure goal for patients with CKD

While almost all guidelines [15, 16] quote a blood pressure goal for a patient with hypertension of <140/90mmHg, in those with CKD, all guidelines recommend a blood pressure goal of <130/80mmHg [16]. The question is: what is the strength of the evidence to support this lower number? Almost all the evidence to support this lower level of blood pressure comes from post hoc, non-pre-specified analyses of large outcome trials. Additionally, many of these studies did not measure or assess albuminuria or proteinuria, a factor that clearly affects outcome [6].

A summary of studies with CVD endpoints that evaluate CKD progression are in Table 1. The Hypertension Optimal Treatment (HOT) trial [17] **(Ib/A)** and the United Kingdom Prospective Diabetes Study (UKPDS) 38 [18] **(Ib/A)** were some of the first studies to randomize blood pressure to two different levels and examine CVD outcomes. While the HOT primary outcome did not support the lower BP goal, the diabetes subgroup did support the lower goal, as did the results of the UKPDS. In fact, these are the main trials that drive lower blood pressure in those with diabetes. Lastly, the ALLHAT evaluated progression of CKD as a post hoc analysis based on stage of nephropathy and found no difference among drug groups slowing progression to ESRD; however, blood pressure values in all groups were above 130mmHg [19] **(IIa/B)**. These analyses for the most part, however, are post hoc and the definitive answer about blood pressure goals in those with diabetes is evident from the ACCORD trial results. This randomized long-term, appropriately powered outcome trial, demonstrates that a blood pressure well below 130/80mmHg is not associated with a lower cardiovascular event rate **(Ib/A)**. It did demonstrate, however, a stroke benefit on secondary analyses. This trial taken together with all previous studies now suggests that all patients with hypertension should have a blood pressure goal well below 140/90mmHg, approaching 130/80mmHg. Only those with high risk for stroke or those who have proteinuric (>300mg/day) kidney disease should have their blood pressure lowered below 130/80mmHg **(IIa/B)** [20].

Table 1. A summary of outcome trials focused on kidney outcomes.

CV trials	Achieved systolic BP (mmHg) at trial end	CKD progression slowed in lower BP group
Post hoc analyses NOT pre-specified		
HOT*	136	YES
UKPDS*	144	NA
ALLHAT	134	NA
Trials Primary CKD outcome#		
MDRD*^	132	NO*^
AASK*	128	NO
AIPRI	136	-
RENAAL	140	-
IDNT	140	-
Benazapril Advanced Nephropathy Trial	128	-
ABCD	132	-
REIN-2*	130	NO

NA = not assessed in trial; * = randomized to different levels of blood pressure; # = focused on kidney disease progression as a primary endpoint;^ = outcome showed no difference after main trial completed with 2.6 years for follow-up but long-term follow-up of more than a decade showed a significant benefit on slowed progression in the lower blood pressure group.

In patients with CKD, the evidence for a lower blood pressure to reduce the rate of both kidney disease progression and CVD events is also not uniform. In order to understand the data fully on CKD progression and blood pressure level, one needs to be aware of the natural decline in kidney function. Decline of GFR begins at age 30 at a rate varying from 0.6 to 1.1mL/min per year. This age-related loss in GFR is directly proportional to blood pressure levels and early interventions that lower blood pressure in CKD patients markedly slows kidney function loss [21] **(IIa/B)**.

There are many prospective trials focused on kidney disease progression but only three have randomized to different levels of blood pressure control (Table 1). All retrospective analyses show a benefit on slowing of nephropathy at levels below a systolic blood pressure of 130mmHg; however, the prospective studies tell a different story. The first trial to randomize individuals with advanced nephropathy to two different levels of blood pressure was the Modification of Diet in Renal Disease (MDRD) Study. In this study, patients with CKD and high rates of protein excretion, were randomly assigned to a low blood pressure group with a goal mean arterial pressure (MAP) <92mmHg and a high blood pressure group (goal MAP <107mmHg) for 4 years. At the end of the study, patients randomized to the low target blood pressure group did not have a significantly slower reduction in GFR decline, compared to patients assigned to the higher target blood pressure group [22] **(Ib/A)**. However, a continued follow-up of these subjects beyond the initial 3 years of the trial showed that 7 years following randomization, the risks of kidney failure, and the composite outcome of kidney failure and all-cause mortality were lower in the low target blood pressure group [23].

A second trial that prospectively randomized patients to two different blood pressure levels was the African American Study of Kidney Disease and Hypertension (AASK) [24] **(Ib/A)**. African American patients with hypertensive kidney disease (GFR between 20 and 65ml/min/1.73m^2) and an average urine protein excretion <1g/day were randomized to a low blood pressure goal (MAP ≤92mmHg) or a usual one (MAP 102-107mmHg). At the end of the study, no benefit of the lower blood pressure goal was noted in reducing the decline in GFR compared to the usual goal. Recent analysis also demonstrated that after a 10-year follow-up, CKD progression while slowed was not stopped [25]. The reasons for this may be related to the observation that masked hypertension and non-dipping was prevalent in more than two thirds of the cohort studied [26, 27]. However, another finding in this trial is that those with proteinuria of >300mg/day had a much stronger trend favoring the lower blood pressure compared to those with microalbuminuria or normoalbuminuria **(IIa/B)**.

Lastly, the only other study to randomize levels of blood pressure was the Ramipril Efficacy in Nephropathy (REIN-2) trial [28] **(Ib/A)**. This trial included patients with non-diabetic CKD; however, the outcome was limited by the fact that the sample size was small and duration of follow-up short.

Taken together, these findings suggest that those with high levels of proteinuria, i.e. >300mg/day, garner greater benefit by further lowering of blood pressure to levels below a systolic pressure of 130mmHg. The evidence comes from a meta-analysis showing that lower levels of systolic blood pressure slow nephropathy progression in non-diabetic kidney disease [29] **(Ia/A)**. In this meta-analysis by the ACE Inhibition in Progressive Renal Disease (AIPRI) Study Group, a systolic blood pressure range of 110-129mmHg was associated with the lowest risk of CKD progression, in patients with urine protein excretion >1g/day [29].

Among other trials that did not randomize the level of blood pressure, retrospective analyses did show a benefit of lower pressures as well, although the average systolic blood pressure in the trials was between 138-141mmHg. The Irbesartan Diabetic Nephropathy Trial (IDNT) included subjects with diabetic nephropathy with median urine protein excretion of 2.9g/day and mean creatinine 1.65mg/dL. Median patient follow-up was 2.6 years. Follow-up achieved SBP most strongly predicted renal outcomes. Systolic blood pressure above 149mmHg was associated with a 2.2-fold increase in the risk for doubling serum creatinine or ESRD compared with systolic pressure below 134mmHg. They also noted that progressive lowering pressure to 120mmHg was associated with improved kidney and patient survival, an effect independent of baseline renal function. Below this threshold, all-cause mortality increased [30] **(Ib/A)**. Similar findings were noted in the RENAAL trial where those with the highest pulse pressure garnered the greatest CKD benefit if systolic pressure was lowered to levels below a mean of 134mmHg [31] **(Ib/A)**.

In spite of the relatively modest data supporting a lower blood pressure goal for CKD progression, all guidelines, to date, support the lower goal. In the United States, estimates of those achieving the goal of 140/90mmHg among the general population is over 50%; however, the 130/80mm Hg goal for those with diabetes is approximately 34% [32, 33]. Data from NHANES III demonstrates that blood pressure control rates in patients with CKD was even lower, as only 11% of hypertensives with elevated serum creatinine levels had a blood pressure of less than 130/85mmHg [34]. A review of the NHANES 2003-2004 data shows some improvement but still well below the 50% mark [8].

In patients with kidney disease, achievement of blood pressure goals is more difficult and requires even more antihypertensive agents. It is noteworthy that in people with CKD, to achieve these lower levels of blood pressure will require an average of three to four different antihypertensive agents in moderate to high doses, Figure 1.

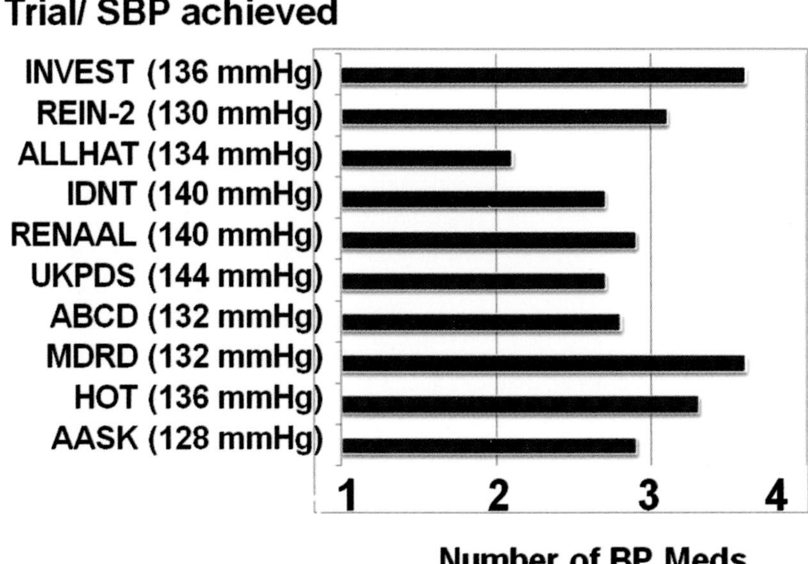

Figure 1. Average number of antihypertensive medications needed to attain blood pressure reduction in clinical trials.

Albuminuria and cardiorenal endpoints

Microalbuminuria

Microalbuminuria is a predictor of CVD morbidity and mortality in individuals with and without diabetes [35-37]. It was assumed to be also an early marker of diabetic nephropathy but is now found to not reflect nephropathy [38]. However, increases of microalbuminuria over time into the macroalbuminuria range, i.e. >300mg/d, is clearly indicative of nephropathy. Without specific interventions 40% of patients with type 1 diabetes and 20% to 30% of those with type 2 diabetes and microalbuminuria will progress to macroalbuminuria over the next 10 to 15 years [39] **(IIa/B)**.

The presence of macroalbuminuria or clinical proteinuria indicates presence of nephropathy. In its totality, the trial data indicate that people with proteinuria especially those >1g per day should have a systolic blood pressure value below 130mm Hg to maximally slow CKD progression [13] .

Studies have consistently demonstrated that early changes in proteinuria predict long-term CKD outcomes in patients with and without diabetes [40-42]. The application of these outcomes to the bedside is to lower blood pressure to goal and ideally reduce proteinuria to levels >30% below the starting value but ideally reduce it by 50% or more [6, 14, 40]. Reduction in microalbuminuria is associated with a lower CVD event rate but no study, to date, in patients with CKD and microalbuminuria has shown a slowed nephropathy outcome by lowering microalbuminuria [11, 43]. The link between reduction of microalbuminuria with RAAS blockers and reduction of CVD endpoints is still uncertain. An analysis of the LIFE trial showed a reduced risk of the composite endpoint of cardiovascular death, myocardial infarction, or stroke among participants who had a substantial reduction in microalbuminuria at the 1-year follow-up [44] **(Ib/A)**.

Agents that block the renin-angiotensin-aldosterone (RAAS) system are the best agents to reduce or blunt the rise across the spectrum of albuminuria. In the Irbesartan Renal Microalbuminuria (IRMA 2) study, 590 patients with hypertension, type 2 diabetes and GFR microalbuminuria (average range of UAE between 53.4-58.3μg/min), were randomly assigned to receive placebo or irbesartan 150mg or 300mg daily. The primary endpoint was appearance of clinical nephropathy, i.e. albuminuria >200μg/min and at least a 30% increase from the baseline level. After 24 months of follow-up, the approach of the three groups to the endpoint was 14.9%, 9.7%, and 5.2%, respectively, which translates into a 68% reduction in progression to albuminuria between irbesartan 300mg daily and placebo groups [45] **(Ib/A)**.

In the AASK trial, African American patients with hypertensive kidney disease, mean serum creatinine of 2.2mg/dL and 24-hour urine protein excretion of 0.6g/day were randomized to ramipril, amlodipine, or metoprolol. Patients treated with ramipril had a 36% reduction in the secondary composite outcome of 50% reduction of GFR, ESRD or death compared to amlodipine, and a 22% reduction compared to metoprolol. The meta-analysis by the AIPRD Study Group in non-diabetic CKD showed that regimens including an ACE inhibitor were associated with a 31% reduction in progression to ESRD and 30% reduction in the combined endpoint in doubling of serum creatinine or progression to ESRD [29].

Two randomized controlled trials demonstrate angiotensin receptor blockers (ARBs) are effective in reducing proteinuria and slow CKD progression in type 2 diabetic patients with nephropathy. In the Reduction in Endpoints in NIDDM with the Angiotensin II Antagonist Losartan (RENAAL) Study, 1513 type 2 diabetic patients with nephropathy (mean creatinine 1.9mg/dL and median urine albumin-to-creatinine ratio 1237mg/g) were randomized to losartan or placebo. Patients treated with losartan had a 35% reduction in the urinary albumin-to-creatinine ratio while patients in the placebo group tended to have an increase. In addition, treatment with losartan resulted in a 16% reduction in the primary endpoint of doubling of baseline serum creatinine, progression to ESRD or death. The median rate of decline in estimated clearance was 4.4 and 5.2mL/min/1.73m^2/per year in the losartan and placebo group, respectively [46]. A recent post hoc analysis from the aforementioned RENAAL study showed that the combination of the reduction in both albuminuria and SBP results in a most favorable clinical outcome in hypertensive patients with diabetic nephropathy. It was shown that the risk of ESRD had a dependence clearly on albuminuria reduction regardless of change in SBP [47]. In the IDNT study, after a mean follow-up of 2.6 years, proteinuria decreased by 33% in the irbesartan group versus 6% in the amlodipine group and 10%, in the placebo group. Treatment with irbesartan also resulted in a 20% reduction compared to placebo and 23% reduction compared to amlodipine in the primary composite outcome of doubling of baseline serum creatinine, onset of ESRD, or death from any cause. The risk of a doubling of the serum creatinine concentration was 33% lower in the irbesartan group than in the placebo group and 37% lower in the irbesartan group than in the amlodipine group [48].

The role of dual RAAS blockade, i.e. combining an ACE inhibitor and ARBs, in the context of slowing CKD progression is unclear. A recent meta-analysis of all trials evaluating dual RAAS blockade demonstrates an additional 20% reduction in proteinuria over either agent alone [49] **(Ia/A)**. The recent AVOID trial also supports the notion of a renin inhibitor added to a maximally dosed ARB reduces proteinuria by an additional 20-22% [50] **(Ib/A)**. There is no trial, to date, that demonstrates dual RAAS blockade slows nephropathy progression more than achieving blood pressure goal with a single RAAS agent coupled with other medications. Data from one trial that implied protection have many data irregularities [51].

The addition of an aldosterone receptor antagonist in patients with proteinuric nephropathy already receiving an ACE inhibitor or ARB also demonstrates further reduction of urine protein excretion [52-54]. The effects of this blockade on long-term CKD progression also remains untested.

These data taken together suggest that unless proteinuria >300mg/day is present, blood pressure goals should be <140mm Hg systolic. If proteinuria is present, a goal of <130mmHg is much more defensible than if no or microalbuminuria is present. Moreover, the achievement of a goal blood pressure less than 130/80mmHg in patients with kidney disease is difficult and requires both lifestyle modifications, most important of which is sodium restriction [55] and use of appropriately dosed multiple antihypertensive medications (Figure 1). In patients with

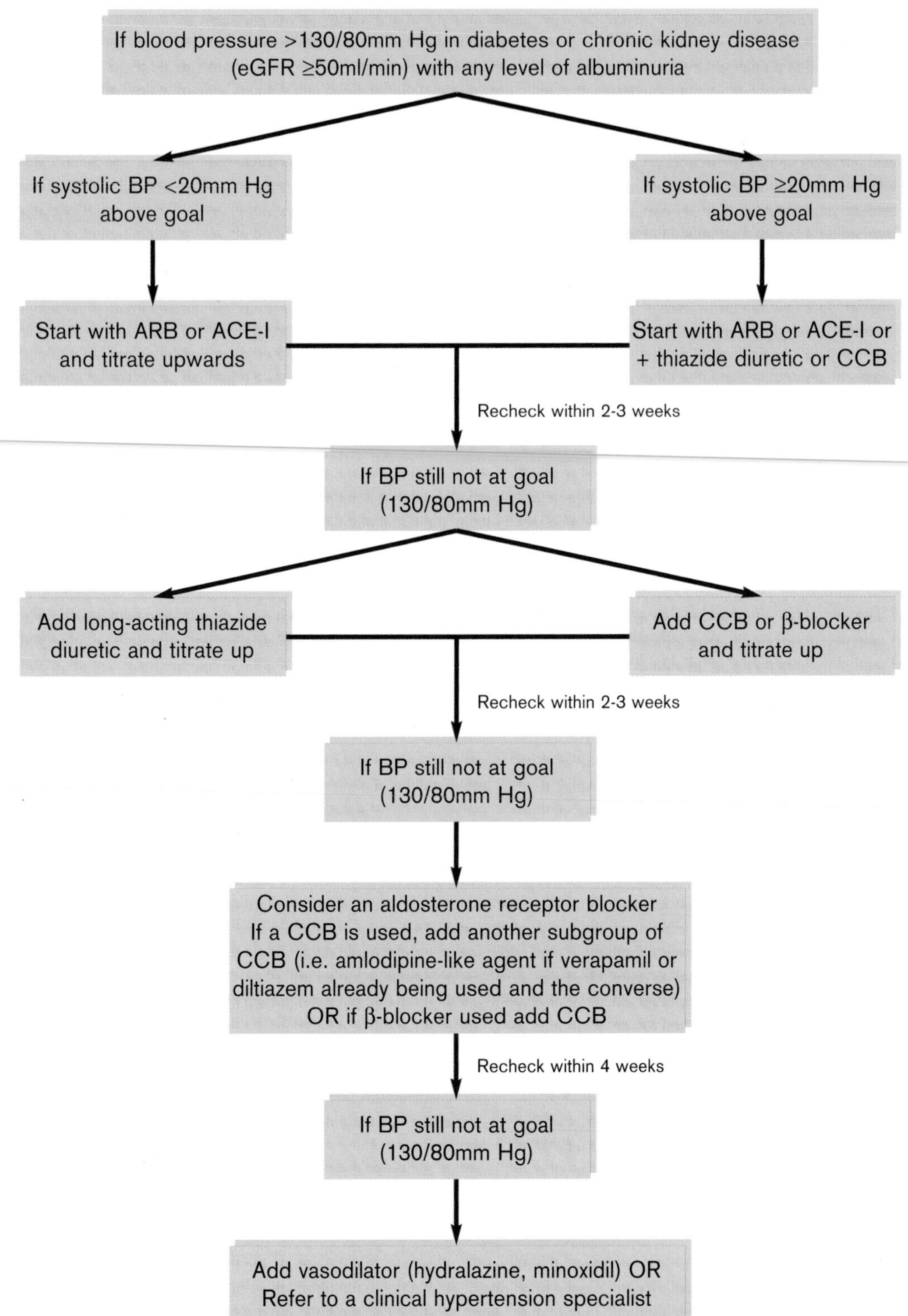

Figure 2. Approach to achieving blood pressure goal in people with various stages of CKD.

proteinuric CKD, the goal should be a reduction in proteinuria of more than 30% from the starting value in addition to blood pressure reduction to goal.

Approach to attain blood pressure goal

There is no optimal approach to attain blood pressure goal, as each treatment needs to be tailored to the patent phenotype and genotype. A few observations are clear, however, in almost all cases of CKD a minimum of two to three appropriately dosed antihypertensive medications are needed to achieve goal, one of which will be a diuretic. The diuretic chosen should be appropriate for level of eGFR, i.e. loop diuretics for those with eGFR <40ml.min [56].

A general approach put forth by an international consensus panel to treat CKD and recently updated for diabetic CKD is shown in Figure 2 [57, 58]. It should be remembered that starting with a fixed dose combination in those whose blood pressure is 20/10mmHg above the guideline goal results in not only achieving goal blood pressure quicker but a reduced likelihood of cardiovascular events [59, 60]. This algorithm has been updated to reflect the recent data from the Avoiding Cardiovascular Events through Combination Therapy in Patients Living with Systolic Hypertension (ACCOMPLISH) trial [60] **(Ib/A)**.

Calcium channel blockers are effective antihypertensive agents in patients with kidney disease. Among patients with advanced proteinuric CKD, current evidence supports the use of non-dihydropyridine CCBs (verapamil, diltiazem) for greater proteinuria reduction among patients with advanced proteinuric nephropathy [61, 62] **(Ia/A)**. Dihydropyridine CCBs do not have the same magnitude of proteinuria reduction unless used in the presence of a RAAS blocker [7, 63, 64]. Guidelines state that dihydropyridine CCBs should not be used as monotherapy in CKD patients with proteinuria but always in combination with an ACE inhibitor or an ARB [5].

The antihypertensive effects of conventional β-blockers, as well as their capability to reduce cardiovascular mortality in high-risk patients, has been well-established [65, 66], but there is no direct evidence that these agents provide additional renoprotective effects. Newer β-blockers with vasodilating properties, such as carvedilol and nebivolol, reduce the risk of microalbuminuria in patients with hypertension and diabetes [67, 68] and mortality in people with ESRD [69]. Moreover, recent findings showing negative effects of β-blockers are relegated to atenolol and not others in the class [70]. These findings suggest that vasodilator β-blockers should be used in patients with CKD when a combination of proper doses of an ACE inhibitor or an ARB regimen with an appropriately selected and dosed diuretic and calcium antagonist is not enough to attain blood pressure goals.

Conclusions

Hypertension is a risk factor for cardiovascular disease (CVD) as well as development and progression of kidney disease. Microalbuminuria is associated with increased risk of CVD disease. Increases of albuminuria over time to a level >300mg indicate the presence of nephropathy and should be addressed urgently. Retrospective analyses show a benefit in slowing nephropathy progression when systolic blood pressure levels are below 130mm Hg among people with >300mg of proteinuria per day. Otherwise most prospective data are supportive of blood pressure levels of <140/90mm Hg. Most people will require a combination of antihypertensive therapy to achieve blood pressure goals and among those with chronic kidney disease a blocker of the renin-angiotensin-aldosterone system should be included since it has been shown to slow nephropathy and reduce CV risk in such patients.

Key points	Evidence level
◆ Increases in albuminuria, over time, to levels >300mg/day indicate presence of nephropathy.	IIa/B
◆ The current recommended lower level of blood pressure of <130/80mmHg is only supported in people with >300mg/ day of proteinuria.	IIa/B
◆ Microalbuminuria is a cardiovascular risk marker and NOT an indicator of kidney disease.	IIa/B
◆ Initial combinations of antihypertensive therapy that include a blocker of the renin-angiotensin system (RAS) with a calcium antagonist slow nephropathy progression to a greater extent than a RAS combined with a diuretic at BP levels around 130/80mmHg.	Ib/A
◆ Patients with diabetic nephropathy (those with >300mg/day of proteinuria) and hypertension should have blood pressure lowered to <130/80mmHg to maximally slow nephropathy progression and should include a RAS blocker.	Ia/A
◆ Combinations of ACE inhibitors with angiotensin receptor blockers can be used in certain subtypes of patients with massive proteinuria >2g/day to further reduce proteinuria by 20-30%.	Ia/B

References

1. MacMahon S, Peto R, Cutler J, *et al.* Blood pressure, stroke, and coronary heart disease. Part 1, Prolonged differences in blood pressure: prospective observational studies corrected for the regression dilution bias. *Lancet* 1990; 335(8692): 765-74.
2. Go AS, Chertow GM, Fan D, McCulloch CE, Hsu CY. Chronic kidney disease and the risks of death, cardiovascular events, and hospitalization *N Engl J Med* 2004; 351(13): 1296-305.
3. Klag MJ, Whelton PK, Randall BL *et al.* Blood pressure and end-stage renal disease in men. *N Engl J Med* 1996; 334(1): 13-8.
4. Hill GS. Hypertensive nephrosclerosis. *Curr Opin Nephrol Hypertens* 2008; 17(3): 266-70.
5. K/DOQI clinical practice guidelines on hypertension and antihypertensive agents in chronic kidney disease. *Am J Kidney Dis* 2004; 43(5 Suppl 1): S1-290.
6. Bakris GL. Slowing nephropathy progression: focus on proteinuria reduction. *Clin J Am Soc Nephrol* 2008; 3 Suppl 1: S3-10.

7. Bakris GL, Weir MR, Shanifar S, *et al.* Effects of blood pressure level on progression of diabetic nephropathy: results from the RENAAL study. *Arch Intern Med* 2003; 163(13): 1555-65.
8. Sarafidis PA, Li S, Chen SC, *et al.* Hypertension awareness, treatment, and control in chronic kidney disease. *Am J Med* 2008; 121(4): 332-40.
9. Coresh J, Selvin E, Stevens LA *et al.* Prevalence of chronic kidney disease in the United States. *JAMA* 2007; 298(17): 2038-47.
10. USRD 2007 ADR/reference tables. Available: http//www.usrds.org-2007.htm 2008. 2008.
11. So WY, Kong AP, Ma RC, *et al.* Glomerular filtration rate, cardiorenal end points, and all-cause mortality in type 2 diabetic patients. *Diabetes Care* 2006; 29(9): 2046-52.
12. Bakris GL. Protecting renal function in the hypertensive patient: clinical guidelines. *Am J Hypertens* 2005; 18(4 Pt 2): 112S-9.
13. Sarafidis PA, Khosla N, Bakris GL. Antihypertensive therapy in the presence of proteinuria. *Am J Kidney Dis* 2007; 49(1): 12-26.
14. Khosla N, Sarafidis PA, Bakris GL. Microalbuminuria. *Clin Lab Med* 2006; 26(3): 635-vii.
15. Mancia G, De BG, Dominiczak A, *et al.* 2007 Guidelines for the Management of Arterial Hypertension: The Task Force for the Management of Arterial Hypertension of the European Society of Hypertension (ESH) and of the European Society of Cardiology (ESC). *J Hypertens* 2007; 25(6): 1105-87.
16. Chobanian AV, Bakris GL, Black HR, *et al.* Seventh report of the Joint National Committee on Prevention, Detection, Evaluation, and Treatment of High Blood Pressure. *Hypertension* 2003; 42(6): 1206-52.
17. Hansson L, Zanchetti A, Carruthers SG, *et al.* Effects of intensive blood-pressure lowering and low-dose aspirin in patients with hypertension: principal results of the Hypertension Optimal Treatment (HOT) randomised trial. HOT Study Group. *Lancet* 1998; 351(9118): 1755-62.
18. Tight blood pressure control and risk of macrovascular and microvascular complications in type 2 diabetes: UKPDS 38. UK Prospective Diabetes Study Group. *BMJ* 1998; 317(7160): 703-13.
19. Rahman M, Pressel S, Davis BR, *et al.* Renal outcomes in high-risk hypertensive patients treated with an angiotensin-converting enzyme inhibitor or a calcium channel blocker vs a diuretic: a report from the Antihypertensive and Lipid-Lowering Treatment to Prevent Heart Attack Trial (ALLHAT). *Arch Intern Med* 2005; 165(8): 936-46.
20. Cushman WC, Evans GW, Byington RP, *et al,* for the ACCORD Study Group. The effects of intensive blood pressure control in type 2 diabetes mellitus. Epub - published on March 14, 2010, www.nejm.org.
21. Bakris GL, Williams M, Dworkin L, *et al.* Preserving renal function in adults with hypertension and diabetes: a consensus approach. National Kidney Foundation Hypertension and Diabetes Executive Committees Working Group. *Am J Kidney Dis* 2000; 36(3): 646-61.
22. Klahr S, Levey AS, Beck GJ, *et al.* The effects of dietary protein restriction and blood-pressure control on the progression of chronic renal disease. Modification of Diet in Renal Disease Study Group. *N Engl J Med* 1994; 330(13): 877-84.
23. Sarnak MJ, Greene T, Wang X, *et al.* The effect of a lower target blood pressure on the progression of kidney disease: long-term follow-up of the Modification of Diet in Renal Disease study. *Ann Intern Med* 2005; 142(5): 342-51.
24. Wright JT, Jr., Bakris G, Greene T, *et al.* Effect of blood pressure lowering and antihypertensive drug class on progression of hypertensive kidney disease: results from the AASK trial. *JAMA* 2002; 288(19): 2421-31.
25. Appel LJ, Wright JT, Jr., Greene T, *et al.* Long-term effects of renin-angiotensin system-blocking therapy and a low blood pressure goal on progression of hypertensive chronic kidney disease in African Americans. *Arch Intern Med* 2008; 168(8): 832-39.
26. Pogue V, Rahman M, Lipkowitz M, *et al.* Disparate estimates of hypertension control from ambulatory and clinic blood pressure measurements in hypertensive kidney disease. *Hypertension* 2009; 53(1): 20-7.
27. Peterson GE, de BT, Gabriel A, *et al.* Prevalence and correlates of left ventricular hypertrophy in the African American Study of Kidney Disease Cohort Study. *Hypertension* 2007; 50(6): 1033-9.
28. Ruggenenti P, Perna A, Loriga G, *et al.* Blood-pressure control for renoprotection in patients with non-diabetic chronic renal disease (REIN-2): multicentre, randomised controlled trial. *Lancet* 2005; 365(9463): 939-46.
29. Jafar TH, Stark PC, Schmid CH, *et al.* Progression of chronic kidney disease: the role of blood pressure control, proteinuria, and angiotensin-converting enzyme inhibition: a patient-level meta-analysis. *Ann Intern Med* 2003; 139(4): 244-52.

30. Pohl MA, Blumenthal S, Cordonnier DJ, *et al.* Independent and Additive Impact of Blood Pressure Control and Angiotensin II Receptor Blockade on Renal Outcomes in the Irbesartan Diabetic Nephropathy Trial: clinical implications and limitations. *J Am Soc Nephrol* 2005; 16(10): 3027-37.
31. Bakris GL, Weir MR, Shanifar S, *et al.* Effects of blood pressure level on progression of diabetic nephropathy: results from the RENAAL study. *Arch Intern Med* 2003; 163(13): 1555-65.
32. Sarafidis PA, Li S, Chen SC, *et al.* Hypertension awareness, treatment, and control in chronic kidney disease. *Am J Med* 2008; 121(4): 332-40.
33. Ong KL, Cheung BM, Man YB, Lau CP, Lam KS. Prevalence, awareness, treatment, and control of hypertension among United States adults 1999-2004. *Hypertension* 2007; 49(1): 69-75.
34. Coresh J, Wei GL, McQuillan G, *et al.* Prevalence of high blood pressure and elevated serum creatinine level in the United States: findings from the third National Health and Nutrition Examination Survey (1988-1994). *Arch Intern Med* 2001; 161(9): 1207-16.
35. Sarafidis PA, Bakris GL. Microalbuminuria and chronic kidney disease as risk factors for cardiovascular disease. *Nephrol Dial Transplant* 2006; 21(9): 2366-74.
36. McCullough PA, Jurkovitz CT, Pergola PE, *et al.* Independent components of chronic kidney disease as a cardiovascular risk state: results from the Kidney Early Evaluation Program (KEEP). *Arch Intern Med* 2007; 167(11): 1122-9.
37. MacIsaac RJ, Jerums G, Cooper ME. New insights into the significance of microalbuminuria. *Curr Opin Nephrol Hypertens* 2004; 13(1): 83-91.
38. Steinke JM, Sinaiko AR, Kramer MS, Suissa S, Chavers BM, Mauer M. The early natural history of nephropathy in Type 1 Diabetes: III. Predictors of 5-year urinary albumin excretion rate patterns in initially normoalbuminuric patients. *Diabetes* 2005; 54(7): 2164-71.
39. American Diabetes Association. Nephropathy in diabetes. *Diabetes Care* 2004; 27: S79-84.
40. Lea J, Greene T, Hebert L, *et al.* The relationship between magnitude of proteinuria reduction and risk of end-stage renal disease: results of the African American study of kidney disease and hypertension. *Arch Intern Med* 2005; 165(8): 947-53.
41. De Zeeuw D, Remuzzi G, Parving HH, *et al.* Proteinuria, a target for renoprotection in patients with type 2 diabetic nephropathy: lessons from RENAAL. *Kidney Int* 2004; 65(6): 2309-20.
42. Atkins RC, Briganti EM, Lewis JB, *et al.* Proteinuria reduction and progression to renal failure in patients with type 2 diabetes mellitus and overt nephropathy. *Am J Kidney Dis* 2005; 45(2): 281-7.
43. Chua DC, Bakris GL. Is proteinuria a plausible target of therapy? *Curr Hypertens Rep* 2004; 6(3): 177-81.
44. Ibsen H, Olsen MH, Wachtell K *et al.* Reduction in albuminuria translates to reduction in cardiovascular events in hypertensive patients: Losartan Intervention for Endpoint Reduction in Hypertension study. *Hypertension* 2005; 45(2): 198-202.
45. Parving HH, Lehnert H, Brochner-Mortensen J, Gomis R, Andersen S, Arner P. The effect of irbesartan on the development of diabetic nephropathy in patients with type 2 diabetes. *N Engl J Med* 2001; 345(12): 870-8.
46. Brenner BM, Cooper ME, de ZD, *et al.* Effects of losartan on renal and cardiovascular outcomes in patients with type 2 diabetes and nephropathy. *N Engl J Med* 2001; 345(12): 861-9.
47. Eijkelkamp WB, Zhang Z, Remuzzi G, *et al.* Albuminuria is a target for renoprotective therapy independent from blood pressure in patients with type 2 diabetic nephropathy: post hoc analysis from the Reduction of Endpoints in NIDDM with the Angiotensin II Antagonist Losartan (RENAAL) trial. *J Am Soc Nephrol* 2007; 18(5): 1540-6.
48. Lewis EJ, Hunsicker LG, Clarke WR, *et al.* Renoprotective effect of the angiotensin-receptor antagonist irbesartan in patients with nephropathy due to type 2 diabetes. *N Engl J Med* 2001; 345(12): 851-60.
49. Kunz R, Friedrich C, Wolbers M, Mann JF. Meta-analysis: effect of monotherapy and combination therapy with inhibitors of the renin angiotensin system on proteinuria in renal disease. *Ann Intern Med* 2008; 148(1): 30-48.
50. Parving HH, Persson F, Lewis JB, Lewis EJ, Hollenberg NK. Aliskiren combined with losartan in type 2 diabetes and nephropathy. *N Engl J Med* 2008; 358(23): 2433-46.
51. Bidani A. Controversy about COOPERATE ABPM trial data. *Am J Nephrol* 2006; 26(6): 629-32.
52. Rossing K, Schjoedt KJ, Smidt UM, Boomsma F, Parving HH. Beneficial effects of adding spironolactone to recommended antihypertensive treatment in diabetic nephropathy: a randomized, double-masked, cross-over study. *Diabetes Care* 2005; 28(9): 2106-12.
53. Epstein M, Williams GH, Weinberger M, *et al.* Selective aldosterone blockade with eplerenone reduces albuminuria in patients with type 2 diabetes. *Clin J Am Soc Nephrol* 2006; 1(5): 940-51.

54. Bomback AS, Kshirsagar AV, Amamoo MA, Klemmer PJ. Change in proteinuria after adding aldosterone blockers to ACE inhibitors or angiotensin receptor blockers in CKD: a systematic review. *Am J Kidney Dis* 2008; 51(2): 199-211.
55. Mailloux LU, Levey AS. Hypertension in patients with chronic renal disease. *Am J Kidney Dis* 1998; 32(5 Suppl 3): S120-41.
56. Brater DC. Diuretic therapy. *N Engl J Med* 1998; 339(6): 387-95.
57. Ruilope L, Kjeldsen SE, de la Sierra A, *et al.* The kidney and cardiovascular risk - implications for management: a consensus statement from the European Society of Hypertension. *Blood Press* 2007; 16(2): 72-9.
58. Bakris GL, Sowers JR. ASH position paper: treatment of hypertension in patients with diabetes - an update. *J Clin Hypertens* (Greenwich) 2008; 10(9): 707-13.
59. Bakris GL, Weir MR. Achieving goal blood pressure in patients with type 2 diabetes: conventional versus fixed-dose combination approaches. *J Clin Hypertens* (Greenwich) 2003; 5(3): 202-9.
60. Jamerson K, Weber MA, Bakris GL, *et al.* Benazepril plus amlodipine or hydrochlorothiazide for hypertension in high-risk patients. *N Engl J Med* 2008; 359(23): 2417-28.
61. Bakris GL, Copley JB, Vicknair N, Sadler R, Leurgans S. Calcium channel blockers versus other antihypertensive therapies on progression of NIDDM associated nephropathy. *Kidney Int* 1996; 50(5): 1641-50.
62. Bakris GL, Mangrum A, Copley JB, Vicknair N, Sadler R. Effect of calcium channel or beta-blockade on the progression of diabetic nephropathy in African Americans. *Hypertension* 1997; 29(3): 744-50.
63. Smith AC, Toto R, Bakris GL. Differential effects of calcium channel blockers on size selectivity of proteinuria in diabetic glomerulopathy. *Kidney Int* 1998; 54(3): 889-96.
64. Bakris GL, Weir MR, Secic M, Campbell B, Weis-McNulty A. Differential effects of calcium antagonist subclasses on markers of nephropathy progression. *Kidney Int* 2004; 65(6): 1991-2002.
65. Bakris GL, Hart P, Ritz E. Beta blockers in the management of chronic kidney disease. *Kidney Int* 2006; 70(11): 1905-13.
66. Turnbull F, Neal B, Ninomiya T, *et al.* Effects of different regimens to lower blood pressure on major cardiovascular events in older and younger adults: meta-analysis of randomised trials. *BMJ* 2008; 336(7653): 1121-3.
67. Bakris GL, Fonseca V, Katholi RE, *et al.* Metabolic effects of carvedilol vs metoprolol in patients with type 2 diabetes mellitus and hypertension: a randomized controlled trial. *JAMA* 2004; 292(18): 2227-36.
68. Schmidt AC, Graf C, Brixius K, Scholze J. Blood pressure-lowering effect of nebivolol in hypertensive patients with type 2 diabetes mellitus: the YESTONO study. *Clin Drug Investig* 2007; 27(12): 841-9.
69. Cice G, Ferrara L, D'Andrea A, *et al.* Carvedilol increases two-year survival in dialysis patients with dilated cardiomyopathy: a prospective, placebo-controlled trial. *J Am Coll Cardiol* 2003; 41(9): 1438-44.
70. Lindholm LH, Carlberg B, Samuelsson O. Should beta blockers remain first choice in the treatment of primary hypertension? A meta-analysis. *Lancet* 2005; 366(9496): 1545-53.

Chapter 15

Hypertension management in diabetes

Deepashree Gupta [1] MD, PGY-3 Resident Physician
Guido Lastra [1, 2] MD, Fellow,
Camila Manrique [1, 2] MD, Fellow
James R. Sowers [1, 2, 3] MD, Professor and Division Director of Endocrinology, Diabetes and Metabolism; Professor of Medicine, Physiology and Pharmacology
1 Department of Internal Medicine, University of Missouri-Columbia, Columbia, Missouri, USA
2 Division of Endocrinology, Diabetes and Metabolism, University of Missouri-Columbia, Columbia, Missouri, USA
3 Department of Physiology and Pharmacology, University of Missouri-Columbia, Columbia, Missouri, USA

Introduction

Hypertension is an important risk factor for coronary artery disease (CAD), heart failure, cerebrovascular disease, chronic kidney disease (CKD) and peripheral vascular disease (PVD) [1-2]. According to the National Health and Nutrition Examination Survey data (NHANES III) spanning over approximately 10 years, the prevalence of hypertension in Americans increased from 42 million (1988-1994) to almost 70 million (1999-2004) [3]. Contemporaneously, the obesity epidemic is driving the rapid expansion of type 2 diabetes mellitus (DM) across the globe; type 2 DM is an established independent risk factor for cardiovascular disease (CVD) and CKD. Hence, the risk of CVD and CKD in persons with hypertension escalates even further in the presence of DM and other risk factors like obesity, dyslipidemia, smoking, family history of premature coronary heart disease, physical inactivity and age (older than 55 for men and 65 for women) [4-5]; the clustering of these independent CVD risk factors is now termed the cardiometabolic syndrome (CMS) [6-7].

Hypertension can be classified as either essential (primary) or secondary; essential hypertension is when no specific medical cause can be found to explain the patient's high blood pressure. Ninety-five percent of hypertensive Americans are thought to have essential hypertension, while secondary hypertension accounts for the remaining 5% of cases [8]. However, many patients in the United States with hypertension have obesity which enhances the risk for CVD [7] and CKD [8]. Additionally, overweight and obesity states are associated with increased inflammation and hyperaldosteronism, which likely contribute to increased CVD and CKD with coexistence of overweight, obesity and hypertension.

It has been reported that more than 50% of patients with newly diagnosed type 2 DM present with coexisting hypertension [9]. Also, approximately 50% of the 75 million Americans with hypertension have insulin resistance (IR), higher fasting and post-prandial insulin levels [10-11] and will develop type 2 DM over a 10- to 15-year period [12-14]. These data indicate that these two common chronic diseases frequently coexist. Moreover, even though each disease has its independent natural history, their coexistence tends to exacerbate CVD and renal disease risk afforded by each clinical entity [15-16]. In this regard, up to 75% of CVD in diabetes may be attributable to coexisting hypertension [17]. Diabetics with hypertension also have a significantly higher risk of developing retinopathy and nephropathy than those who are normotensive [18]. Adequate treatment of hypertension not only decreases the risk of CAD, CKD, heart failure, strokes, PVD and microvascular complications in diabetic patients, but may also decrease new onset of insulin resistance/type 2 DM in hypertensive individuals.

Pathophysiology

Excess adiposity is critical to the development of the CMS. Adipose tissue is now considered to be an active endocrine organ and dysfunctional adipocytes in obesity are known to produce excess proinflammatory adipokines. These adipocyte-derived cytokines in turn activate the tissue and systemic renin-angiotensin-aldosterone system (RAAS) and lead to a chronic low-grade inflammatory state and insulin resistance (IR) in peripheral tissues [19, 20]. Fatty acid (FA) elevation [21], related to IR, hypertension, hyperglycemia [22] and atherogenic dyslipidemia also contribute to inappropriate activation of circulating and/or local RAAS in the CMS and trigger excessive oxidative stress in numerous tissues. RAAS actions in the CMS appear to be largely mediated through increased production of angiotensin II (Ang II) and aldosterone and activation of Ang II type 1 receptor (AT1 R) [23]. Excessive oxidative stress can decrease insulin sensitivity in vascular tissue [24] and vascular dysfunction is implicated in the pathogenesis of macrovascular and microvascular complications, including retinopathy, nephropathy, neuropathy, and CVD in diabetic patients [25].

Insulin metabolic signaling plays an important role in proper glucose transport and glucose homeostasis in conventional insulin-sensitive tissues. It is important for normal cardiovascular physiological responses, for example, by enhancing vasodilation (promoting the endothelial nitric oxide synthase [eNOS] enzyme activity and nitric oxide [NO] bioavailability). Insulin also has antioxidant, anti-inflammatory, and profibrinolytic properties in the kidney and cardiovascular system [26]. Abnormalities in insulin metabolic signaling and associated metabolic and hemodynamic derangements are important mechanisms that contribute to the pathophysiology of the CMS [27]. A direct correlation between fasting insulin levels and blood pressure (BP) has been described [28]. IR raises arterial tone and pressure by increasing the activity of the sympathetic nervous system, decreasing urinary sodium excretion, activating the tissue and systemic RAAS, promoting the generation of reactive oxygen species (ROS), and increasing the expression of AT1 R [29-30]. IR and hypertension are implicated in the pathophysiology of atherosclerosis that results in increased CVD risk; available human studies have shown that improving IR positively affects blood pressure control [31].

Amylin, the major component of islet amyloid, is the second beta-cell-derived hormone important in glucose homeostasis. Amylin is cosynthesized and cosecreted with insulin in response to glucose or nutrient stimuli. Unlike insulin, however, amylin is amyloidogenic and islet amyloid deposition appears to be a factor in the progressive nature of type 2 DM [32]. The islet amyloid results in a diffusion barrier within the islet and its small oligomeric forms are capable of causing apoptosis of islet beta-cells [33]. Hyperamylinemia (HA) can also activate the RAAS [32, 34-35].

The specific genomic actions of aldosterone in the regulation of blood pressure, water, sodium, and potassium homeostasis are well known and are mediated through its interaction with the steroid-type cytoplasmatic mineralocorticoid receptor (MR) [19]. In addition to these actions, aldosterone via 'non-genomic' mechanisms, i.e. mechanisms which do not require gene transcription and are independent of their effect on blood pressure [36], result in insulin resistance and endothelial dysfunction, processes that in turn contribute to maladaptive renal and cardiovascular remodeling [24, 31, 37].

In rodent fat tissue, aldosterone stimulates pro-inflammatory adipokine production leading to reduced insulin receptor expression and impaired insulin-induced glucose uptake [38]. It has also been linked to impaired insulin intracellular signaling [39]. Studies in obese diabetic mice have demonstrated that mineralocorticoid receptor blockade reduced expression of these pro-inflammatory and prothrombotic factors and increased the expression of adiponectin in heart and adipose tissue, which is protective against adipokines [40]. Human adipocytes produce a yet unidentified mineralocorticoid-releasing factor that by paracrine or endocrine mechanisms stimulate adrenal aldosterone production [41-42]. The epoxy-keto derivative of linoleic acid is a free fatty acid that strongly stimulates aldosterone production and it is present in obese persons with increased levels of free fatty acids [42]. Hence, obesity is thought to be associated with increased aldosterone production, and elevated levels of aldosterone in turn promote development of the metabolic syndrome.

A recent study suggests that mineralocorticoids influence the adipocyte biology in white adipose tissue. It was seen in rodent models that aldosterone promotes the development of adipose-type phenotype in a time- and dose-dependent manner, which is associated with induction of peroxisome proliferator-activated receptor-γ mRNA. All these changes were reversed by spironolactone, suggesting a key role for MR activation in glucose homeostasis and differentiation of adipose tissue with potential implications on insulin sensitivity [43-44].

Oxidative stress

The systemic and local tissue RAAS stimulate the reduced form of nicotinamide adenine dinucleotide phosphate (NADPH) oxidase enzyme. NADPH oxidase is a membrane-bound electron transport complex that catalyzes the production of superoxide from oxygen and NADPH. It is a multisubunit enzyme composed of three cytosolic ($p40^{phox}$, $p47^{phox}$ and $p67^{phox}$) and two membrane-bound components (Nox 2 [$P91^{phox}$] and $p22^{phox}$), plus the small proteins Rac 1 and Rac 2, which are essential to NADPH oxidase assembly. 'Phox' stands for phagocytic oxidase and Rac 1 or Rac 2 (Rac stands for Rho-related C3 botulinum toxin substrate) is a Rho guanosine triphosphatase (GTPase).

Activation of NADPH oxidase involves the assembly in the plasma membrane of membrane-bound and cytosolic components of the NADPH oxidase system, which are disassembled in the resting state. Activation starts with the phosphorylation of one of the cytosolic components and their translocation to the plasma membrane where electron transfer between gp 91 and O_2 molecules leads to formation of superoxide ($O_2^{\cdot}$) and ROS [45]. Ang II via AT1 R can promote this pathway by stimulating intracellular pathways that result in translocation of cytosolic subunits to the plasma membrane and direct phosphorylation of membrane-bound subunit p22 phox via protein kinase C activation and activation of Rac 1 by association with caveolin 1 [46-47].

ROS cause uncoupling of the endothelial nitric oxidase synthase (eNOS) enzyme with resultant decrease in the antioxidant and vasodilator NO and overactivity of superoxide. This in turn leads to endothelial dysfunction and increased peripheral vascular resistance, hence playing an important role in the development of essential hypertension. Endothelial dysfunction due to imbalance between superoxide and NO is also the starting point of the morphologic and functional changes observed in various organ systems like the heart and kidney.

Patients with essential hypertension are more prone than normotensive individuals to develop impaired glucose tolerance, IR and type 2 DM; this may be explained, in part, by the inhibitory action of angiotensin II on insulin-induced relaxation and glucose transport in vascular and skeletal muscle tissue, respectively. Ang II interferes with insulin signaling through phosphatidylinositol 3-kinase (PI3K) and its downstream protein kinase B (Akt) signaling pathways by stimulation of RhoA (the small G protein family – guanosine triphosphateases) activity and oxidative stress. RhoA and ROS inhibition of PI3K/Akt signaling results in decreased endothelial cell production of NO (impaired vasodilation), increased myosin light chain activation (causing vasoconstriction), and reduced insulin-stimulated glucose transport in skeletal muscle [28].

Evidence-based management of hypertension

The American Diabetes Association (ADA) recommends a multifactorial approach for the management of the CMS. This includes lifestyle modification, a BP <130/80mm Hg, LDL <70mg/dL, glycemic control (glycated hemoglobin A1c <7%), low-dose aspirin (75-162mg/day) and reduction of albuminuria/proteinuria by >30% within 6 months of starting treatment. In addition, the Seventh Report of the Joint National Committee on Prevention, Detection, Evaluation, and Treatment of High Blood Pressure (JNC 7), as well as the 2007 treatment guidelines from the ADA, recommend a blood pressure goal of <130/80mm Hg in diabetic patients to maximally reduce the risk of cardiovascular disease and death and the progression of diabetic complications [48-52]. It was seen in the Systolic Hypertension in the Elderly Program (SHEP) study that aggressive systolic blood pressure (SBP) lowering decreased CVD more in diabetics than non-diabetics [53] **(Ib/A)**. This was a randomized, double-blind, placebo-controlled trial that began in March 1985, and had an average follow-up of 4.5 years. It comprised a total of 4736 men and women aged 60 years or older with isolated systolic hypertension at 16 clinical centers in the United States. Patients were randomly assigned to receive treatment with 12.5mg/d of chlorthalidone (step 1) (either 25mg/d of atenolol or 0.05mg/d of reserpine [step 2] could be added according to blood pressure response) or placebo. A total of 85 and 132 participants in the active treatment and placebo groups, respectively, had ischemic strokes (adjusted relative risk [RR], 0.63; 95% confidence interval [CI], 0.48-0.82) and 9 and 19 had hemorrhagic strokes (adjusted RR, 0.46; 95% CI, 0.21-1.02). Treatment effect was observed within 1 year for hemorrhagic strokes but was not seen until the second year for ischemic strokes. Both hemorrhagic and ischemic (including lacunar) stroke incidence significantly decreased in participants attaining study-specific systolic blood pressure goals.

The degree of blood pressure control appears to be more important in determining outcomes. Indeed, for approximately every 10mm Hg decrease in SBP, the risk of any complication of diabetes is reduced by 12% [54-55]. Studies show a significant slowing in the decline in glomerular filtration rate (GFR) especially in patients with proteinuria with optimal blood pressure control [56-58]. The blood pressure arm of the Action to Control Cardiovascular Risk in Diabetes (ACCORD) trial, still ongoing, evaluated the impact of intensive blood pressure lowering (SBP <120mm Hg) compared to conventional antihypertensive treatment on CVD risk in type 2 diabetics [59]. This is a randomized, multicenter, double 2 × 2 factorial design study involving 10,251 middle-aged and older participants with type 2 diabetes who are at high risk for CVD events because of existing CVD or additional risk factors. ACCORD evaluated the effects of three medical treatment strategies to reduce CVD morbidity and mortality. All participants were initially included in the glycemic control arm, which tested the hypothesis that a therapeutic strategy that targets an HbA1c level of <6.0% would reduce the rate of CVD events more than a strategy that targets an HbA1c of 7.0%-7.9%. The lipid trial included 5518 of the participants, who received either fenofibrate or placebo in a double-masked fashion to test the hypothesis that, in the context of good glycemic control, the use of a fibrate in combination with a statin is more effective to reduce the rate of CVD events relative to use of a statin plus a placebo. The blood pressure trial included the remaining 4733 participants and tests the hypothesis that a therapeutic strategy that targets a SBP of <120mm Hg in the context of good glycemic control will reduce the rate of CVD events more effectively than a strategy that targets a SBP of <140mm Hg. The primary outcome was the first occurrence of a major CVD event, specifically non-fatal myocardial infarction, non-fatal stroke, or cardiovascular death. The glycemia trial was terminated early due to higher mortality in the intensive compared with the standard glycemia treatment strategies [60]. However, in the blood pressure arm of the ACCORD study, lowering blood pressure to below 130mmHg systolic, while decreasing stroke, did not reduce overall cardiovascular disease mortality in high-risk patients with type 2 diabetes. These results are discussed in more detail in Chapter 1.

Non-pharmacologic intervention

In all diabetic patients with BP >130/80mm Hg, lifestyle modification should be strongly encouraged. The changes recommended by the JNC 7 include weight loss, an increase in regular physical activity, smoking cessation, adoption of the DASH (Dietary Approaches to Stop Hypertension) dietary plan, reduction in alcohol intake (less than two drinks per day in men and one drink per day in women and lighter weight individuals), as well as sodium intake (less than 2.4g/d) [48].

Sodium intake restriction to levels below the current recommendation of 100mmol per day (equivalent to 2.3g of sodium or 5.8g of sodium chloride) appears to be of paramount importance, as studied by Sacks *et al* in a recent randomized clinical trial including 412 participants randomly assigned to eat either a control diet typical of sodium intake in the United States or the DASH diet [61]. This trial also demonstrated that the DASH diet that emphasizes fruits, vegetables, and low-fat dairy products, includes whole grains, poultry, fish, and nuts, contains only small amounts of red meat, sweets, and sugar-containing beverages, and that contains decreased amounts of total and saturated fat and cholesterol, lowers blood pressure substantially both in people with hypertension and those without hypertension, as compared with a typical diet in the United States **(Ib/A)**.

Pharmacologic approach

If non-pharmacologic measures fail to control blood pressure adequately, antihypertensive medications should be considered. The cardiovascular outcome trials over the past decade indicate that diabetic hypertensives require an average of 2.9 appropriately dosed antihypertensive medications to achieve blood pressure goals, whereas in type 2 diabetics with pre-existing stage 3 or higher kidney disease, the average number of antihypertensives goes up to 3.5. Thus, these medications should have the maximal efficacy, the least adverse effects and preferably be low in cost [62-63].

Current guidelines by the American Diabetes Association (ADA) recommend starting patients on a once daily RAAS blocker, preferably an ACE-I as the first-line therapy. If side effects like cough develop, then treatment should be changed to an equivalent dose of an ARB. The doses of either of these medications should be titrated to the maximum tolerated dose within a month to reach the target BP <130/80mm Hg. If blood pressure goal is not achieved with maximum dose titration of either an ACE-I or an ARB, the option is to add either a low-dose thiazide diuretic (12.5mg of chlorthalidone or hydrochlorothiazide) or a calcium channel blocker (CCB). In patients with an estimated glomerular filtration rate (eGFR) <50ml/min or with hyperkalemia, loop diuretics would be preferred over thiazide diuretics. Also, thiazide diuretics and CCBs should be titrated to their maximum tolerated dose to get blood pressure to the target range. However, in about 20% of cases, a fourth or fifth agent is required; vasodilating β-blockers and α-blockers are useful in this case. More recently, there has been an increasing interest in the use of aldosterone blockers as a fourth-line agent, especially in patients with obesity and obstructive sleep apnea and multiple trials are underway to prove the efficacy of the same [63].

Numerous recent randomized controlled trials have demonstrated the benefit of initiating combination therapy over single drug therapy to control hypertension in patients with diabetes **(Ib/A)**. Three of them are Valsartan-Managing Blood Pressure Aggressively and Evaluating Reductions in hsCRP (Val-MARC) [64], Valsartan/HCTZ Combination Therapy in patients with Moderate to Severe Systolic Hypertension (VALOR) [65], and the Valsartan Effectiveness in Lowering Blood Pressure Comparative Study (VELOCITY) [66]. The Val-MARC study included patients aged 18-75 years with stage 2 hypertension (SBP ≥160mm Hg or diastolic blood pressure [DBP] ≥100mm Hg). Patients were randomized to monotherapy with valsartan 160mg daily (n=836) or to combination therapy with valsartan 160mg daily plus HCTZ 12.5mg (n=832). After 2 weeks, the dose of valsartan was force uptitrated to 320mg daily in all patients who were still symptomatic. Patients remained on this dose of valsartan with or without HCTZ for 6 weeks, after which, if blood pressure remained uncontrolled, patients previously on monotherapy were allowed HCTZ 12.5mg at the physician's discretion, and the dose of HCTZ in the combination therapy arm could be raised to 25mg until week 12. The VALOR trial enrolled a total of 767 patients with stages 2 and 3 systolic hypertension (SBP ≥160mm Hg and ≤200mm Hg), with or without other CVD risk factors. After a 2-week washout (if previously treated) and a 2-week placebo run-in, they were randomized to either monotherapy with valsartan 80mg or valsartan 160mg, both administered once daily. At the end of 4 weeks of monotherapy, patients were force-titrated to once-daily dosing with valsartan 160mg, valsartan 160mg plus HCTZ 12.5mg, or valsartan 160mg plus HCTZ 25mg for an additional 4 weeks. The primary objective of VALOR was to evaluate the incremental benefit of valsartan plus HCTZ 12.5mg or 25mg on sitting SBP. VELOCITY was a 6-week, multi-center, randomized, double-blind, parallel-group treatment regimen study which included 648 adults with hypertension (age=52.6±10 yrs; 54% male; baseline BP=161/98mm Hg). Participants in the three groups were initiated on valsartan 80mg, valsartan 160mg or valsartan/HCTZ (160/12.5mg) for the first 2 weeks and were then titrated according to the study design.

Collectively, these studies demonstrated more effective blood pressure lowering in hypertensive patients with and without diabetes with valsartan/HCTZ than with valsartan only. In addition, while switching patients to a combination therapy as a second-line strategy did lower blood pressure more than monotherapy, the initial use of combination therapy offered an incremental systolic blood pressure reduction of nearly 3mm Hg [55]. Given the fact that blood pressure lowering may be more difficult in diabetic patients, partly because the goal in this patient population is lower (SBP <130mm Hg) compared to non-diabetics (SBP <140mm Hg), under-treatment of hypertension in diabetics is common [67]. Hence, fixed combination treatment can increase patient compliance by simplifying the regimen as well as cause greater blood pressure reductions more rapidly than monotherapy [68].

Angiotensin-converting enzyme inhibitor (ACE-I)/angiotensin receptor blocker (ARB)

It is now well documented that both ACE-Is and ARBs have cardioprotective and renoprotective effects [69-70]. As previously discussed, hypertension increases the risk of development of new type 2 DM and antihypertensives that produce RAAS blockade, in particular ACE-Is and ARBs, have been related to a reduced incidence of type 2 DM **(Ib/A)**. The Prospective Randomized Open Blinded Endpoint (PROBE) trial which compared the effect of captopril versus conventional therapy (β-blockers and diuretics) on CVD-related morbidity and mortality, failed to demonstrate a significant difference in overall CVD morbidity and mortality in the ACE-I-treated group but a significant reduction of 30% in the incidence of type 2 DM was observed after a follow-up of 6.1 years [71]. The PROBE study suggests that RAAS inhibition is particularly beneficial in patients with type 2 DM, and that the reduction observed in the incidence of type 2 DM could lead to a further reduction of CVD in the long term.

The Heart Outcomes Prevention Evaluation Study (HOPE) trial also demonstrated similar outcomes with the incidence of new-onset diabetes being 34% lower in the ramipril-treated group as compared to placebo [72]. In this study, a total of 9297 high-risk patients (55 years of age or older) who had evidence of vascular disease or diabetes plus one other cardiovascular risk factor and who were not known to have a low ejection fraction or heart failure were randomly assigned to receive ramipril (10mg once per day orally) or matching placebo for a mean of 5 years. There was a decreased incidence of adverse cardiovascular events (by 22%) including heart failure, myocardial infarction and stroke. These beneficial effects of ramipril in the HOPE study, however, appear to be independent of blood pressure reduction [70, 73]. The secondary outcome of decreased incidence of new-onset type 2 DM (102 vs. 155; relative risk, 0.66; $p<0.001$) found in this study is thought to be mediated by improved insulin sensitivity, a decrease in hepatic clearance of insulin, an anti-inflammatory effect of ACE inhibition, improved blood flow to the pancreas [74], or an effect on abdominal fat [75].

Other studies that have demonstrated decreased incidence of new-onset diabetes with the use of ACE-Is and ARBs include ALLHAT [76-77], SOLVD [78] and LIFE [79]. The Antihypertensive and Lipid-Lowering Treatment to Prevent Heart Attack Trial (ALLHAT) was a randomized, double-blind, active-controlled clinical trial conducted from February 1994 through March 2002 which included a total of 33,357 participants aged 55 years or older with hypertension and at least one more cardiovascular risk factor from 623 North American centers. The objective was to compare treatment with a calcium channel blocker or an angiotensin-converting enzyme inhibitor with a diuretic in lowering the incidence of coronary heart disease (CHD) or other cardiovascular disease (CVD) events. Participants were randomly assigned to receive chlorthalidone, 12.5 to 25mg/d (n=15,255); amlodipine 2.5 to 10mg/d (n=9048); or lisinopril, 10 to 40mg/d (n=9054) for planned follow-up of approximately 4 to 8 years. In this study, thiazide-type diuretics were superior in preventing one or more major forms of CVD, suggesting that this class of medications should be preferred as first-line antihypertensive therapy. Given the large sample size in ALLHAT, almost all differences in follow-up blood pressure and biochemical measurements were statistically significant. Among individuals classified as non-diabetic at baseline (fasting serum glucose less than 126mg/dL), the incidence of diabetes (fasting serum glucose ≥126mg/dL) at 4 years was 11.6% in the chlorthalidone group, 9.8% in the amlodipine group, and 8.1% in the lisinopril group. These metabolic differences, however, did not translate into a higher incidence of cardiovascular events or all-cause mortality in the chlorthalidone group.

In the Effect of Enalapril on Mortality and the Development of Heart Failure in Asymptomatic Patients with Reduced Left Ventricular Ejection Fractions (SOLVD investigators) study, patients were randomly assigned to receive either placebo (n=2117) or enalapril (n=2111) at doses of 2.5 to 20mg per day in a double-blind randomized controlled trial. Follow-up in this study averaged 37.4 months. The reduction in mortality from cardiovascular causes was larger in the ACE-I-treated group, but it was not statistically significant (298 deaths in the placebo group vs. 265 in the enalapril group; risk reduction, 12%; 95% CI, -3 to 26%; p=0.12). The total number of deaths and cases of heart failure was lower in the enalapril group than in the placebo group (630 vs. 818; risk reduction, 29%; 95% CI, 21 to 36%; p <0.001). In addition, fewer patients given enalapril died or were hospitalized for heart failure (434 in the enalapril group; vs. 518 in the placebo group; risk reduction, 20%; 95% CI, 9 to 30%; p <0.001) **(Ib/A)**.

The Losartan Intervention for Endpoint Reduction in Hypertension (LIFE) study was a double-masked, randomized, parallel-group trial in 9193 participants aged 55-80 years with essential hypertension (sitting blood pressure 160-200/95-115mm Hg) and left ventricle hypertrophy (LVH). Participants were assigned to either once daily losartan-based or atenolol-based antihypertensive treatment for at least 4 years and until 1040 patients had a primary cardiovascular event (death, myocardial infarction, or stroke). Blood pressure fell by 30·2/16·6 (SD 18·5/10·1) and 29·1/16·8mm Hg (19·2/10·1) in the losartan and atenolol groups, respectively. The primary composite endpoint occurred in 508 losartan (23·8 per 1000 patient-years) and 588 atenolol patients (27·9 per 1000 patient-years; relative risk 0·87, 95% CI 0·77-0·98, p=0·021). Two hundred and four losartan and 234 atenolol patients died from cardiovascular disease (0·89, 0·73-1·07, p=0·206); 232 and 309, respectively, had fatal or non-fatal stroke (0·75, 0·63-0·89, p=0·001); and myocardial infarction (non-fatal and fatal) occurred in 198 and 188, respectively (1·07, 0·88-1·31, p=0·491); hence, losartan conferred cardioprotective benefits independent of its antihypertensive effect **(Ib/A)**. New-onset diabetes was 25% less frequent in the group treated with losartan relative to the atenolol-treated participants.

In the Candesartan in Heart Failure Assessment of Reduction in Mortality and Morbidity (CHARM) study, the use of candesartan versus placebo in patients with cardiac failure was also associated with fewer new diagnoses of type 2 DM [80]. Importantly, however, in these studies, the primary outcome being looked at was not the effect of ACE-Is and ARBs on the incidence of type 2 DM, but cardiovascular outcomes.

On the other hand, the Diabetes Reduction Assessment with Ramipril and Rosiglitazone Medication (DREAM) trial, which specifically analyzed the incidence of type 2 DM, demonstrated that the use of ramipril was not associated with a significant reduction in the incidence of type 2 DM but resulted in significantly increased regression to normoglycemia relative to placebo thus suggesting a beneficial effect of RAAS blockade on glucose homeostasis [81] **(Ib/A)**. This was a double-blinded, randomized clinical trial with a 2-by-2 factorial design where 5269 participants without CVD but with impaired fasting glucose (after an 8-hour fast) or impaired glucose tolerance were randomly assigned to receive ramipril (up to 15mg per day) or placebo (and rosiglitazone or placebo) and were followed for a median of 3 years. The effects of ramipril on the development of diabetes or death, whichever came first (the primary outcome), and on secondary outcomes, including regression to normoglycemia were studied. The incidence of the primary outcome did not differ significantly between the ramipril group (18.1%) and the placebo group (19.5%; hazard ratio for the ramipril group, 0.91; 95% CI, 0.81 to 1.03; p=0.15). Participants receiving ramipril were more likely to have regression to normoglycemia than assigned to placebo (hazard ratio, 1.16; 95% CI, 1.07 to 1.27; p=0.001). At the end of the study, the median fasting plasma glucose level was not significantly lower with ramipril (102.7mg per deciliter [5.70mmol/L]) relative to placebo (103.4mg per deciliter [5.74mmol/L], p=0.07), although glycemia 2 hours after an oral glucose load was significantly lower with ramipril (135.1mg per deciliter [7.50mmol/L] vs. 140.5mg per deciliter [7.80mmol/L], p=0.01).

Serum creatinine and potassium levels should be monitored, as ACE-Is can cause elevations in serum creatinine (which usually stabilize) and potassium levels. In the event of hyperkalemia, it is prudent to review all potassium containing food/over the counter substances that the patient might be taking as observational data demonstrate that these lifestyle changes can cause potassium reductions of up to 0.6mEq/L [63].

Thiazide diuretics

The JNC 7 report recommends thiazide diuretics as the first-line agents in most patients with uncomplicated hypertension, not associated with other high-risk conditions [48]; however, in diabetics with hypertension, they are considered as good adjuvants to ACE-Is/ARBs. In the Antihypertensive and Lipid-Lowering Treatment to Prevent Heart Attack Trial (ALLHAT), high-risk hypertensive patients receiving a thiazide-like diuretic (chlorthalidone) experienced fewer overall cardiovascular events than those on other agents (amlodipine and lisinopril) [41] **(Ib/A)**. Thiazide diuretics may lead to several metabolic derangements, including hypomagnesemia, hyperuricemia, hypercholesterolemia, hypertriglyceridemia and hypokalemia. In addition, they not only worsen glycemic status in diabetics but can lead to the development of new onset type 2 DM in people with impaired fasting glucose [82-84]. The mechanism behind hyperglycemia caused by thiazides is thought to be at least partially related to hypokalemia and recent data suggest that the treatment of thiazide-induced hypokalemia may reverse glucose intolerance and possibly prevent the development of diabetes [85].

However, two recent cardiovascular outcome trials have demonstrated that even though diuretics worsen glycemic control, cardiovascular event rates in people being treated with them were not higher [86-87]. This observation was confirmed in the diabetic subgroup in the ALLHAT trial which had the greatest worsening of glycemic control but no significant difference in cardiovascular event rate [86]. The Systolic Hypertension in the Elderly Program (SHEP) trial revealed the long-term beneficial effect of the antihypertensive effect of chlorthalidone on cardiovascular risk despite worsening of glycemic control [87]. This study analyzed the long-term mortality rate of subjects included in the Systolic Hypertension in the Elderly Program, in which 4732 patients were randomized to stepped-care therapy with 12.5

to 25mg/day of chlorthalidone or matching placebo. After a mean follow-up of 14.3 years, the cardiovascular mortality rate was lower in the chlorthalidone-treated group (19%) compared to placebo-treated participants (19% vs 22%; adjusted hazard ratio 0.854, 95% CI 0.751-0.972). Diabetes at baseline (n=799) was associated with increased cardiovascular and total mortality (and total mortality rate). Interestingly, diabetes that developed during therapy with chlorthalidone did not have significant associations with cardiovascular nor total mortality, and treatment with the diuretic in diabetic patients was associated with lower long-term mortality (cardiovascular and total). These results suggest that long-term chlorthalidone-based treatment improves both cardiovascular and total mortality, especially among type 2 diabetics **(Ib/A)**.

Calcium channel blockers (CCBs) and β-blockers

A recent review of major randomized clinical trials including the ALLHAT concluded that CCBs were associated with a 39% reduction in stroke and 28% reduction in major cardiovascular events [88] **(Ib/A)**. Also, long-acting CCBs are the drugs of choice in patients with hypertension and stable angina in whom β-blockers are contraindicated [89].

On the other hand, β-blockers should not be used as first-line therapy for hypertension management in people of any age group [90] unless there are compelling indications like CAD, post-myocardial infarction [91] or congestive heart failure (CHF) [92] **(IIa/B)**. This has been supported by the findings of the landmark Anglo-Scandinavian Cardiac Outcomes Trial (ASCOT) [93]. The ASCOT was an independent, investigator-led study set up to compare different treatment strategies in the prevention of cardiovascular disease in patients who were hypertensive but were not considered conventionally dyslipidemic. A total of 19,257 patients were enrolled in Ireland, the Nordic countries (Denmark, Finland, Iceland, Norway, and Sweden) and the United Kingdom between February 1998 and May 2000. In the blood pressure-lowering arm (ASCOT-BPLA), patients were randomized to amlodipine or atenolol, to be followed by the addition of perindopril or bendroflumethiazide (BFZ), respectively. An α-blocker, doxazosin, could be added as a third drug to either combination. The two regimens were administered in six steps in order to reach blood pressure goal (<140/<90mm Hg SBP/DBP for non-diabetic patients, or <130/<80mm Hg for diabetic patients). If target blood pressures were not achieved after step six, another drug could be added that was not from one of the antihypertensive drug classes used in the other limb of the trial. In addition, using a 2 x 2 factorial design, a subset of 10,305 patients was also randomized to the addition of atorvastatin 10mg or placebo (lipid-lowering arm - LLA). The ASCOT-LLA was stopped early after a significant benefit was seen in the reduction of cardiovascular events in patients treated with atorvastatin. ASCOT-BPLA was also stopped early in December 2004, following the recommendation of its Data Safety Monitoring Board, due to significant differences in cardiovascular events and total mortality favoring the amlodipine-based regimen.

β-blockers, like thiazide diuretics, have been associated with metabolic derangements like hyperglycemia, especially in patients with diabetes or obesity [40] and, hence, should not be combined [94]. Vasodilating β-blockers like carvedilol and nebivolol, however, are better tolerated and metabolically neutral compared to the vasoconstricting agents [95] and are thought to not affect or even improve insulin sensitivity [96]. They can be especially useful in hypertensive patients with tachycardia not controlled by more than two agents [97].

α-blockers

α-blockers have beneficial metabolic effects like improved insulin sensitivity, elevated high-density lipoprotein cholesterol, and lowered low-density lipoprotein cholesterol [98-99], but paradoxically their use (doxazosin) was associated with excess cardiovascular events compared with patients treated with thiazide-like diuretics in the ALLHAT trial [100]. They are also the major culprits in causing orthostatic hypotension especially in diabetics with autonomic dysfunction and, hence, should be used as only the fourth- or fifth-line agents in hypertension management.

Aldosterone antagonists (spironolactone and eplerenone)

As discussed above, elevated levels of aldosterone have been associated with hypertension, insulin resistance, abnormal glucose metabolism and endothelial dysfunction [11, 24, 101-103]. Excessive aldosterone levels are also associated with CVD independent of their effect on blood pressure [104].

The RALES (Randomized Aldactone Evaluation Study) was a double-blind study which enrolled 1663 patients who had severe heart failure and a left ventricular ejection fraction of no more than 35% and who were being treated with an angiotensin-converting-enzyme inhibitor, a loop diuretic, and in most cases, digoxin. A total of 822 patients were randomly assigned to receive 25mg of spironolactone daily, and 841 to placebo. The primary endpoint was death from all causes. The trial was discontinued early, after a mean follow-up period of 24 months, because an interim analysis determined that spironolactone was efficacious. There were 386 deaths in the placebo group (46%) and 284 in the spironolactone group (35%; relative risk of death, 0.70; 95% CI, 0.60 to 0.82; $p<0.001$). This 30% reduction in the risk of death among patients in the spironolactone group was attributed to a lower risk of death from progressive heart failure as well as sudden death from cardiac causes. The frequency of hospitalization for worsening heart failure was 35% lower in the spironolactone group than in the placebo group (relative risk of hospitalization, 0.65; 95% CI, 0.54 to 0.77; $p<0.001$). In addition, patients who received spironolactone had a significant improvement in symptoms of heart failure, as assessed on the basis of the New York Heart Association functional class ($p<0.001$) [105] **(Ib/A)**.

Subsequently, EPHESUS (Eplerenone Post-Acute Myocardial Infarction Heart Failure Efficacy and Survival Study) demonstrated that treatment with eplerenone, a selective mineralocorticoid receptor antagonist, reduced mortality after myocardial infarction **(Ib/A)** [106]. Patients were randomly assigned to eplerenone (25mg per day initially, titrated to a maximum of 50mg per day; 3313 patients) or placebo (3319 patients) in addition to optimal medical therapy. The study continued until 1012 deaths occurred. The primary endpoints were death from any cause and death from cardiovascular causes or hospitalization for heart failure, acute myocardial infarction, stroke, or ventricular arrhythmia. During a mean follow-up of 16 months, there were 478 deaths in the eplerenone group and 554 deaths in the placebo group (relative risk, 0.85; 95% CI, 0.75 to 0.96; p=0.008). Of these deaths, 407 in the eplerenone group and 483 in the placebo group were attributed to cardiovascular causes (relative risk, 0.83; 95% CI, 0.72 to 0.94; p=0.005). The rate of the other primary endpoints, death from cardiovascular causes or hospitalization for cardiovascular events, was reduced by eplerenone (relative risk, 0.87; 95% CI, 0.79 to 0.95; p=0.002), as was the secondary endpoint of death from any cause or any hospitalization (relative risk, 0.92; 95% CI, 0.86 to 0.98; p=0.02). There was also a reduction in the rate of sudden death from cardiac causes (relative risk, 0.79; 95% CI, 0.64 to 0.97; p=0.03).

In diabetic patients with hypertension resistant to therapy, it is not uncommon to find primary aldosteronism (PA), and its prevalence is as high as 14% in some studies [107]. It has been demonstrated that surgical excision of aldosterone-producing tumors, as well as medical therapy with spironolactone in patients with PA, significantly reduces blood pressure and normalizes insulin sensitivity [108]. Aldosterone blockade can also inhibit adipokine production and stimulate adiponectin production as discussed above, further improving insulin sensitivity [19].

MR blockers, such as spironolactone or eplerenone, have been demonstrated to significantly reduce proteinuria – a marker of endothelial dysfunction and predictor of CVD – in type 2 diabetic patients already treated with angiotensin-converting enzyme inhibitors (ACE-Is) or angiotensin receptor blockers (ARBs) [109]. In a significant proportion of patients, aldosterone levels can remain elevated despite chronic pharmacologic RAAS blockade with ACE-Is or ARBs due to incomplete RAAS inhibition (a phenomenon known as aldosterone escape); this is associated with increased frequency of proteinuria, which can be reduced by MR antagonism [110]. Beneficial effects also have been reported in cardiac tissue in a recent study in patients with type 2 DM and microalbuminuria already treated with enalapril; it was seen that coronary perfusion measured by adenosine-stimulated myocardial perfusion reserve was improved by eplerenone as compared with patients assigned to receive hydrochlorothiazide. These effects were independent of changes in blood pressure [111]. Nonetheless, the combined use of ACE-Is or ARBs and spironolactone is limited by a small but significant risk of hyperkalemia.

Conclusions

Uncontrolled hypertension in diabetics significantly increases the risk of CVD and this problem is often undertreated in this patient population due to various reasons. There are multiple ongoing studies to understand more about the pathophysiology of end organ damage in patients with hypertension and diabetes and there have been several exciting findings recently like the effects of aldosterone in the CMS. There has emerged a consensus among experts that target blood pressure should be <130/90mm Hg in diabetics with multiple modalities discussed and this should be the goal of every physician when managing a diabetic patient. A summary of the current recommendations for the management of hypertension in type 2 DM is shown below.

Key points	Evidence level
◆ Non-pharmacologic approaches like weight loss, exercise, a DASH diet, a reduction in salt and alcohol intake and smoking cessation should be tried in all patients.	Ib/A
◆ If these fail, pharmacologic agents should be considered. It has been found that it takes an average of 2.9 appropriately dosed antihypertensive medications to achieve BP goals in diabetics and in those with pre-existing stage 3 or higher kidney disease, the average number of antihypertensives goes up to 3.5.	
◆ Current guidelines by the ADA recommend starting patients on a once daily RAS blocker, preferably an ACE-I as the first-line therapy; if side effects like cough develop with the same, then treatment should be changed to an equivalent dose of an ARB. The doses of either of these medications should be titrated to the maximum tolerated dose within a month to reach the target BP <130/80mm Hg.	Ib/A
◆ If the BP goal is not achieved with maximum dose titration of either an ACE-I or an ARB, the option is to add either a low-dose thiazide diuretic (12.5mg of chlorthalidone or hydrochlorothiazide) or a calcium channel blocker (CCB). Again, thiazide diuretics and CCBs should be titrated to their maximum tolerated dose to get BP in the target range and the combination of ACE-I/ARB, thiazide diuretic and/or CCB usually works well for the majority of patients.	Ib/A
◆ β-blockers should not be used as first-line therapy for hypertension management in people of any age group unless there are compelling indications like CAD, post-myocardial infarction or CHF. α-blockers can also be added as fourth- or fifth-line agents but come with significant side effects like orthostatic hypotension.	Ib/A
◆ With the new trials with aldosterone antagonists showing significant decrease in CVD morbidity and mortality, there are now the preferred third/fourth-line agents in addition to ACE-Is/ARBs, CCBs or thiazides. There is, however, a slightly increased risk of hyperkalemia with their concomitant use with ACE-Is/ARBs.	Ib/A

References

1. Whitworth JA, World Health Organization, and International Society of Hypertension Writing Group. World Health Organization (WHO)/International Society of Hypertension (ISH) Statement on Management of Hypertension. *J Hypertens* 2003; 21: 1983-92.
2. Cutler JA, *et al.* Trends in hypertension prevalence, awareness, treatment, and control rates in United States adults between 1988-1994 and 1999-2004. *Hypertension* 2008; 52(5): 818-27.

3. National Center for Health Statistics, National Health and Nutrition Examination Survey. Accessed April 19th 2006.
4. Stamler J, Stamler R, Neaton J. Blood pressure, systolic and diastolic, and cardiovascular risks: US population data. *Arch Intern Med* 1993; 153: 598-615.
5. Wilson P, *et al.* Prediction of coronary heart disease using risk factor categories. *Circulation* 1998; 97: 1837-47.
6. Sowers JR. Obesity as a cardiovascular risk factor. *Am J Med* 2003; 115 suppl 8a: 37s-41.
7. Sowers JR. Metabolic risk factors and renal disease. *Kidney Int* 2007; 71: s12-8.
8. Wang Y, Wang Q. The prevalence of prehypertension and hypertension among US adults according to the new Joint National Committee Guidelines: new challenges of the old problem. *Arch Intern Med* 2004; 164: 21-6.
9. Arauz-Pacheco C, Parrott MA, Raskin P. The treatment of hypertension in adult patients with diabetes. *Diabetes Care* 2002; 25: 134-47.
10. Whaley-Connell A, Sowers JR. Hypertension and insulin resistance. *Hypertension* 2009; 54 (3): 462-4.
11. Lastra G, Manrique C, Sowers JR. The role of aldosterone in cardiovascular disease in people with diabetes and hypertension: an update. *Current Diabetes Reports* 2008; 8: 203-7.
12. McFarlane SI, Banerji MS, Jr. Insulin resistance and cardiovascular disease. *J Clin Endocrinol Metab* 2001; 86: 713-8.
13. Expert Panel on Detection, Evaluation and Treatment of High Blood Cholesterol in Adults; Executive Summary of the Third Report of the National Cholesterol Education Program (NCEP). Expert Panel on Detection, Evaluation, and Treatment of High Blood Cholesterol in Adults (Adult Treatment Panel III). *JAMA* 2001; 285: 2486-97.
14. Expert Committee on the Diagnosis and Classification of Diabetes Mellitus; Report of the Expert Committee on the Diagnosis and Classification of Diabetes Mellitus. *Diabetes Care* 2003; 26(suppl 1): s5-20.
15. The National High Blood Pressure Education Program Working Group; National High Blood Pressure Education Program Working Group Report on Hypertension in Diabetes. *Hypertension* 1994; 23: 145-58.
16. Sowers JR, Epstein M. Diabetes mellitus and associated hypertension, vascular disease, and nephropathy: an update. *Hypertension* 1995; 25(pt 1): 869-79.
17. Sowers JR, Epstein M, Frohlich ED. Diabetes, hypertension, and cardiovascular disease: an update. *Hypertension* 2001; 37: 1053-9.
18. Manrique C, Lastra G, Gardner M, Sowers JR: The renin angiotensin aldosterone system in hypertension: roles of insulin resistance and oxidative stress. *Med Clin North Am* 2009; 93(3): 569-82.
19. Sowers JR, Whaley-Connell A, Epstein M. Narrative review: the emerging clinical implications of the role of aldosterone in the metabolic syndrome and resistant hypertension. *Ann Intern Med* 2009; 150(11): 776-83.
20. Pickup JC. Inflammation and activated innate immunity in the pathogenesis of type 2 diabetes. *Diabetes Care* 2004; 27: 813-23.
21. Ran J, Hirano T, Adachi M. Angiotensin II type 1 receptor blocker ameliorates overproduction and accumulation of triglyceride in the liver of zucker fatty rats. *Am J Physiol Endocrinol Metab* 2004; 287: e227-32.
22. Vidotti DB, *et al.* High glucose concentration stimulates renin activity and angiotensin II generation in mesangial cells. *Am J Physiol Renal Physiol* 2004; 286: f1039-45.
23. Mehta PK, Griendling KK. Angiotensin II cell signaling: physiological and pathological effects in the cardiovascular system. *Am J Physiol Cell Physiol* 2007; 292: 82-97.
24. Engeli S, Negrel R, Sharma AM. Physiology and pathophysiology of the adipose tissue renin-angiotensin system. *Hypertension* 2000; 35: 1270-7.
25. Manrique C, Lastra G, Sowers JR. Hypertension and the cardiometabolic syndrome. *J Clin Hypertens* 2005; 7: 471-6.
26. Dandona P, *et al.* Insulin as an anti-inflammatory and antiatherosclerotic hormone. *Clin Cornerstone* 2003; (suppl 4): p. s13-20.
27. Sowers JR. Update on the cardiometabolic syndrome. *Clin Cornerstone* 2001; 4: 17-23.
28. Sowers JR. Insulin resistance and hypertension. *Am J Physiol Heart Circ Physiol* 2004; 286: h1597-602.
29. Hayden MR. Global risk reduction of reactive oxygen species in metabolic syndrome, type 2 diabetes mellitus, and atheroscleropathy. *Med Hypotheses Res* 2004; 1: 171-85.
30. Nickenig G, *et al.* Insulin induces upregulation of vascular AT1 receptor gene expression by posttranscriptional mechanisms. *Circulation* 1998; 98: 2453-60.

31. Cooper SA, Whaley-Connell A, *et al.* Renin angiotensin-aldosterone system and oxidative stress in cardiovascular insulin resistance. *Am J Physiol Heart Circ Physiol* 2007; 293: h2009-23.
32. Hayden MR, *et al.* Type 2 diabetes mellitus as a conformational disease. *JOP* 2005; 6: 287-302.
33. Butler AE, *et al.* Increased beta cell apoptosis prevents adaptive increase in beta-cell mass in mouse model of type 2 diabetes: evidence for role of islet amyloid formation rather than direct action of amyloid. *Diabetes* 2003; 52: 2304-14.
34. Hayden MR, Tyagi SC. 'A' is for amylin and amyloid in type 2 diabetes mellitus. *JOP* 2001; 2: 124-39.
35. Hayden MR, Tyagi SC. Islet redox stress: the manifold toxicities of insulin resistance, metabolic syndrome and amylin derived islet amyloid in type 2 diabetes mellitus. *JOP* 2002; 3: 86-108.
36. Funder JW. The nongenomic actions of aldosterone. *Endocr Rev* 2005; 26: 313-21.
37. Schiffrin EL. Effects of aldosterone on the vasculature. *Hypertension* 2006; 47: 312-8.
38. Ehrhart-Bornstein M, Arakelyan K, *et al.* Fat cells may be the obesity-hypertension link: human adipogenic factors stimulate aldosterone secretion from adrenocortical cells. *Endocr Res* 2004; 30: 865-70.
39. Corry DB, Tuck ML. The effect of aldosterone on glucose metabolism. *Curr Hypertens Rep* 2003; 5: 106-9.
40. Guo C, Ricchiuti V, *et al.* Mineralocorticoid receptor blockade reverses obesity-related changes in expression of adiponectin, peroxisome proliferator-activated receptor-gamma, and proinflammatory adipokines. *Circulation* 2008; 117: 2253-61.
41. Lamounier-Zepter V, Ehrhart-Bornstein M. Fat tissue metabolism and adrenal steroid secretion. *Curr Hypertens Rep* 2006; 8: 30-4.
42. Goodfriend TL, Ball DL, *et al.* Epoxy-keto derivative of linoleic acid stimulates aldosterone secretion. *Hypertension* 2004; 43: 358-63.
43. Campion J, Maestro B, *et al.* Aldosterone impairs insulin responsiveness in U-937 promonocytic cells via downregulation of its own receptor. *Cell Biochem Funct* 2002; 20: 237-45.
44. Caprio M, Feve B, *et al.* Pivotal role of the mineralocorticoid receptor in corticosteroid-induced adipogenesis. *Faseb J* 2007; 21: 2185-94.
45. Umeki S. Mechanisms for the activation/electron transfer of neutrophil NADPH-oxidase complex and molecular pathology of chronic granulomatous disease. *Ann Hematol* 1994; 68(6): 267-77.
46. Zuo I, *et al.* Microtubules regulate angiotensin II type 1 receptor and Rac1 localization in caveolae/lipid rafts: role in redox signaling. *Arterioscler Thromb Vasc Biol* 2004; 24: 1223-8.
47. Zuo I, *et al.* Caveolin 1 is essential for activation of Rac-1 and NADPH oxidase after angiotensin II type 1 receptor stimulation in vascular smooth muscle cells: role in redox signaling and vascular hypertrophy. *Arterioscler Thromb Vasc Biol* 2005; 25: 1824-30.
48. Bakris GL, Weir MR, *et al.* Effects of blood pressure level on progression of diabetic nephropathy: results from the RENAAL study. *Arch Intern Med* 2003; 163: 1555-65.
49. Mancia G, *et al.* 2007 Guidelines for the Management of Arterial Hypertension: the Task Force for the Management of Arterial Hypertension of the European Society of Hypertension (ESH) and the European Society of Cardiology (ESC). *J Hypertens* 2007; 25(6): 1105-87.
50. Kidney Disease Outcomes Quality Initiative (K/DOQI), K/DOQI Clinical Practice Guidelines on Hypertension and Antihypertensive Agents in Chronic Kidney Disease. *Am J Kidney Dis* 2004; 43(5 suppl 2): s1-290.
51. American Diabetes Association. Standards of Medical Care in Diabetes. *Diabetes Care* 2007; 30 (suppl 1): s4-41.
52. Chobanian AV, Bakris GL, *et al.* National High Blood Pressure Education Program Coordinating Committee. Seventh Report of the Joint National Committee on Prevention, Detection, Evaluation and Treatment of High Blood Pressure. *Hypertension* 2003; 42: 1206-52.
53. Curb JD, Pressel MS, *et al.* Effect of diuretic-based antihypertensive treatment on cardiovascular disease risk in older diabetic patients with isolated hypertension. *JAMA* 1996; 276: 1886-92.
54. Bakris GL. The importance of blood pressure control in the patient with diabetes. *Am J Med* 2004; 116(suppl 5a): 30s-8.
55. Sowers JR, Lastra G, *et al.* Initial combination therapy compared with monotherapy in diabetic hypertensive patients. *J Clin Hypertens* (Greenwich) 2008; 10: 668-76.
56. Ritz E, Dikow R. Hypertension and antihypertensive treatment of diabetic nephropathy. *Nat Clin Prac Nephrol* 2006; 2: 562-7.
57. Peterson JC, Adler S, *et al.* Blood pressure control, proteinuria, and the progression of renal disease: the Modification of Diet in Renal Disease study. *Ann Intern Med* 1995; 123: 754-62.

58. Klahr S, Levey AS, *et al.* Modification of Diet in Renal Disease Study Group. The effects of dietary protein restriction and blood-pressure control on the progression of chronic kidney disease. *N Engl J Med* 1994; 330: 877-84.
59. Cushman WC, Evans GW, Byington RP, *et al,* for the ACCORD Study Group. The effects of intensive blood pressure control in type 2 diabetes mellitus. Epub - published on March 14, 2010, www.nejm.org.
60. The Action to Control Cardiovascular Risk in Diabetes Study Group; Effects of Intensive Glucose Lowering in Type 2 Diabetes. *N Engl J Med* 2008; 358: 2545-59.
61. Sacks FM, Svetkey LP, *et al.* Effects on blood pressure of reduced dietary sodium and the Dietary Approaches to Stop Hypertension (DASH) diet. *N Engl J Med* 2001; 344: 3-10.
62. Chua DC, Bakris GL. Is proteinuria a plausible target of therapy? *Curr Hypertension Rep* 2004; 6(3): 177-81.
63. Bakris GL, Sowers JR. Ash position paper: treatment of hypertension in patients with diabetes - an update. *J Clin Hypertens* 2008; 10(9): 707-13.
64. Ridker PM, Danielson E, *et al.* Val-MARC investigators. Valsartan, blood pressure reduction, and c-reactive protein: primary report of the Val-MARC trial. *Hypertension* 2006; 48: 73-9.
65. Lacourcire Y, Poirier L, *et al.* Antihypertensive efficacy and tolerability of two fixed-dose combinations of valsartan and hydrochlorothiazide compared with valsartan monotherapy in patients with stage 2 or 3 systolic hypertension: an 8-week, randomized, double-blind, parallel-group trial. *Clin Ther* 2005; 27: 1013-21.
66. Jamerson KA, Zappe DH, *et al.* The time to blood pressure control by initiating antihypertensive therapy with a higher dose of valsartan (160mg) or valsartan/hydrochlorothiazide compared to low-dose valsartan (80mg) in the treatment of hypertension: the VELOCITY study (Ash abstract p400). *J Clin Hypertens* (Greenwich) 2007; 9(suppl a): a166-7.
67. Malik S, Lopez V, *et al.* Undertreatment of cardiovascular risk factors among persons with diabetes in the United States. *Diabetes Res Clin Pract* 2007; 77: 126-33.
68. Basile J, Black HR, *et al.* The role of therapeutic inertia and the use of fixed-dose combination therapy in the management of hypertension. *J Clin Hypertens* (Greenwich) 2007; 9: 636-45.
69. The Heart Outcomes Prevention Evaluation Study Investigators. Effects of an angiotensin-converting-enzyme inhibitor, ramipril on cardiovascular events in high-risk patients. *N Engl J Med* 2000; 342: 145-53.
70. The Heart Outcomes Prevention Evaluation Study Investigators. Effects of ramipril on cardiovascular and microvascular outcomes in people with diabetes mellitus: results of the HOPE study and MICRO-HOPE substudy. *Lancet* 2000; 355: 253-9.
71. Hansson L, *et al.* Effect of angiotensin-converting-enzyme inhibition compared with conventional therapy on cardiovascular morbidity and mortality in hypertension: the Captopril Prevention Project (CAPPP) randomized trial. *Lancet* 1999; 353(9153): 611-6.
72. Yusuf S, Gerstein H, Hoogwerf B, Pogue J, Bosch J, Wolffenbuttel BHR, Zinman B; for the HOPE Study Investigators. Ramipril and the development of diabetes *JAMA* 2001; 286 (15): 1882-5.
73. Zanella MT, Kohlmann OJ, Ribeiro AB. Treatment of obesity hypertension and diabetes syndrome. *Hypertension* 2001; 38: 705-8.
74. Carlsson PO, Berne C, Jansson L. Angiotensin II and the endocrine pancreas: effects on islet blood flow and insulin secretion in rats. *Diabetologia* 1998; 41: 127-33.
75. Engeli S, Gorzelniak K, *et al.* Co-expression of renin-angiotensin system genes in human adipose tissue. *J Hypertens* 1999; 17: 555-60.
76. The ALLHAT Officers and Coordinators for the ALLHAT Collaborative Research Group. Major Outcomes in High-risk Hypertensive Patients Randomized to Angiotensin-converting Enzyme Inhibitor or Calcium Channel Blocker vs Diuretic: the Antihypertensive and Lipid-lowering Treatment to Prevent Heart Attack Trial (ALLHAT). *JAMA* 2002; 288(23): 2981-97.
77. The ALLHAT Officers and Coordinators for the ALLHAT Collaborative Research Group. Major Cardiovascular Events in Hypertensive Patients Randomized to Doxazosin vs Chlorthalidone: the Antihypertensive and Lipid-lowering Treatment to Prevent Heart Attack Trial (ALLHAT). *JAMA* 2000; 283(15): 1967-75.
78. The SOLVD Investigators. Effect of enalapril on mortality and the development of heart failure in asymptomatic patients with reduced left ventricular ejection fractions. *N Engl J Med* 1992; 327(10): 685-91.
79. Dahlof B, *et al.* Cardiovascular morbidity and mortality in the Losartan Intervention for Endpoint Reduction in Hypertension Study (LIFE): a randomised trial against atenolol. *Lancet* 2002; 359(9311): 995-1003.
80. Pfeffer MA, *et al.* Effects of candesartan on mortality and morbidity in patients with chronic heart failure: the CHARM-overall programme. *Lancet* 2003; 362(9386): 759-66.

81. Bangalore S, *et al.* Effect of ramipril on the incidence of diabetes. *N Engl J Med* 2006; 355(15): 1551-62.
82. Sarafidis PA, Bakris GL. Antihypertensive therapy and the risk of new-onset diabetes. *Diabetes Care* 2006; 29(5): 1167-9.
83. Elliott WJ, Meyer PM. Incident diabetes in clinical trials of antihypertensive drugs: a network meta-analysis. *Lancet* 2007; 369(9557): 201-7.
84. Mancia G, Grassi G, Zanchetti A. New-onset diabetes and antihypertensive drugs. *J Hypertens* 2006; 24(1): 3-10.
85. Zillich AJ, Garg J, *et al.* Thiazide diuretics, potassium, and the development of diabetes: a quantitative review. *Hypertension* 2006; 48: 219-24.
86. Whelton PK, Barzilay J, *et al.* Clinical outcomes in antihypertensive treatment of type 2 diabetes, impaired fasting glucose concentration, and normoglycemia: Antihypertensive and Lipid-lowering Treatment to Prevent Heart Attack Trial (ALLHAT). *Arch Intern Med* 2005; 165(12): 1401-9.
87. Kostis JB, Wilson AC, *et al.* Long-term effect of diuretic-based therapy on fatal outcomes in subjects with isolated systolic hypertension with and without diabetes. *Am J Cardiol* 2005; 95(1): 29-35.
88. Black HR. Calcium channel blockers in the treatment of hypertension and prevention of cardiovascular disease: results from major clinical trials. *Clin Cornerstone* 2004; 6: 53-66.
89. National High Blood Pressure Education Program. The Sixth Report of the Joint National Committee on Prevention, Detection, Evaluation, and Treatment of High Blood Pressure. *Arch Intern Med* 1997; 157: 2413-46.
90. Khan N, McAlister F. Re-examining the efficacy of beta-blockers for the treatment of hypertension: a meta-analysis. *Can Med Assoc J* 2006; 174: 1737-42.
91. Braunwald E, Antman E, Beasley J. ACC/AHA 2002 Guideline Update for the Management of Patients with Unstable Angina and Non-ST-Segment Elevation Myocardial Infarction - Summary Article: A Report of the American College of Cardiology/American Heart Association Task Force on Practice Guidelines (Committee on the Management of Patients with Unstable Angina). *J Am Coll Cardiol* 2002; 40: 1366-74.
92. Hunt S, Abraham W, *et al.* ACC/AHA 2005 Guideline Update for the Diagnosis and Management of Chronic Heart Failure in the Adult: a Report of the American College of Cardiology/American Heart Association Task Force on Practice Guidelines (Writing Committee to Update the 2001 Guidelines for the Evaluation and Management of Heart Failure): Developed in Collaboration with the American College of Chest Physicians and the International Society for Heart and Lung Transplantation: endorsed by the Heart Rhythm Society. *Circulation* 2005; 112: e154-235.
93. The National Collaborating Centre for Chronic Conditions, Hypertension: Management of Hypertension in Adults in Primary Care (partial update of NICE clinical guideline 18, published August 2004), June 2006. Accessed from http://www.nice.org.uk/full guideline on October 16, 2006.
94. Manrique C, Johnson M, Sowers JR. Thiazide diuretics alone or with β-blockers impair glucose metabolism in hypertensive patients with abdominal obesity. *Hypertension* 2010; 55(1): 15-17.
95. Hart PD, Bakris GL. Should beta-blockers be used to control hypertension in people with chronic kidney disease? *Semin Nephrol* 2007; 27(5): 555-64.
96. Bell D. Advantages of a third-generation beta-blocker in patients with diabetes mellitus. *Am J Cardiol* 2004; 93: 49b-52.
97. Bakris GL, Williams M, *et al.* Preserving renal function in adults with hypertension and diabetes: a consensus approach. National Kidney Foundation Hypertension and Diabetes Executive Committees Working Group. *Am J Kidney Dis* 2000; 36(3): 646-61.
98. Anderson PE, Lithell H. Metabolic effects of doxazosin and enalapril in hypertriglyceridemic, hypertensive men: relationship to changes in skeletal muscle blood flow. *Am J Hypertens* 1996; 9: 323-33.
99. Lithell H. Hyperinsulinemia, insulin resistance, and the treatment of hypertension. *Am J Hypertens* 1996; 9: s150-4.
100. ALLHAT. Diuretic versus alpha-blocker as first-step antihypertensive therapy. Final results from the Antihypertensive and Lipid-lowering Treatment to Prevent Heart Attack Trial (ALLHAT). *Hypertension* 2003; 2: 239-46.
101. Nistala R, Wei Y, Sowers J, Whaley-Connell A. Renin-angiotensin-aldosterone system-mediated redox effects in chronic kidney disease. *Translational Research* 2009: 153(3): 102-13.

102. Whaley-Connell A, Habibi J, Wei Y, Gutweiler A, Jellison J, Wiedmeyer CE, Ferrario CM, Sowers JR. Mineralocorticoid receptor antagonism attenuates glomerular filtration barrier remodeling in the transgenic Ren2 rat. *Am J Physiol Renal Physiol* 2009; 296: F1013-22.
103. Wei Y, Whaley-Connell AT, Habibi J, Rehmer J, Rehmer N, Patel K, Hayden M, DeMarco V, Ferrario CM, Ibdah JA, Sowers JR. Mineralocorticoid receptor antagonism attenuates vascular apoptosis and injury via rescuing protein kinase B activation. *Hypertension* 2009; 53(2):158-65.
104. Rossi G, Boscaro M, Funder JW. Aldosterone as a cardiovascular risk factor. *Trends Endocrinol Metab* 2005; 16: 104-7.
105. Pitt B, Zannad F, *et al.* The effect of spironolactone on morbidity and mortality in patients with severe heart failure. Randomized Aldactone Evaluation Study investigators. *N Engl J Med* 1999; 341: 709-17.
106. Pitt B, Remme W, *et al.* Eplerenone Post-acute Myocardial Infarction Heart Failure Efficacy and Survival Study investigators. Eplerenone, a selective aldosterone blocker, in patients with left ventricular dysfunction after myocardial infarction. *N Engl J Med* 2003. 348: 1309-21.
107. Umpierrez GE, *et al.* Primary aldosteronism in diabetic suspects with resistant hypertension. *Diabetes Care* 2007; 30: 1699-703.
108. Catena C, Lapena R, *et al.* Insulin sensitivity in patients with primary aldosteronism: a follow-up study. *J Clin Endocrinol Metab* 2006; 91: 3457-63.
109. Epstein M, Williams GH, *et al.* Selective aldosterone blockade with eplerenone reduces albuminuria in patients with type 2 diabetes. *Clin J Am Soc Nephrol* 2006. 1: 940-51.
110. Sato A, Hayashi K, *et al.* Effectiveness of aldosterone blockade in patients with nephropathy. *Hypertension* 2003; 41: 64-8.
111. Joffe HV, Kwong RY, *et al.* Beneficial effects of eplerenone versus hydrochlorothiazide on coronary circulatory function in patients with diabetes mellitus. *J Clin Endocrinol Metab* 2007; 92: 2552-8.

Index

BP = blood pressure

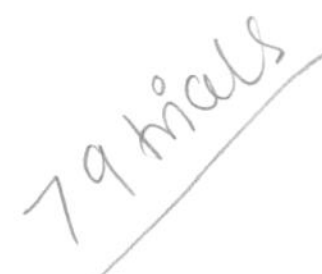
79 trials